DAVI-ELLEN CHABNER

Medical Terminology

A SHORT COURSE

9TH EDITION

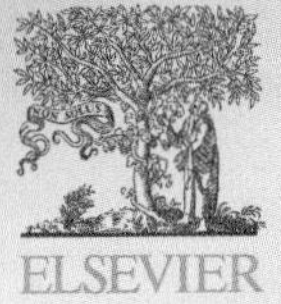

Elsevier
3251 Riverport Lane
St. Louis, Missouri 63043

MEDICAL TERMINOLOGY: A SHORT COURSE, NINTH EDITION ISBN: 978-0-323-47991-2

Library of Congress Control Number: 2022931120

Senior Content Strategist: Linda Woodard
Senior Content Development Manager: Luke Held
Content Development Specialist: Rae Robertson
Publishing Services Manager: Julie Eddy
Senior Project Manager: Abigail Bradberry
Design Direction: Amy Buxton

Printed in Canada

Last digit is the print number: 9 8 7 6 5 4 3 2

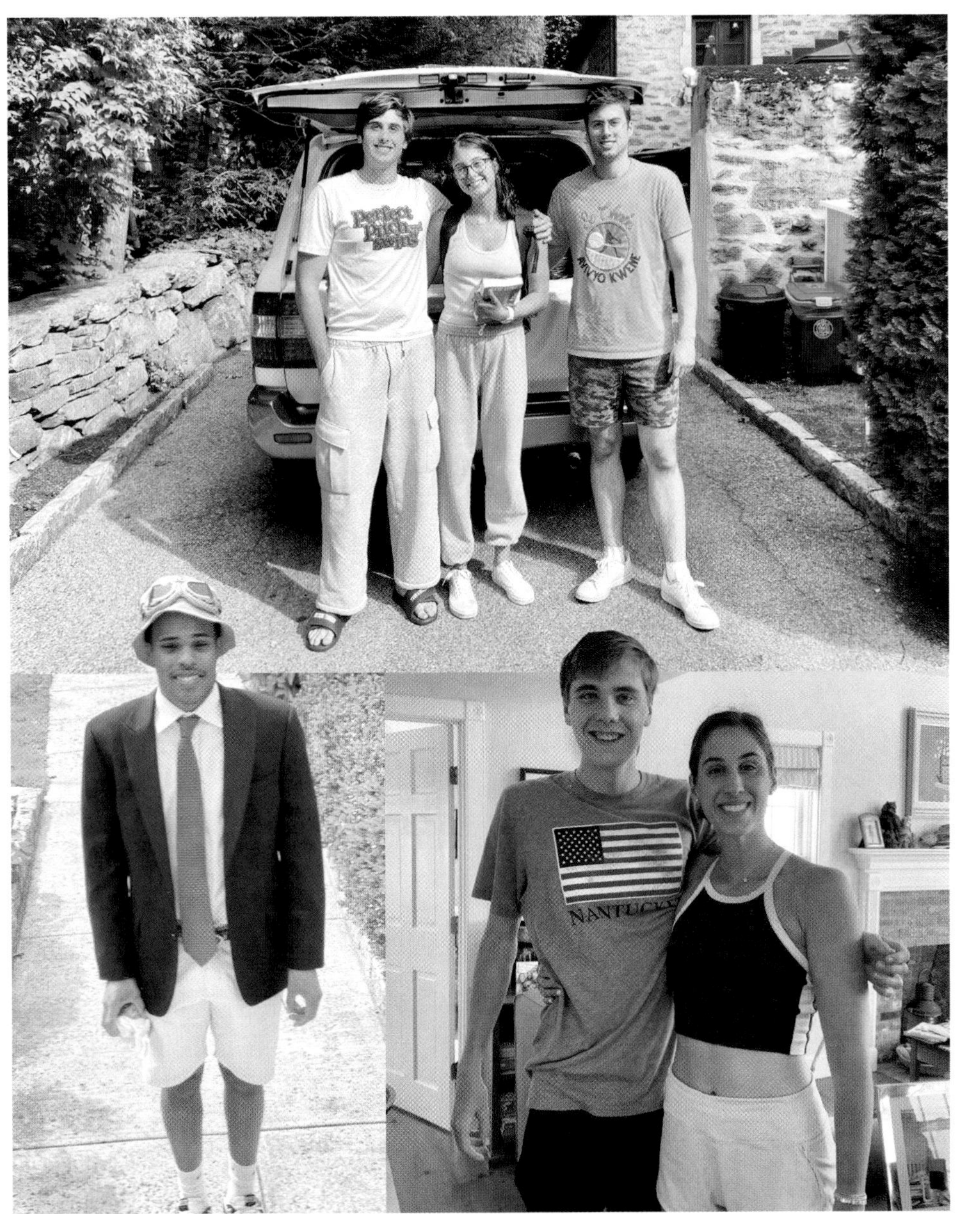

To Solomon, Louisa, Gus, Amari, Ben, and Bebe
You are my hope for the future!

Preface to the 9th Edition

I wrote the first edition of *Medical Terminology: A Short Course* almost 35 years ago with the hope that it would fill a specific niche in the education of allied health professionals. My goal was to present a comprehensive introduction and overview of medical terminology in a straightforward and easy manner for students who had no previous background in biology or medicine.

It is gratifying to know that this book is now widely used in colleges, career schools, universities, hospitals, and other medical settings in the United States and abroad, where allied health workers use medical language and interpret it for patients and their families. There is no doubt that the method used in *Medical Terminology: A Short Course* takes potentially complicated subject matter and makes it manageable and understandable. In this ninth edition, the text has been updated and carefully reviewed for clarity, simplicity, and practicality, but its essential elements remain. Here are its important features:

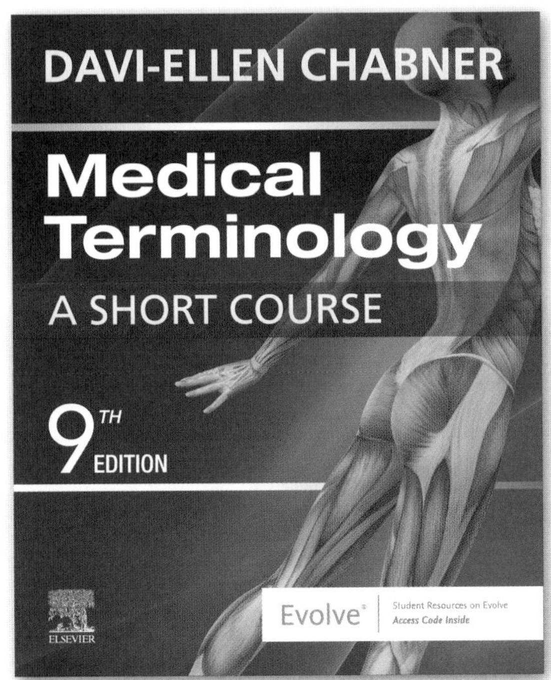

WORKBOOK-TEXT FORMAT. In this book, you learn by doing. On nearly every page you are writing and interacting with medical terminology. You complete exercises (and check your answers), label diagrams, test your understanding with review sheets, and practice pronunciation. The best path to success is to write terms and their meanings as you test yourself. I really believe this method of learning will work for you!

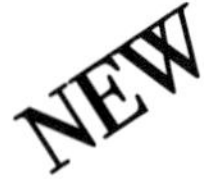

CURRENT MEDICAL TOPICS EXPLAINED. Complex topics, such as immunity and vaccines, are presented in clear and simple langage. A new appendix teaches the basics of immunology and explains how different types of vaccines work in the body. Spotlights throughout the book provide insight and explantion on current and essential issues in medicine.

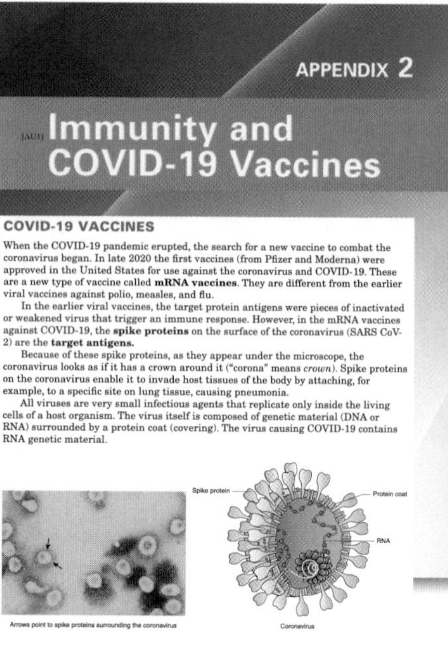
APPENDIX 2

Immunity and COVID-19 Vaccines

COVID-19 VACCINES

When the COVID-19 pandemic erupted, the search for a new vaccine to combat the coronavirus began. In late 2020 the first vaccines (from Pfizer and Moderna) were approved in the United States for use against the coronavirus and COVID-19. These are a new type of vaccine called **mRNA vaccines**. They are different from the earlier viral vaccines against polio, measles, and flu.

In the earlier viral vaccines, the target protein antigens were pieces of inactivated or weakened virus that trigger an immune response. However, in the mRNA vaccines against COVID-19, the **spike proteins** on the surface of the coronavirus (SARS CoV-2) are the **target antigens**.

Because of these spike proteins, as they appear under the microscope, the coronavirus looks as if it has a crown around it ("corona" means *crown*). Spike proteins on the coronavirus enable it to invade host tissues of the body by attaching, for example, to a specific site on lung tissue, causing pneumonia.

All viruses are very small infectious agents that replicate only inside the living cells of a host organism. The virus itself is composed of genetic material (DNA or RNA) surrounded by a protein coat (covering). The virus causing COVID-19 contains RNA genetic material.

Arrows point to spike proteins surrounding the coronavirus

Coronavirus

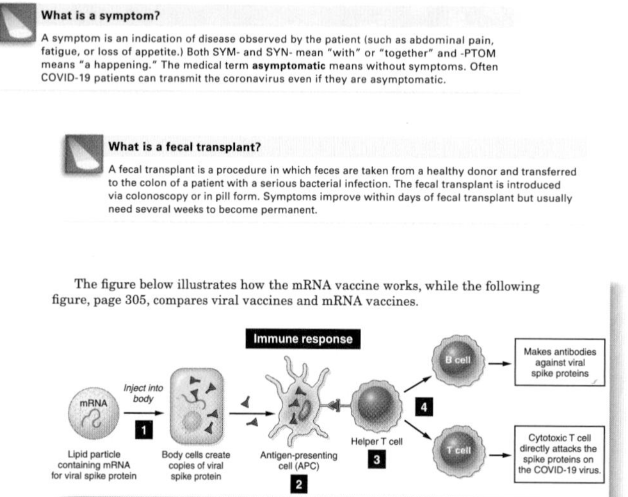
What is a symptom?

A symptom is an indication of disease observed by the patient (such as abdominal pain, fatigue, or loss of appetite.) Both SYM- and SYN- mean "with" or "together" and -PTOM means "a happening." The medical term **asymptomatic** means without symptoms. Often COVID-19 patients can transmit the coronavirus even if they are asymptomatic.

What is a fecal transplant?

A fecal transplant is a procedure in which feces are taken from a healthy donor and transferred to the colon of a patient with a serious bacterial infection. The fecal transplant is introduced via colonoscopy or in pill form. Symptoms improve within days of fecal transplant but usually need several weeks to become permanent.

The figure below illustrates how the mRNA vaccine works, while the following figure, page 305, compares viral vaccines and mRNA vaccines.

EASY TO READ AND UNDERSTAND. Explanations of terms are worded simply and clearly, and repetition reinforces learning throughout the text. Answers to questions are located easily so that you can check and correct your responses while gaining additional explanation of terminology.

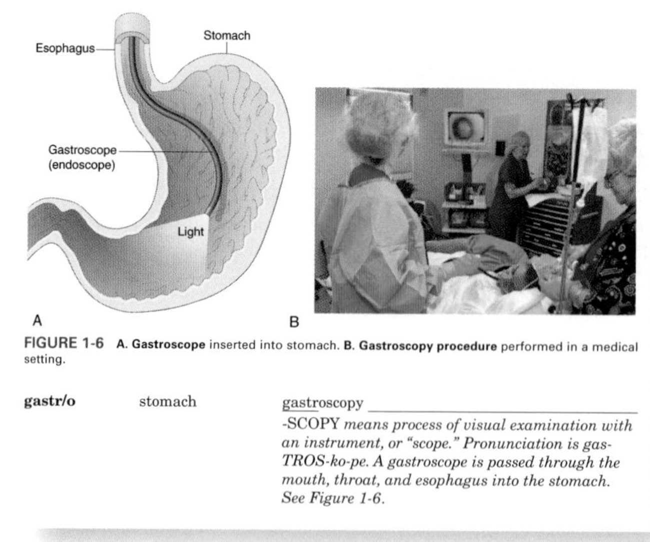

FIGURE 1-6 **A. Gastroscope** inserted into stomach. **B. Gastroscopy procedure** performed in a medical setting.

gastr/o	stomach	gastroscopy ____________
		-SCOPY *means process of visual examination with an instrument, or "scope." Pronunciation is gas-TROS-ko-pe. A gastroscope is passed through the mouth, throat, and esophagus into the stomach. See Figure 1-6.*

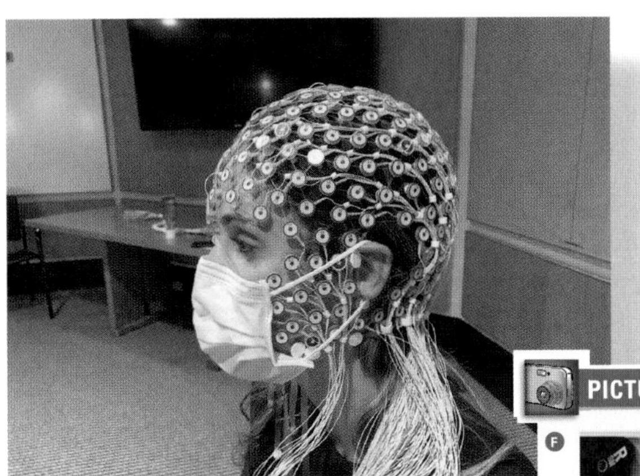

DYNAMIC ILLUSTRATIONS AND PHOTOGRAPHS. Medical terms come alive with images on nearly every page! Learning is reinforced by seeing parts of the body diseases, conditions and real medical procedures. At the end of each chapter, "Picture Shows" highlight key images and allow you to apply your knowledge of terminology.

PICTURE SHOW

F

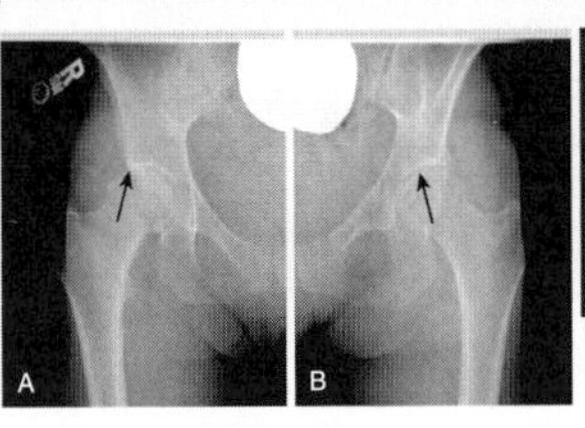

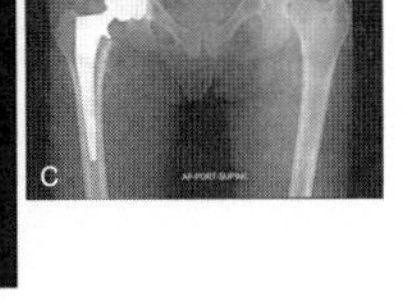

1. The image in *A* shows degeneration of the hip (pelvic) joint with narrowed joint spaces (see arrow). The image in *B* shows a normal hip for comparison (see arrow). The patient with the hip changes has arthralgia, stiffness, and joint tenderness. Your diagnosis?
   a. osteoarthritis
   b. gastroenteritis
   c. hyperthyroidism
   d. osteogenic sarcoma

NOTE: The image in C shows a **THR (total hip replacement)** as treatment for this condition.

INTRODUCTION TO BODY SYSTEMS. The Body Systems Resource, beginning on page 217, begins with the following five sections:

Anatomy—shows full-color images of each body system, labeled for easy reference with combining forms for each body part.

Terminology—repeats each combining form and gives a medical term illustrating the use of the combining form. Definitions are in the *Mini-Dictionary* at the end of the book.

Pathology—presents explanations of disease conditions related to each body system.

Diagnostic and Treatment Procedures—explains and defines common examples for each body system.

Matching Exercises—tests your understanding of the material, with answers included.

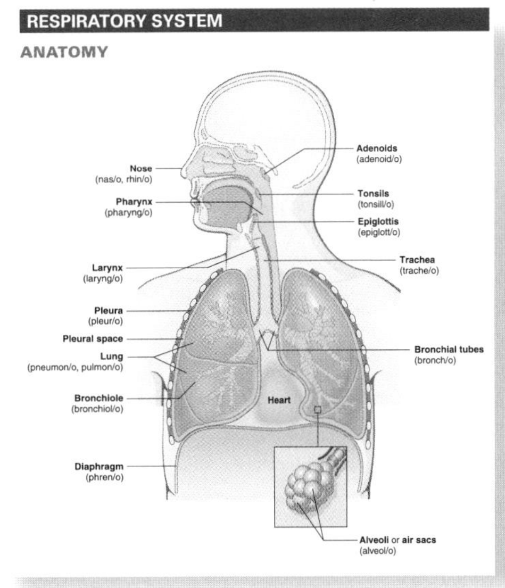

PRACTICAL APPLICATIONS. Throughout the text, and on the Student Evolve website, you will find exciting images, medical case reports, and vignettes that illustrate terminology in the context of stories about patients and procedures.

CASE REPORTS

CASE 2 *Gynecology*

Ms. Sessions has had **dysmenorrhea** and **menorrhagia** for several months. She is also **anemic.** Because of the presence of a **large fibroid,** as seen on a pelvic **ultrasound (sonogram)** (see Figure 5-7, *A*), a **hysterectomy** was recommended. After it was removed, the uterus was opened to reveal multiple fibroids (**leiomyomas**) bulging into the uterine cavity and displaying a firm, white appearance. See Figure 5-7, *B*.

FIGURE 5-7 **A, Pelvic sonogram. B, Fibroids (leiomyomas).** These are benign tumors of the uterus.

anemic ____________

dysmenorrhea ____________

fibroids ____________

hysterectomy ____________

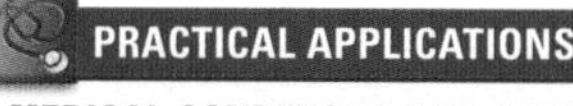

PRACTICAL APPLICATIONS

MEDICAL CONDITIONS AND SPECIALISTS

Match the following physician specialists with the condition each would treat.

cardiologist	gastroenterologist	neurologist	urologist
dermatologist	gynecologist	oncologist	
endocrinologist	hematologist	ophthalmologist	

1. Cerebrovascular accident ____________
2. Skin cancer ____________
3. Dysentery ____________
4. Anemia ____________
5. Lung cancer ____________
6. Prostate gland enlargement ____________
7. Hyperglycemia ____________
8. Cataract (clouding of the lens of the eye) ____________
9. Heart attack ____________
10. Abnormal bleeding of the uterus from the vagina ____________

WHAT'S YOUR DIAGNOSIS?

Case Study

This 7 year-old boy presents with fever, sore throat, runny nose, and persistent fatigue [feeling of being tired all the time]. Physical examination reveals multiple bruises [contusions] of his lower extremities and arms, an erythematous [red] pharynx [throat] with white plaques on the tonsils, and pale gums, lips, and nail beds. CBC [complete blood count] was performed. Increasing fever prompted immediate admission to the children's ward of the hospital.

During the course of admission, the patient's pharyngitis was monitored and subsided. Tonsillitis was ruled out. Fatigue and contusions on his arms and legs were noted and addressed with the parents while taking his social history. A lab hematologist reviewed the high WBC [white blood cell] count, and a WBC differential [percentages of the various types of these cells] shows immature cells. A bone marrow biopsy confirms the diagnosis of WBC malignancy.

IN PERSON: GALLBLADDER STONES

This first-person narrative describes the symptoms and treatment of a 46-year-old woman with gallbladder stones.

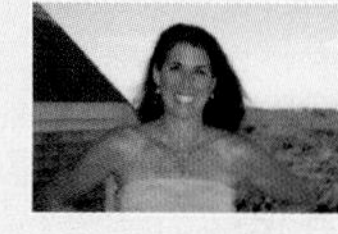

Everyone enjoys a little dessert after dinner, but when the ice cream or a creamy tart leads to pain, most would avoid it. I loved sweets, and despite the revenge they took on my waistline, I still would not pass up an ice cream cone—until my gallbladder decided it had had enough. After several late nights spent doubled over in pain, I tried to steer clear of fatty foods but could not resist the temptation of frozen yogurt.

With one hand I pushed my cart through the supermarket; with the other hand I fed myself some delicious low-fat (not nonfat) frozen yogurt. I never dreamed that the attendant at the quick-service window actually gave me soft-serve ice cream. Within 10 minutes of eating the questionable yogurt, I broke out into a sweat; a wave of nausea took me over, and a knifelike pain stabbed me in my right upper quadrant. It hurt even more when I pressed my hand on the area in an attempt to brace the pain.

Several months earlier, after a similar painful episode, I had undergone an ultrasound of my gallbladder, and the surgeon then recommended cholecystectomy. The US showed multiple stones in my gallbladder. Most of the stones were just the right size to lodge in the common bile duct and cause blockage of the outflow of bile that occurs after a fatty meal. When I heard the ultrasound results, I swore off all fatty foods.

I just did not imagine that ice cream masquerading as "low-fat yogurt" would be the straw that broke the camel's back! Soon enough, I abandoned my shopping cart and apologized to the manager of the store for vomiting all over aisle 4. The unrelenting pain did not cease when I vomited—it only intensified. I have no idea how I made it home and into bed. I managed to call my surgeon and arrange for "semiemergent" surgery the next morning.

Dr. Fernandez and his team performed a laparoscopic cholecystectomy and relayed to me as I came out of anesthesia that I no longer had a "bag of marbles" for a gallbladder. I had a gassy, distended feeling in my abdomen over the 2 weeks after surgery (carbon dioxide gas is injected into the abdomen before surgery to allow space between abdominal organs). I felt "tight as a drum" for the first few days, and then day by day it went away. My four tiny incisions healed just fine, and in about 2 weeks I was feeling back to normal. Now I can eat ice cream to my heart's content, only suffering the padding on my waistline, not the stabbing pain just above. Without missing a beat, my liver now delivers the bile into my small intestine right after I eat a fatty meal. The bile emulsifies (breaks down) the fat. I just don't have a storage bag to hold bile in reserve.

I've had an appendectomy, my wisdom teeth removed, and now I gave up my gallbladder! How many more "useless" body parts are there to go?

Elizabeth Chabner is the CEO/founder of Masthead, a company devoted to bringing innovative products to patients with breast cancer. She is a physician, swimmer, cross country skier, and the proud mother of four children ages 18-23.

IN PERSON. These compelling first-person narratives describe procedures and conditions from a uniquely personal perspective. After reading each story, medical terms take on new meaning as you experience intimately how it feels to be in a patient's "shoes," living through a diagnosis, disease, and treatment.

TERMINOLOGY CHECKUP. This interactive and enhanced feature recaps and reinforces key concepts and easily confused terms in each chapter.

TERMINOLOGY CHECKUP

Before you leave this chapter, here are important concepts that you should thoroughly understand. In your own words, write the answers on the lines provided. Confirm your answers on the next page. Check the box next to each item when you know you've "got" it!

☐ 1. What is the difference between **endocrine glands** and **exocrine glands.** Give an example of each.

☐ 2. What is the difference between a **diagnosis** and a **prognosis?**

☐ 3. What is the difference between a **carcinoma** and a **sarcoma?** Give an example of each.

REFERENCE GUIDE FOR MEDICAL AND HOSPITAL WORK. This book is also a useful resource. Diagnostic Tests and Procedures (radiological imaging, nuclear medicine scans, clinical procedures, and laboratory tests) are found in *Appendix 3*. Abbreviations, symbols, acronyms, and eponyms are located in *Appendix 4*. A handy Quick Drug Reference *is located in Appendix 5*. The *Mini-Dictionary* helps you study each chapter and also will be a reference for you in the workplace. Each definition has been crafted carefully to explain terms using plain, nontechnical language.

ALSO AVAILABLE

Student Evolve Website (access included with text purchase)

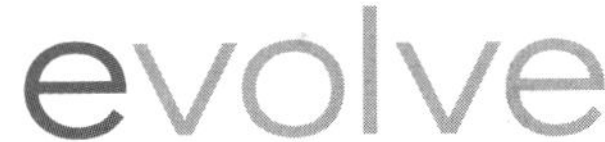

The Evolve website included with this new edition contains additional exercises and activities to test and expand your understanding. In the Audio Resource section you can hear the proper pronunciation with each medical term in the book.

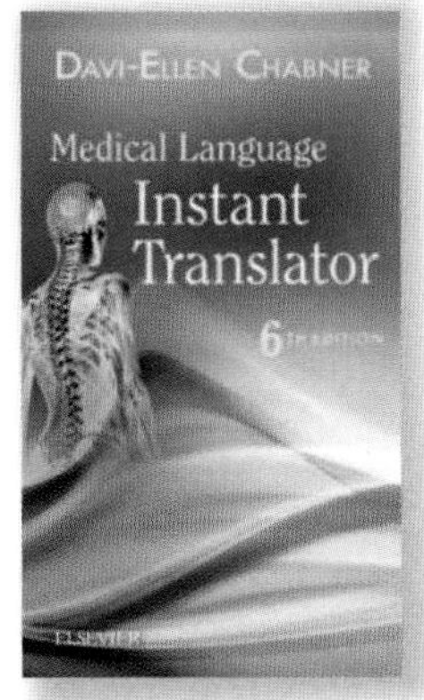

Medical Language Instant Translator (for sale separately)

My *Medical Language Instant Translator* is a uniquely useful resource for all allied health professionals and students of medical terminology. It is a pocket-sized medical terminology reference with convenient information at your fingertips!

Medical Terminology: A Short Course is exactly what you need to begin your medical career—whether in an office, hospital, or other medical setting. Use this handy book in a classroom with an instructor, or study it on your own. The combination of visually reinforced hands-on learning plus easily accessible reference material will mean success for you in your allied health career.

My more comprehensive workbook-text, *The Language of Medicine, 12th edition,* may be of interest to you as you continue your study of medical terminology. It can also serve as a valuable reference in the workplace.

I still experience the thrill and joy of teaching new students. I love being in the classroom (in person or virtually) and feel privileged to continue to write this text. I am available for help at any time. Please communicate your comments, questions, and suggestions to me at chabner.medterm@gmail.com. For technical assistance, please contact technical.support@elsevier.com.

Most of all, I hope this book brings you excitement and enthusiasm for the medical language. It can ignite your imagination for new challenges and make your job more interesting. Work hard and have fun learning medical terminology!

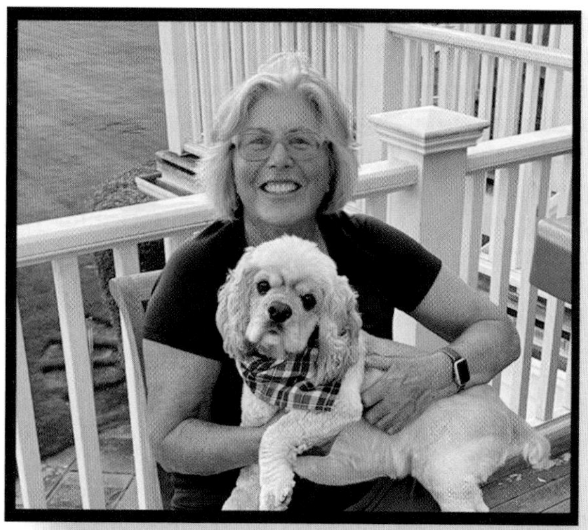

Davi-Ellen Chabner

Acknowledgments

It is impossible to publish another edition of this book without the assistance and hard work of my extraordinary and exceptional editor, Maureen Pfeifer. On virtually every aspect of this edition, she has listened, advised, and delivered the best possible solutions … with great intelligence, thoughtfulness, and careful attention to detail. We are a TEAM! Thank you, Maureen, for not only being a superb cross-country working partner, but my loyal friend, as well.

I appreciate the support and advocacy of Linda Woodard, Senior Content Strategist at Elsevier. She is always responsive to my concerns and willing to find solutions! Luke Held, Senior Content Development Manager, continues to be a reliable resource and support for my books. Thanks, Luke, for being "in my corner." I am also grateful to Rae Robertson, Content Development Specialist, for her coordination and oversight of this edition.

Abigail Bradberry, Senior Project Manager, facilitated the complex production of this edition. I appreciate her hard work and flexibility in all aspects of the project. Thank you, Abbie! Special thanks to Amy Buxton for directing the design and Kim Denando for creating the layout and cover for this edition! I appreciate your expertise, creativity, and responsiveness.

Thanks also to other members of the Elsevier team: Julie Eddy, Publishing Services Manager, Book Production; and Kevin Herrin, Team Manager, Multimedia. Thank you to the sales team for your continued support and promotion of my projects.

Jim Perkins, assistant professor of medical illustration, Rochester Institute of Technology, was responsible for the excellent, first-rate individual drawings that illustrate this edition. As always, he has done an outstanding job.

I am particularly grateful to the In Person contributors who shared their personal medical stories. Thanks so much to Ruthellen Sheldon, Cathy Ward, Elizabeth Chabner, Sidra DeKoven Ezrahi, and Nancy J. Brandwein.

I appreciate the valuable suggestions of the instructors who reviewed *Medical Terminology: A Short Course* for this new edition. They are listed with their credentials on page xv. Their helpful comments are incorporated in this text.

My class at Partners in Career and Workforce Development (PCWD), Partners Healthcare System has been an important resource for this edition. My students' enthusiasm and questions continue to inspire me. I appreciate them, and their commitment to a career in healthcare.

Teachers and students worldwide continue to contact me with insights and questions. Thank you!

My husband, Bruce A. Chabner, MD, and my daughter, Elizabeth Chabner, MD, MPH, are always available for expert medical advice and consultation. I am grateful for their availability no matter what else is going on in their busy lives and work. Special thanks for Dan L. Longo, MD, whom I continue to rely on for his infallible medical knowledge as well as his unwavering friendship.

Bruce and I think continuously of our friends and family who are in the throes of medical issues ... real time. Their positive attitudes and courage give deeper meaning to our daily lives.

Davi-Ellen Chabner

Reviewers

Bruce A. Chabner, MD
Clinical Director, Emeritus
Allen Distinguished Investigator
Massachusetts General Hospital
Cancer Center
Professor of Medicine
Harvard Medical School
Boston, Massachusetts

Elizabeth Chabner, MD, MPH
CEO/Founder Masthead Inc.
Scarsdale, New York

Dan L. Longo, MD
Deputy Editor
New England Journal of Medicine
Professor of Medicine
Harvard Medical School
Boston, Massachusetts

Darci Brown, PAC, MSPAS
Director of Clinical Education, Assistant Professor
Misericordia University Physician Assistant Program
Misericordia University
Dallas, Pennsylvania

Rosalie Griffith, MSN, RN, MAEd
Nursing Success Coordinator
Chesapeake College
Wye Mills, Maryland

Emily L. McClung, RN, MSN
Instructor
Hiram College
Hiram, Ohio

Deborah Harris O' Brien, PhD, Licensed Psychologist
Associate Professor
Trinity Washington University
Washington, DC

Sean F. Peck, MEd, EMT-P
Associate Faculty-Allied Health
Arizona Western College
Yuma, Arizona

Constance Phillips, MA, MPH
Director, Biomedical Laboratory and Clinical Sciences
Boston University School of Medicine/Metropolitan College
Boston, Massachusetts

Dona Powell, BS in Education
Instructor
Technical Education Center, Osceola
Kissimmee, Florida

Mary M. Prorok, RN, MSN
Instructor
South Hills School of Business & Technology
Altoona, Pennsylvania

Julie M. Weldon, RN, MSN
Education Coordinator and Adjunct Faculty
Mercy Medical Center—Des Moines
Mercy College of Health Sciences
Des Moines, Iowa

Contents

CHAPTER 1	**BASIC WORD STRUCTURE**	**1**
	In Person: Living with Type 1 Diabetes	22
CHAPTER 2	**ORGANIZATION OF THE BODY**	**49**
	In Person: CT and MRI	67
CHAPTER 3	**SUFFIXES**	**87**
	In Person: Gallbladder Stones	108
CHAPTER 4	**PREFIXES**	**131**
	In Person: Total Knee Replacement (TKR)	151
CHAPTER 5	**MEDICAL SPECIALISTS AND CASE REPORTS**	**177**
	In Person: Living with Crohn's	197
APPENDIX 1	**BODY SYSTEMS**	**217**
APPENDIX 2	**IMMUNITY AND COVID-19 VACCINES**	**297**
APPENDIX 3	**DIAGNOSTIC TESTS AND PROCEDURES**	**307**
APPENDIX 4	**ABBREVIATIONS, ACRONYMS, SYMBOLS, EPONYMS, AND PLURALS**	**329**
APPENDIX 5	**QUICK DRUG REFERENCE**	**349**
APPENDIX 6	**ALLIED HEALTH CAREERS**	**353**
GLOSSARY 1	**MINI-DICTIONARY**	**363**
GLOSSARY 2	**WORD PARTS**	**399**
GLOSSARY 3	**ENGLISH → SPANISH TERMS**	**417**
ILLUSTRATION CREDITS		**427**
INDEX		**431**

CHAPTER 1

Basic Word Structure

Chapter Sections

Word Analysis 2
Combining Forms, Suffixes, and Prefixes 5
In Person: Living with Type 1 Diabetes 22
Exercises and Answers 23
Pronunciation of Terms 34
Practical Applications 38
Picture Show 40
Review 44
Terminology CheckUp 47

CHAPTER OBJECTIVES

- To divide medical terms into component parts
- To analyze, pronounce, and spell medical terms using common combining forms, suffixes, and prefixes

WORD ANALYSIS

If you work in a medical setting, you use medical words every day. In addition, you hear medical terms spoken in your doctor's office, read about health issues, and make daily decisions about your own health care and the health care of your family. Terms such as arthritis, electrocardiogram, hepatitis, and anemia describe conditions and tests that are familiar. Other medical words are more complicated, but as you work in this book, you will begin to understand them even if you have never studied biology or science.

Medical words are like individual jigsaw puzzles. Once you divide the terms into their component parts and learn the meaning of the individual parts, you can use that knowledge to understand many other new terms.

For example, the term HEMATOLOGY is divided into three parts:

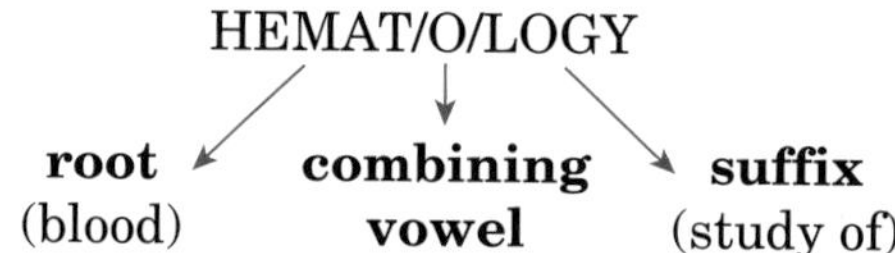

When you analyze a medical term, begin at the *end* of the word. The ending is called a **suffix.** All medical terms contain suffixes. The suffix in HEMATOLOGY is -LOGY, which means study of. Next, look at the beginning of the term. HEMAT is the word **root.** The root gives the essential meaning of the term. The root HEMAT means blood.

The third part of this term, which is the letter O, has no meaning of its own but is an important connector between the root (HEMAT) and the suffix (-LOGY). It is called a **combining vowel.** The letter O is the combining vowel usually found in medical terms.

Now put together the meanings of the suffix and the root: HEMATOLOGY means study of blood.

Another familiar medical term is ELECTROCARDIOGRAM. You probably know this term, often abbreviated as ECG (or sometimes EKG). This is how you divide it into its parts:

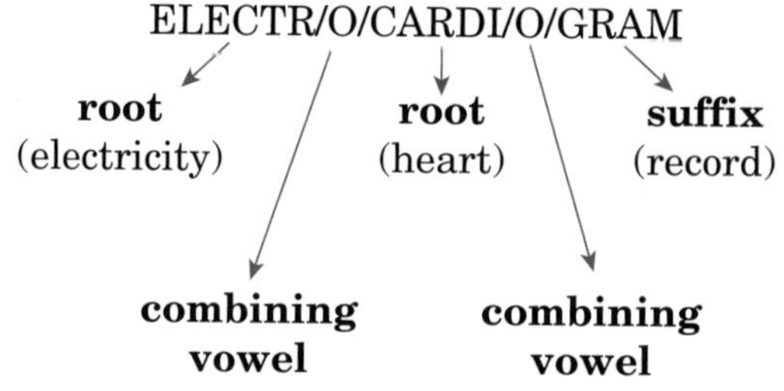

Start with the **suffix** at the end of the term. The suffix -GRAM means a record.

Now look at the beginning of the term. ELECTR is a word **root,** and it means electricity.

This medical term has two roots. The second root is CARDI, meaning heart. Whenever you see CARDI in other medical terms, you will know that it means heart.

Read the meaning of medical terms from the suffix, back to the beginning of the term, and then across. Broken down this way, ELECTROCARDIOGRAM means record of the electricity in the heart. It is the electrical current flowing within the heart that causes the heart muscle to contract, pumping blood throughout the body. The sound made by contraction and relaxation of the heart muscle is called the heartbeat.

Notice the two combining vowels in ELECTROCARDIOGRAM. Looking for the O in medical terms will help you divide the term into its parts. One combining vowel (O) lies between two roots (ELECTR and CARDI) and another between the root (CARDI) and the suffix (-GRAM).

The combining vowel *plus* the root is called a **combining form.** For example, there are two combining forms in the word ELECTROCARDIOGRAM. These combining forms are ELECTR/O, meaning electricity, and CARDI/O, meaning heart.

Notice how the following medical term is analyzed. Can you locate the two combining forms in this term?

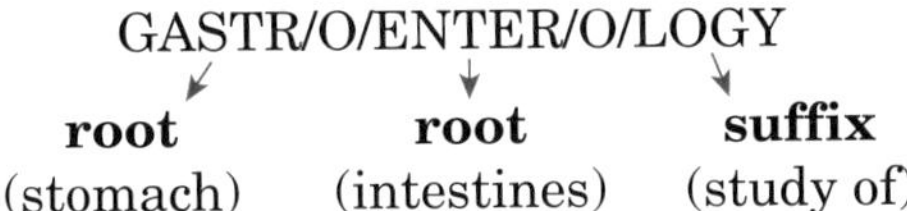

The two combining forms are GASTR/O and ENTER/O. The entire word (reading from the suffix, back to the beginning of the term, and across) means study of the stomach and the intestines. Here are other words that are divided into component parts:

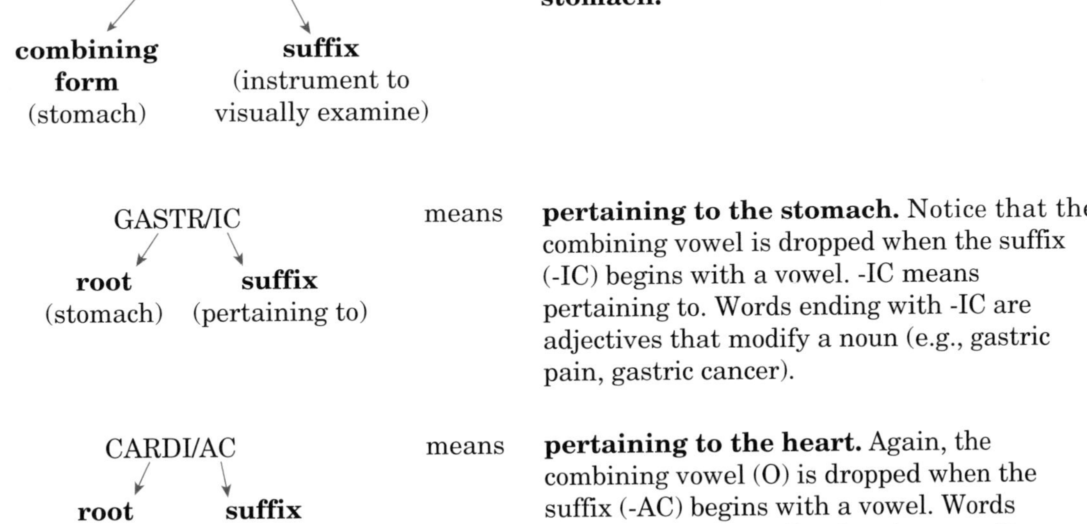

GASTR/O/SCOPE means **instrument to visually examine the stomach.**

GASTR/IC means **pertaining to the stomach.** Notice that the combining vowel is dropped when the suffix (-IC) begins with a vowel. -IC means pertaining to. Words ending with -IC are adjectives that modify a noun (e.g., gastric pain, gastric cancer).

CARDI/AC means **pertaining to the heart.** Again, the combining vowel (O) is dropped when the suffix (-AC) begins with a vowel. Words ending in -AC are adjectives (e.g., cardiac care, cardiac arrest).

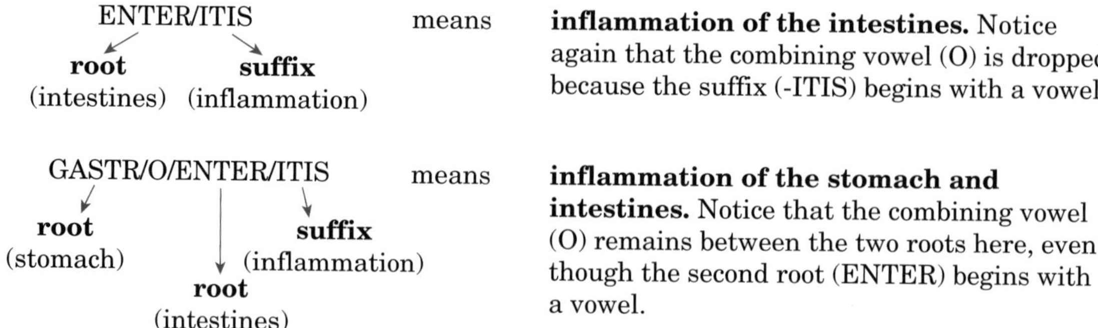

ENTER/ITIS means **inflammation of the intestines.** Notice again that the combining vowel (O) is dropped because the suffix (-ITIS) begins with a vowel.

GASTR/O/ENTER/ITIS means **inflammation of the stomach and intestines.** Notice that the combining vowel (O) remains between the two roots here, even though the second root (ENTER) begins with a vowel.

In addition to roots, suffixes, combining forms, and combining vowels, many medical terms have a word part attached to the *beginning* of the term. This is called a **prefix,** and it can change the meaning of a term in important ways. For example, watch what happens to the meaning of the following medical terms when the prefix changes:

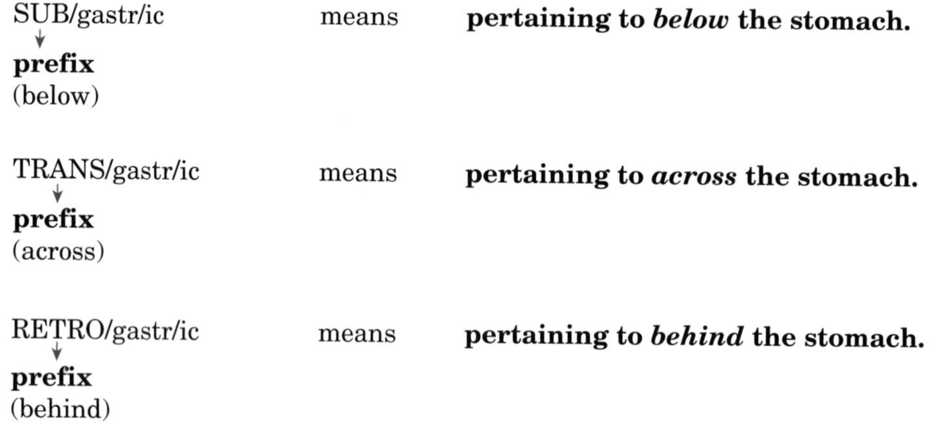

SUB/gastr/ic means **pertaining to *below* the stomach.**

TRANS/gastr/ic means **pertaining to *across* the stomach.**

RETRO/gastr/ic means **pertaining to *behind* the stomach.**

Let's **REVIEW** the important word parts:

1. **Root**—gives the essential *meaning* of the term.
2. **Suffix**—is the word *ending.*
3. **Prefix**—is a small part added to the *beginning* of a term.
4. **Combining vowel**—*connects* roots to suffixes and roots to other roots.
5. **Combining form**—is the combination of the *root* and the *combining vowel.*

Some important rules to **REMEMBER** are:

1. **Read** the meaning of medical words from the suffix to the beginning of the word and then across.
2. **Drop** the combining vowel before a suffix that starts with a vowel.
3. **Keep** the combining vowel between word roots, even if the second root begins with a vowel.

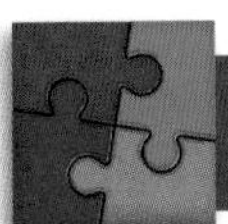

COMBINING FORMS, SUFFIXES, AND PREFIXES

Presented in this section are lists of combining forms, suffixes, and prefixes that are commonly found in medical terms. Write the meaning of the medical term on the line that is provided. Some terms will be more difficult to understand even after you know the meanings of individual word parts. For these, more extensive explanations are given in *italics*. To check your work, see the **Mini-Dictionary** beginning on page 363, which contains meanings of all terms used in this book.

In your study of medical terminology, you will find it helpful to practice writing terms and their meanings many times. You'll succeed when you follow these simple steps:

1. Complete **Exercises** beginning on page 23 for this chapter, and faithfully check your answers on pages 31 to 33.
2. Fill in the meanings in the **Pronunciation of Terms** list on pages 34 to 37.
3. Apply your knowledge in the **Practical Applications** and **Picture Show** features beginning on page 38.
4. Complete the **Review** of word parts beginning on page 44, and check your answers.
5. Make sure you understand the key medical terminology concepts in the **Terminology CheckUp** on page 47.

COMBINING FORMS

Notice that the **combining form** is in **bold** type, while the root in the medical term is underlined.

Combining Form	Meaning	Medical Term	Meaning
aden/o	gland	adenoma ____ -OMA *means tumor or mass.* adenitis ____ -ITIS *means inflammation.*	
arthr/o	joint	arthritis ____	
bi/o	life	biology ____ -LOGY *means study of.* biopsy ____ -OPSY *means (process of) viewing. Living tissue is removed and viewed under a microscope.*	
carcin/o	cancer, cancerous	carcinoma ____	
cardi/o	heart	cardiology ____	

cephal/o	head	cephalic ____________________ -IC *means pertaining to. If an infant is born with the head delivered first, it is a* ***cephalic*** *presentation.*
cerebr/o	cerebrum, largest part of the brain	cerebral ____________________ -AL *means pertaining to. Figure 1-1 shows the cerebrum and its functions.*
		cerebrovascular accident (CVA) ____________ -VASCULAR *means pertaining to blood vessels; a CVA is commonly known as a* ***stroke.***

What happens in a stroke?

Blood, containing oxygen and nutrients that are necessary to keep cells alive and functioning, is prevented from reaching areas of the cerebrum, and brain cells die. Depending on the location and extent of reduced blood flow, signs and symptoms may include loss of movement (paralysis), loss of speech (aphasia), weakness, and changes in sensation.

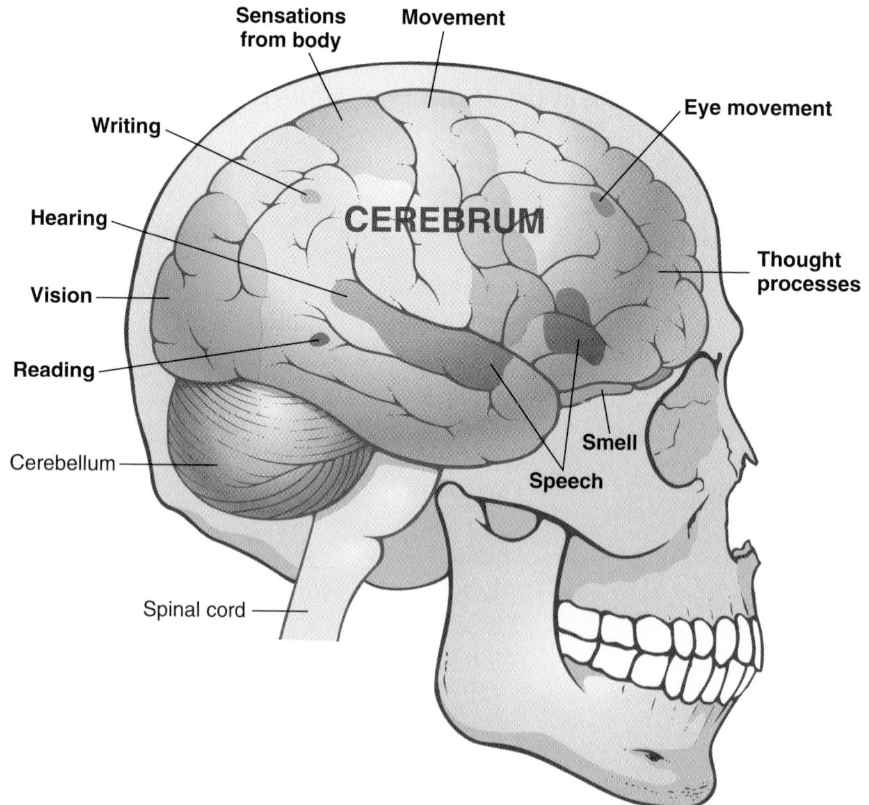

FIGURE 1-1 Functions of the cerebrum.

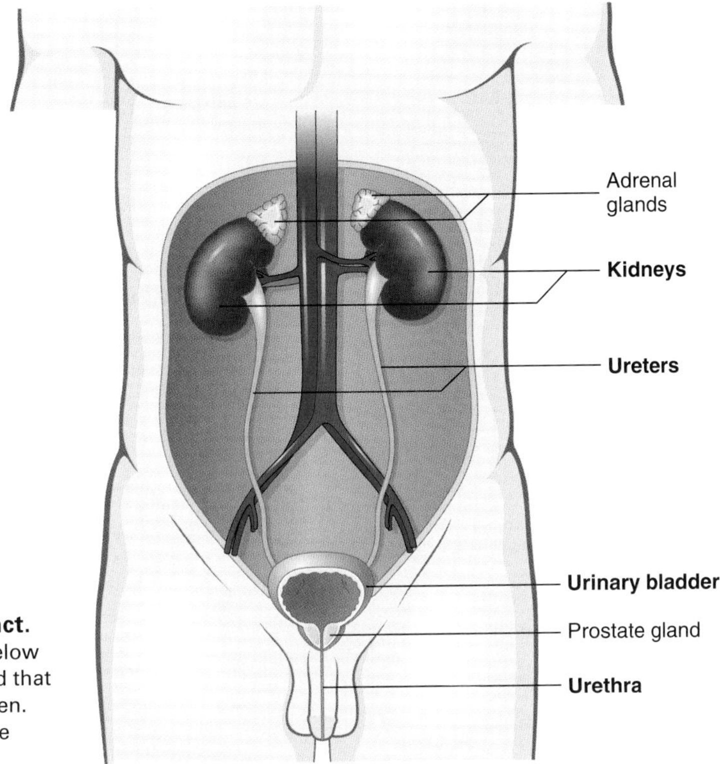

FIGURE 1-2 Male urinary tract. Note that the prostate gland lies below the urinary bladder. It secretes fluid that combines with sperm to form semen. Semen leaves the body through the urethra during ejaculation.

1

cyst/o urinary bladder

cystoscope ____________________

-SCOPE *means instrument to visually examine. Figure 1-2 shows the urinary bladder and urinary tract in a male. Figure 1-3 shows a cystoscope placed through the urethra into the urinary bladder of a female during cystoscopy.*

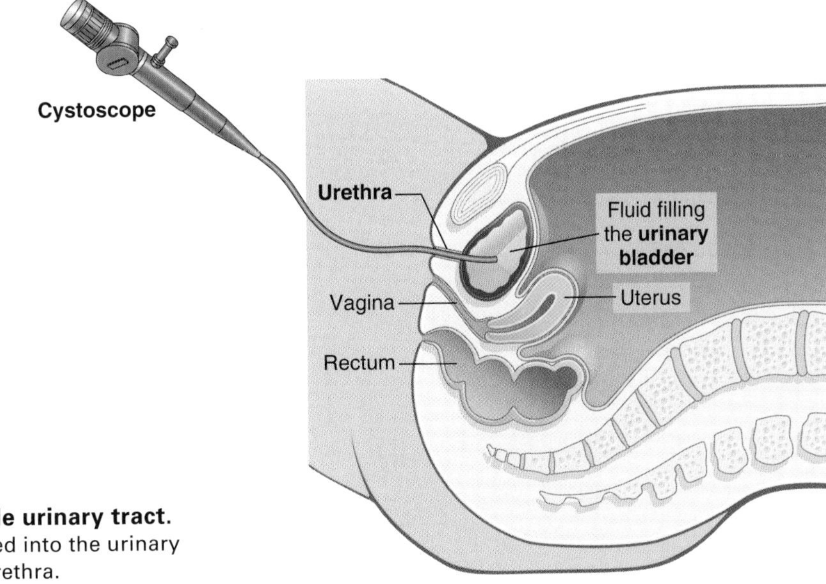

FIGURE 1-3 Female urinary tract. A **cystoscope** is placed into the urinary bladder through the urethra.

cyt/o	cell	cytology ______________________
derm/o	skin	dermal ______________________
dermat/o	skin	dermatitis ______________________
electr/o	electricity	electrocardiogram (ECG) ______________________ -GRAM *means record. EKG is an older abbreviation for this test.*

1

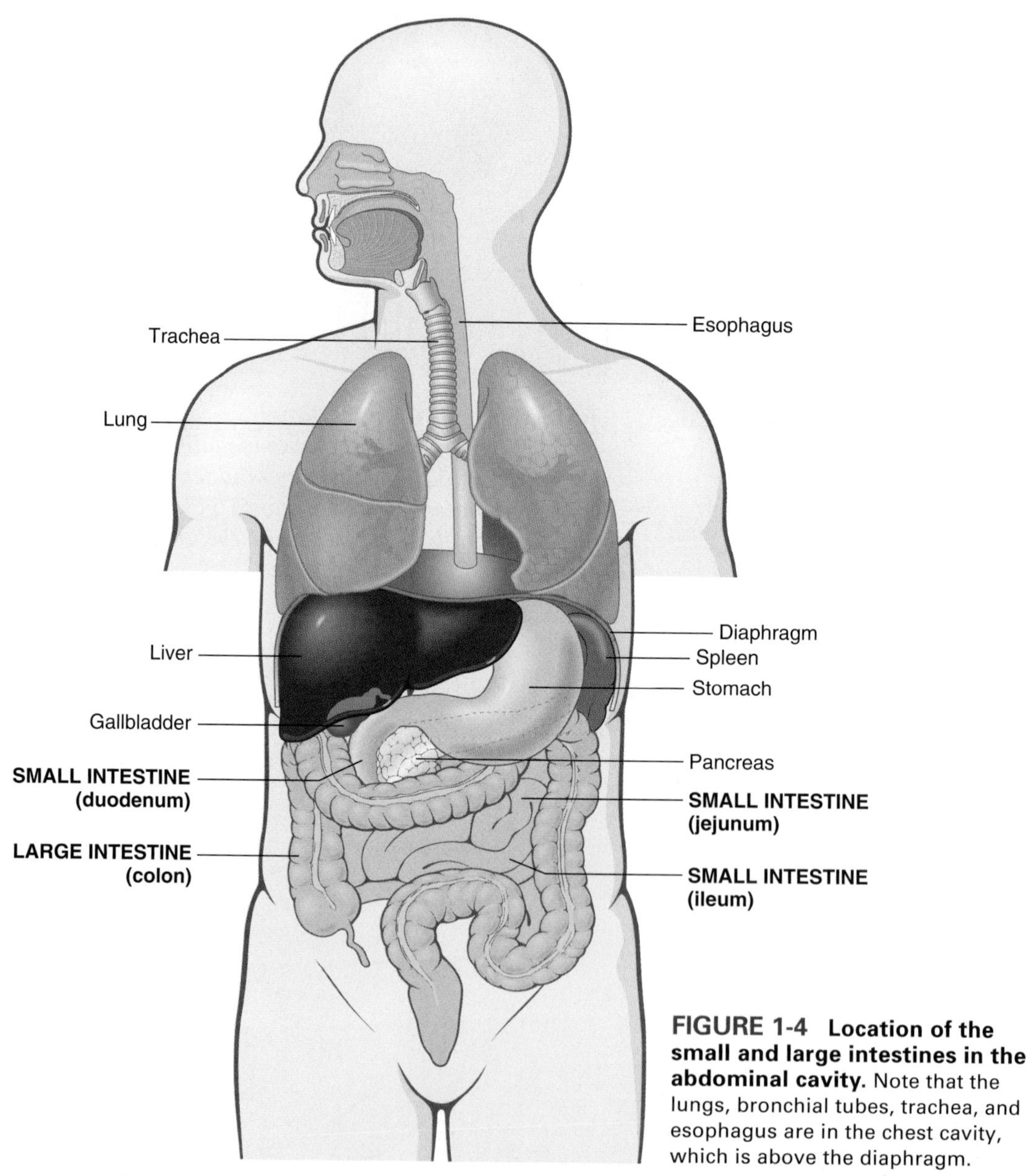

FIGURE 1-4 Location of the small and large intestines in the abdominal cavity. Note that the lungs, bronchial tubes, trachea, and esophagus are in the chest cavity, which is above the diaphragm.

encephal/o	brain	electroencephalogram (EEG) ____________ *This record is helpful in determining whether a patient has a seizure disorder, such as epilepsy.*
enter/o	intestines (often the small intestine)	enteritis ____________ *Figure 1-4 shows the small and large intestines.* ENTER/O *describes the small intestine and sometimes intestines in general.* COL/O *and* COLON/O *are combining forms for the large intestine (colon).*
erythr/o	red	erythrocyte ____________ -CYTE *means cell. Figure 1-5 shows the three major types of blood cells.*

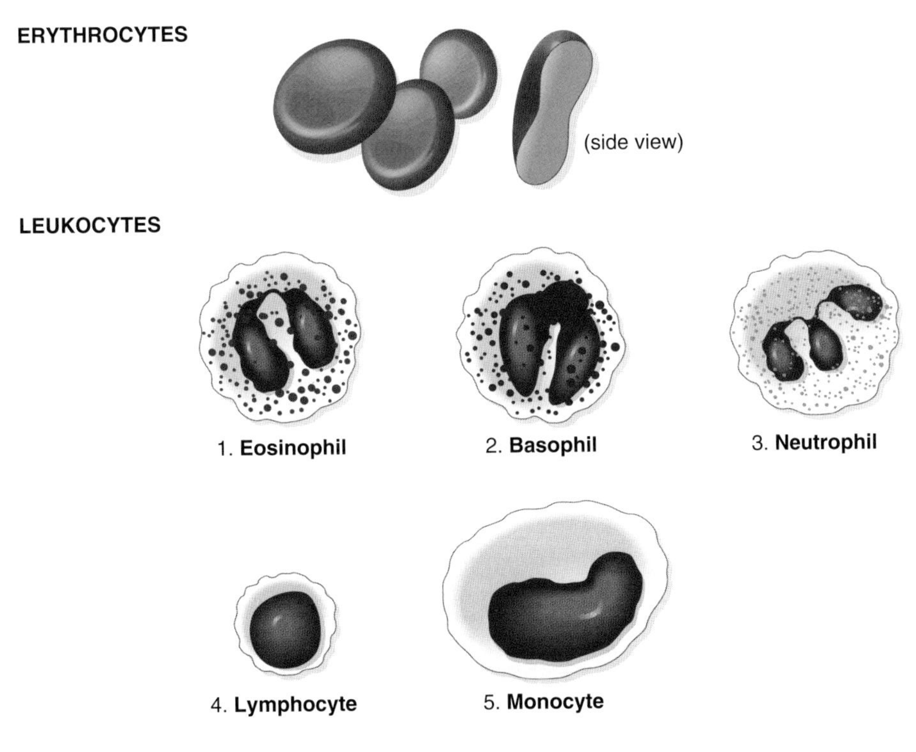

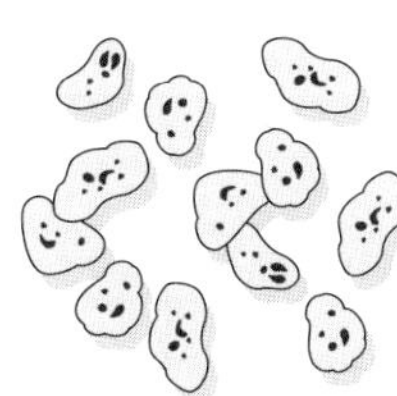

FIGURE 1-5 **Blood cells: *erythrocytes*** (carry oxygen), ***leukocytes*** (five different types help fight disease), and ***thrombocytes*** or ***platelets*** (help blood to clot).

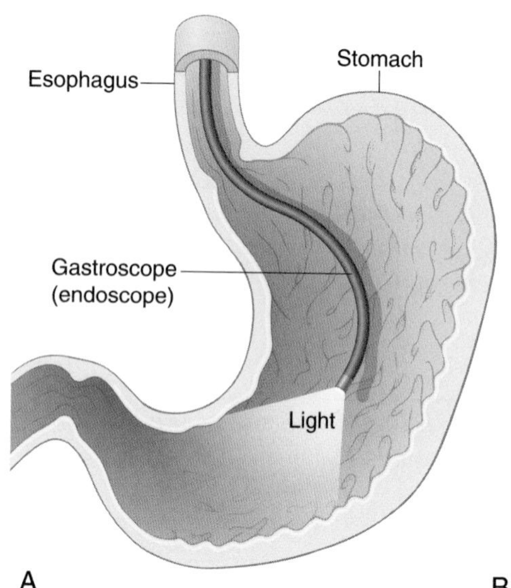

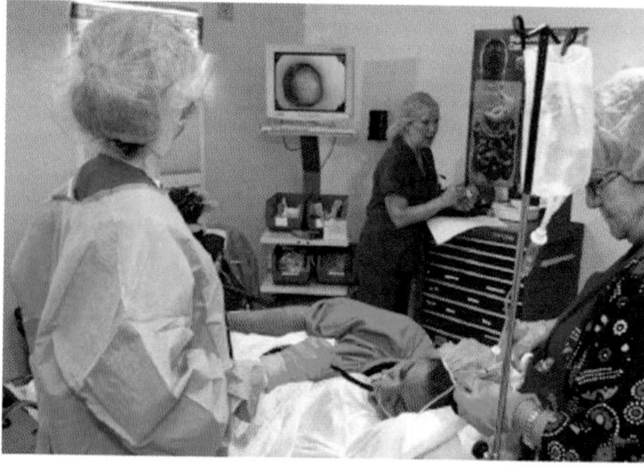

FIGURE 1-6 **A. Gastroscope** inserted into stomach. **B. Gastroscopy procedure** performed in a medical setting.

1

gastr/o	stomach	gastroscopy ______________ -SCOPY *means process of visual examination with an instrument, or "scope." Pronunciation is gas-TROS-ko-pe. A gastroscope is passed through the mouth, throat, and esophagus into the stomach. See Figure 1-6.*
gnos/o	knowledge	diagnosis ______________ -SIS *means state of;* DIA- *means complete. A diagnosis is the complete knowledge gained after testing and examining the patient. The plural of diagnosis is diagnoses.*
		prognosis ______________ PRO- *means before. A prognosis is a prediction (before knowledge) that is made after the diagnosis. It forecasts the outcome of treatment.*

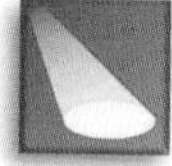

Plurals

Terms ending in -is (diagnosis, prognosis) form their plural by dropping the -is and adding -es. See Appendix 4, page 346, for other rules on formation of plurals.

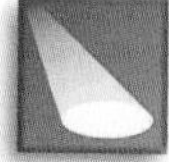

Gynecology: Be careful about spelling this term!

The combining form is **gynec/o**. A **gynecologist** specializes in diseases of the female reproductive organs. Gynecology involves both surgical and internal medicine expertise, and is often practiced with **obstetrics** (care of pregnant women and delivery of a fetus).

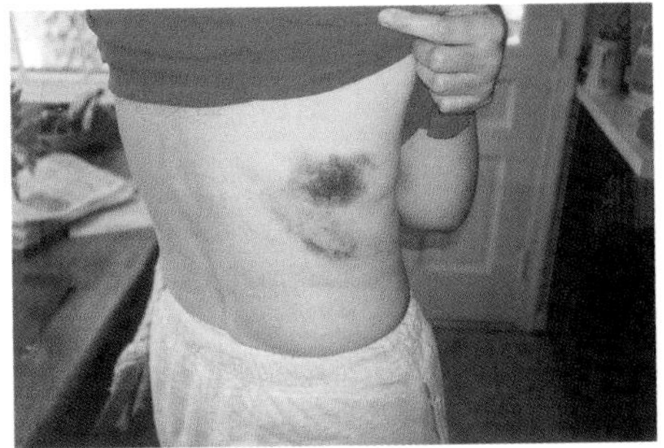

FIGURE 1-7 Hematoma from broken ribs.

gynec/o	woman, female	gynecology ______________________
hem/o, hemat/o	blood	hemoglobin ______________________ -GLOBIN *means protein. Hemoglobin is the protein in red blood cells (erythrocytes) that helps carry oxygen in the blood.* hematoma ______________________ -OMA *means mass or tumor. In this term, -oma indicates a mass or swelling containing blood. A hematoma is a mass of blood trapped in tissues of the skin or in an organ. It often results from trauma and is commonly called a bruise, or "black-and-blue" mark. Figure 1-7 shows a hematoma.*
hepat/o	liver	hepatitis ______________________ *This condition is often caused by different types of viruses: hepatitis A virus, hepatitis B virus, or hepatitis C virus.*

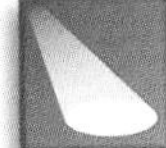

What is a virus?

A virus is a very small particle containing genetic material surrounded by a protein coat. Viruses infect cells and use the components of the host cell to make copies of themselves. Because viruses are different from bacteria, they cannot be killed by antibiotics. This is why the development of vaccines is crucial to the elimination of viral diseases. Examples of viral diseases are hepatitis, AIDS (caused by human immunodeficiency virus), and COVID-19 (caused by coronavirus). See Figure 1-8.

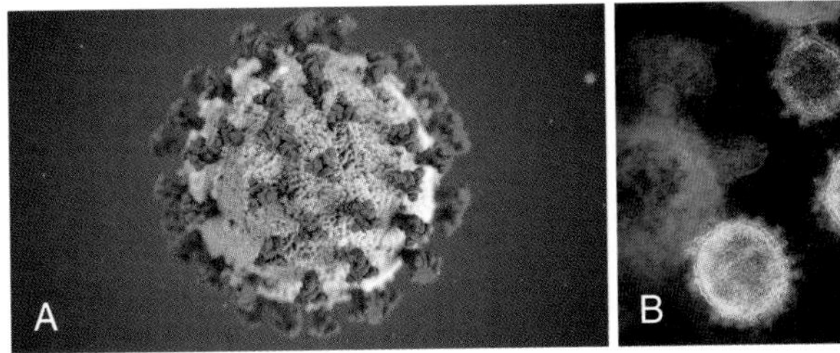

FIGURE 1-8 **A. Representation of a coronavirus** with protruding spikes. The name corona means crown and describes a group of viruses that have crown-like spikes on their surfaces. **B. Electron micrograph of coronaviruses.**

lapar/o	abdomen (area between the chest and hip)	laparotomy ______________ *-TOMY means cutting into. In an **exploratory laparotomy** the surgeon makes a large incision in the abdominal wall to inspect organs for evidence of disease. See Figure 1-9A. **Laparoscopy** is visual examination of the abdomen using several small incisions for a **laparoscope** and other instruments. See Figure 1-9B. Another combining form for abdomen is* ABDOMIN/O, *as in abdominal.*
leuk/o	white	leukocyte ______________ *Figure 1-5 on page 9 shows five different types of leukocytes.*
nephr/o	kidney	nephrectomy ______________ -ECTOMY *means cutting out—an excision or resection of an organ or other part of the body.*
neur/o	nerve	neurology ______________
onc/o	tumor (cancerous)	oncologist ______________ -IST *means a specialist.*

1

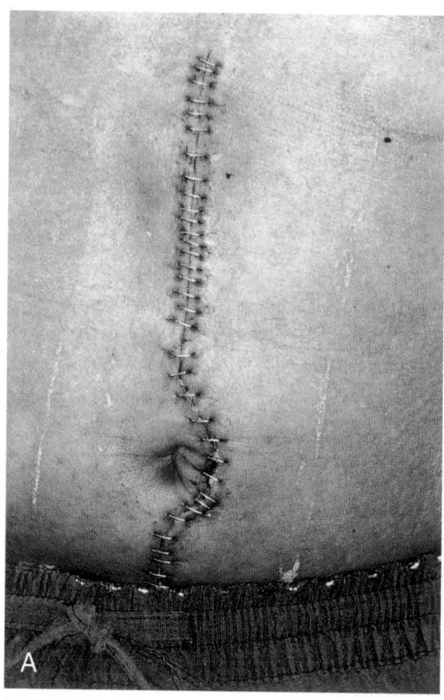

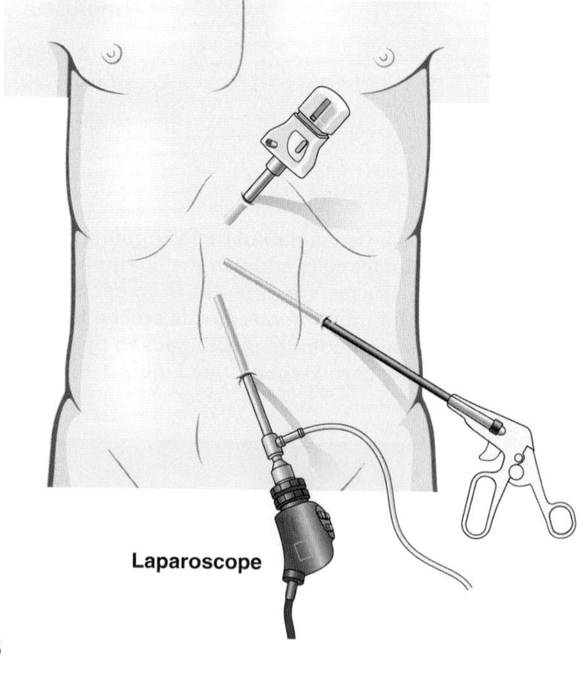

FIGURE 1-9 A, Laparotomy. This large incision was closed with surgical staples. **B, Laparoscopy.** The abdomen is examined making small incisions and using a **laparoscope.**

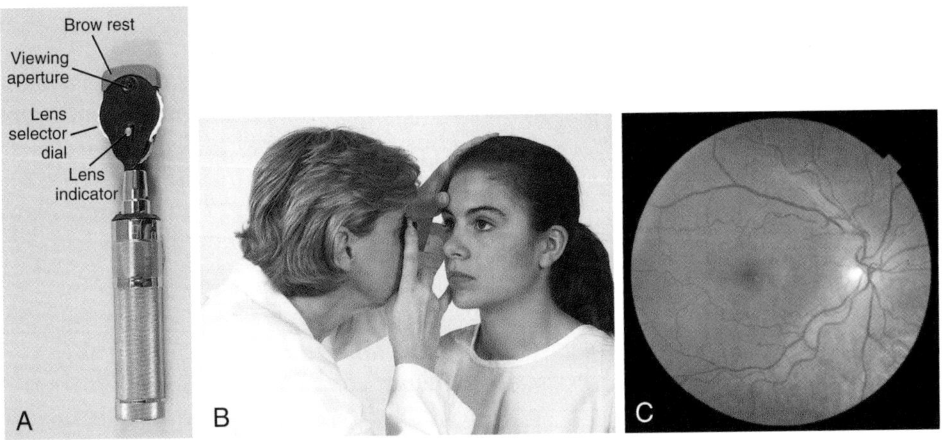

FIGURE 1-10 **A, Ophthalmoscope.** This instrument allows the ophthalmologist to view both the outer and inner areas of the eye. **B, Ophthalmoscopic examination. C, The inner or back area (retina) of a normal eye** as seen through an ophthalmoscope.

ophthalm/o eye

ophthalmoscope ______________________

Figure 1-10A is an image of an ophthalmoscope. Figure 1-10B shows an ophthalmologist, a medical doctor, examining a patient's eye. Figure 1-10C shows the retina, lining the back of the eye (fundus), as seen through an ophthalmoscope.

oste/o bone

osteoarthritis ______________________

Figure 1-11 shows a normal knee joint and a knee joint with osteoarthritis. Degenerative changes with thinning and loss of cartilage occur. Inflammation of the joint membrane occurs late in the disease.

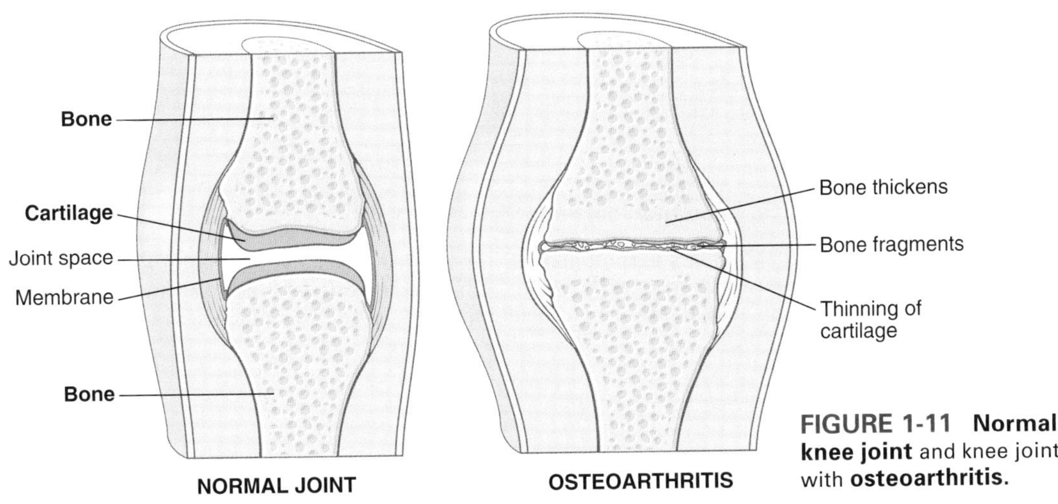

FIGURE 1-11 **Normal knee joint** and knee joint with **osteoarthritis.**

path/o	disease	pathologist ________________ *A pathologist is a medical doctor who views biopsy samples to make a diagnosis and examines dead bodies (in autopsies) to determine the cause of death.* AUT- *means self, and* -OPSY *means (process of) viewing. Thus, an autopsy is an opportunity to see for oneself what caused a patient's death.*
psych/o	mind	psychosis ________________ -OSIS *means abnormal condition. In this serious mental condition, the patient loses touch with reality. Psychotic symptoms include* ***hallucinations*** *(unreal sensory perceptions, such as hearing voices when none are present) and* ***delusions*** *(fixed, false beliefs that can't be changed by logical reasoning).*
ren/o	kidney	renal ________________ *Sometimes there are two combining forms for the same part of the body. Often, one comes from Latin and the other from Greek.* REN- *is the Latin root meaning "kidney," and* NEPHR- *is the Greek root meaning "kidney." The Greek root describes abnormal conditions and procedures, whereas the Latin root is used with* -AL, *meaning "pertaining to."*
rhin/o	nose	rhinitis ________________
sarc/o	flesh	sarcoma ________________ *Sarcomas and carcinomas are both cancerous (malignant) tumors. See Figure 1-12.* ***Sarcomas*** *grow from the fleshy (connective) tissues of the body, such as muscle, fat, bone, and cartilage, whereas* ***carcinomas*** *arise from skin tissue and the linings of internal organs.*

1

Pathologist/medical examiner/coroner

A **medical examiner** (M.E.) is a **pathologist** who specializes in forensic (legal) medicine related to criminal issues. A **coroner,** however, is an elected official (administrator) who investigates any suspicious death. This official may or may not be a medical examiner.

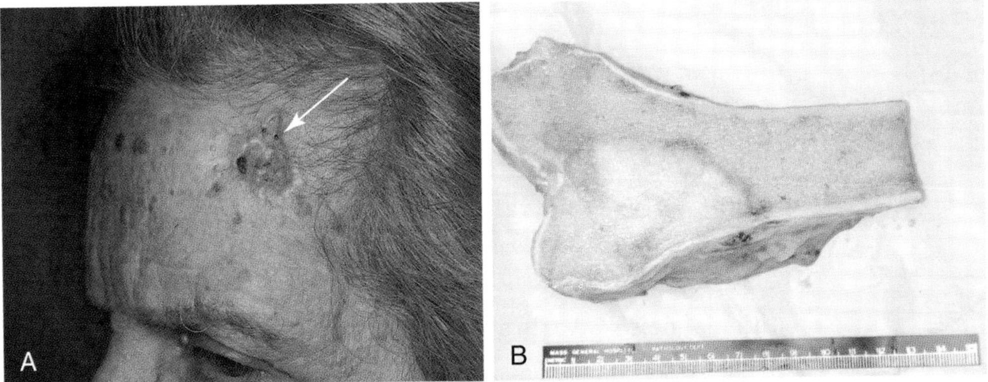

FIGURE 1-12 **A. Basal cell carcinoma.** This type of skin cancer grows from lining or epithelial cells of the skin. Other carcinomas come from cells that line internal organs and glands within the body. **B. Sarcoma of the bone (osteosarcoma).** Sarcomas grow from connective (supportive) tissue such as bone, fat, or muscle.

thromb/o	clotting	thrombocyte ______________
		*A thrombocyte (**platelet**) is a small cell that helps blood to clot. Platelets are shown in Figure 1-5 (see page 9).*
		thrombosis ______________
		*Formation of a **thrombus** (blood clot) occurs when thrombocytes and other clotting factors combine. See Figure 1-13. **Thrombosis** describes the condition of forming a clot (thrombus).*

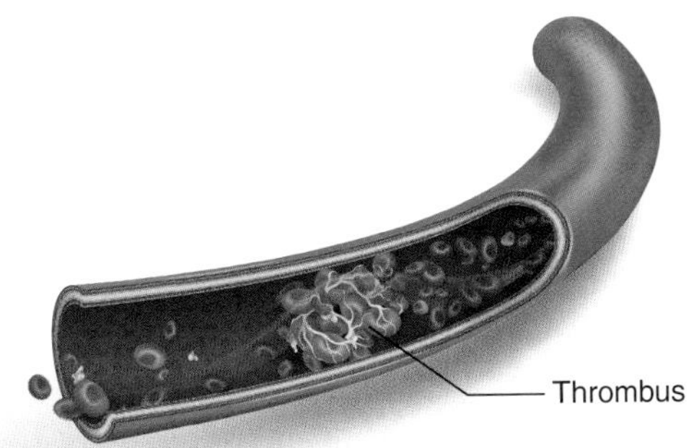

FIGURE 1-13 **Thrombus** (blood clot). (Courtesy iStock #1172668129, urfinguss.)

SUFFIXES

Each suffix is in **bold** in the Suffix column and underlined in the Medical Term column.

Suffix	Meaning	Medical Term	Meaning
-al	pertaining to	neural *Other suffixes meaning pertaining to are listed on page 399 in Glossary of Word Parts.*	
-algia	condition of pain	arthralgia	
-cyte	cell	leukocyte	
-ectomy	cutting out; removal, excision	gastrectomy *In a partial or subtotal gastrectomy, only a portion of the stomach is removed.*	
-emia	blood condition	leukemia *Large numbers of immature, cancerous cells are found in the bloodstream and bone marrow (inner part of bone that makes blood cells).*	
-globin	protein	hemoglobin	
-gram	record	arthrogram *This is an x-ray record of a joint.*	
-ia	condition	neuralgia -IA *means condition and is part of the larger suffix* -ALGIA *meaning condition of pain.*	
-ic	pertaining to	gastric	
-ism	condition, process	hyperthyroidism HYPER- *means excessive. The thyroid gland is in the neck. It secretes the hormone thyroxine, which helps cells burn food to release energy. See Figure 1-14.*	
-itis	inflammation	gastroenteritis	
-logist	specialist in the study of	neurologist	
-logy	study of	nephrology *See Table 1-1 on page 17 for a list of other terms using* -LOGY.	
-oma	tumor, mass	hepatoma *This is a cancerous (malignant) tumor, also called* ***hepatocellular carcinoma.***	

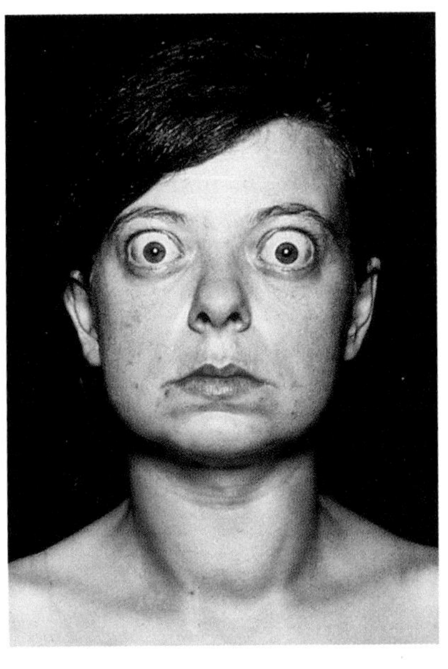

FIGURE 1-14 Hyperthyroidism (Graves disease). The thyroid gland produces too much hormone, which causes signs and symptoms such as rapid pulse, nervousness, excessive sweating, and swelling of tissue behind the eyeball (resulting in exophthalmos, or "bulging" of the eyes). Notice the enlarged thyroid gland in the neck.

-opsy	to view	biopsy ______________________
-osis	abnormal condition	nephrosis ______________________
		leukocytosis ______________________ *This is an increase in numbers of normal white blood cells as a response to infection.*

1

TABLE 1-1	TERMS USING *-LOGY* (STUDY OF)
Cardiology	Study of the heart
Dermatology	Study of the skin
Endocrinology	Study of the endocrine glands
Gastroenterology	Study of the stomach and intestines
Gynecology	Study of women and women's diseases
Hematology	Study of the blood
Neurology	Study of the nerves and the brain and spinal cord
Oncology	Study of tumors (cancerous or malignant diseases)
Ophthalmology	Study of the eye
Pathology	Study of disease
Psychology	Study of the mind and mental disorders
Rheumatology	Study of joint diseases (RHEUMAT/O = flow or watery discharge, which was once thought to cause aches and pains, especially in joints)
Urology	Study of the urinary tract (surgical specialty)

-scope	instrument to visually examine	gastroscope ______________
		laparoscope ______________
-scopy	process of visual examination	laparoscopy ______________ *Small incisions are made near the navel, and instruments are inserted into the abdomen for viewing organs and performing procedures such as tying off the fallopian (uterine) tubes. See Figure 1-15.*
		arthroscopy ______________ *See Figure 1-16.*
-sis	state of	prognosis ______________
-tomy	process of cutting into; incision	neurotomy ______________

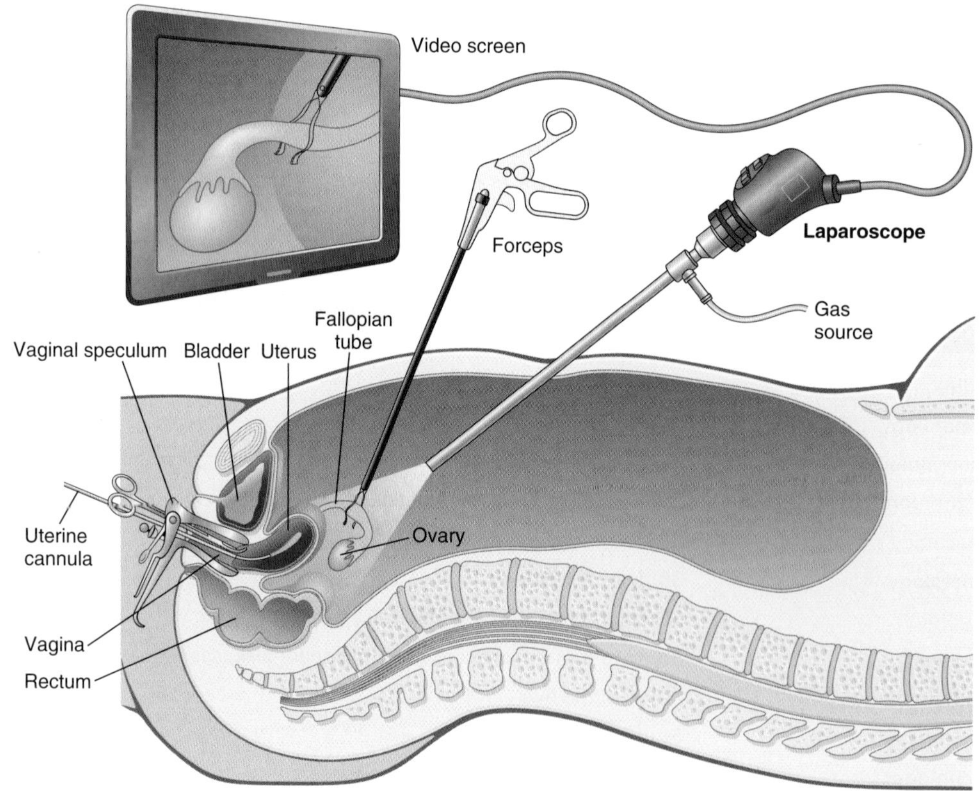

FIGURE 1-15 Laparoscopy for tubal ligation (interruption of the continuity of the fallopian tubes) as a means of preventing future pregnancy. The vaginal speculum keeps the vaginal cavity open. The uterine cannula is a tube placed into the uterus to manipulate the uterus during the procedure. Forceps are used for grasping or manipulating tissue.

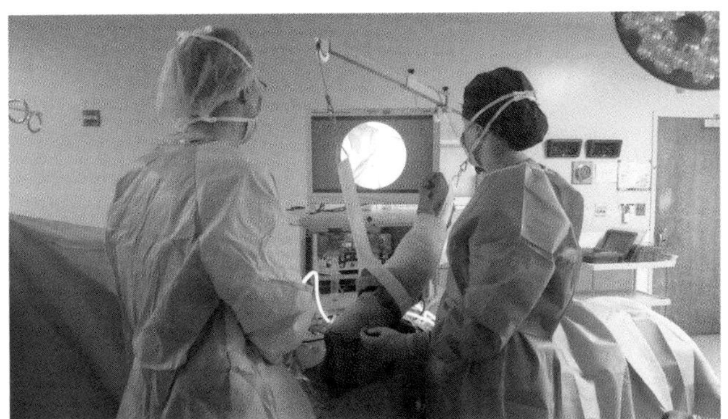

FIGURE 1-16 Arthroscopy of the shoulder. A surgeon (orthopedist) performs an arthroscopic examination to make a diagnosis or treat disease of the joints.

PREFIXES

Each prefix is in **bold** type in the Prefix column and underlined in the Medical Term column.

Prefix	Meaning	Medical Term	Meaning
a-, an-	no, not	anemia ________ *Literally, anemia means a condition of "no blood." Actually, it is a decrease in the number of red blood cells or in hemoglobin, the protein that helps in their ability to carry oxygen.*	
aut-	self	autopsy ________ *Viewing and examining a dead body with one's own (self) eyes. Here the root* OPS- *(viewing) is embedded in the suffix* -OPSY *(process of viewing).*	
dia-	complete, through	diagnosis ________ *In this term,* DIA- *means complete.*	
		diameter ________ *The suffix* -METER *means measurement.* DIA- *means through in this term.*	
dys-	bad, painful, difficult, abnormal	dysentery ________ *The suffix* -Y *means condition or process.*	

Where is the root?

Some suffixes can contain roots. In the term anemia, notice that the root EM- (from HEM, meaning blood) is embedded in the suffix -EMIA.

endo-	within	endocrine glands ________________ CRIN/O *means to secrete (to form and give off). Examples of endocrine glands are the thyroid gland, pituitary gland, adrenal glands, ovaries, and testes. All of these glands secrete hormones* ***within*** *the body and into the bloodstream.* endocardium ________________ *The valves and chambers within the heart are lined with endocardium. The suffix* -UM *indicates a structure.*
epi-	above, upon, on	epigastric ________________
exo-	outside	exocrine glands ________________ *Examples of exocrine glands are sweat, tear, and mammary (breast) glands, which secrete substances to the* ***outside*** *of the body.*
hyper-	excessive, more than normal, too much	hyperglycemia ________________ GLYC/O *means sugar. Hyperglycemia may be a sign of diabetes mellitus. Mellitus means "sweet."*
hypo-	below, less than normal, under	hypoglycemia ________________ *This condition results from too much insulin in the bloodstream. Symptoms are weakness, headache, and hunger.*
pan-	all	pandemic ________________ *DEM/O means people. COVID-19 is a* ***pandemic*** *disease that, in 2020, spread all through the world, causing millions of infections and deaths. An* ***epidemic*** *refers to a disease that has spread to many people, but within a limited or confined area.*
peri-	surrounding	pericardium ________________

Hyperglycemia and diabetes

People with hyperglycemia lack insulin (**type 1 diabetes**) or have ineffective insulin (**type 2 diabetes**). Insulin is a hormone normally released by the pancreas, an endocrine gland near the stomach. Insulin allows sugar to leave the bloodstream and enter cells. When insulin is either absent or not working, sugar remains in the blood, resulting in hyperglycemia and diabetes. See ***In Person: Living with Type 1 Diabetes*** on page 22.

pro-	before, forward	prostate gland ________________ *This exocrine gland "stands" (-STATE) before or in front of the urinary bladder in males (see Figure 1-17).*
re-	back	resection ________________ -SECTION *means cutting into an organ, but* RESECTION *means removing some or all of an organ in the sense of cutting back or away. The Latin* resectio *means "a trimming or pruning."*
retro-	behind	retrogastric ________________
sub-	below, under	subhepatic ________________
trans-	across, through	transdermal ________________
		transurethral ________________ *The urethra is a tube that leads from the urinary bladder to the outside of the body.*

Transurethral resection of the prostate gland (TURP)

This is a surgical procedure to remove noncancerous (benign) growth of the prostate gland. Pieces of the enlarged gland are removed through the urethra. See Figure 1-17.

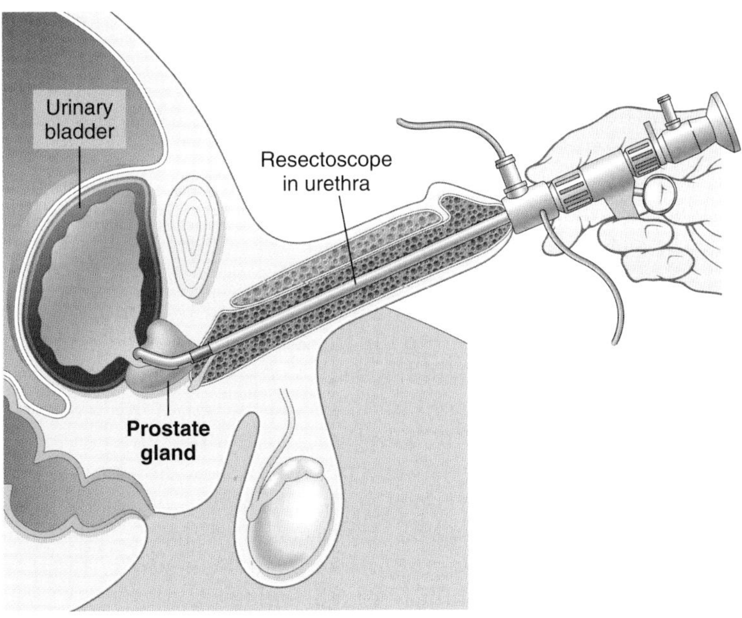

FIGURE 1-17 Transurethral resection of the prostate (TURP). The resectoscope contains a light, valves for controlling irrigating fluid, and an electrical loop that cuts tissue and seals blood vessels.

IN PERSON: LIVING WITH TYPE 1 DIABETES

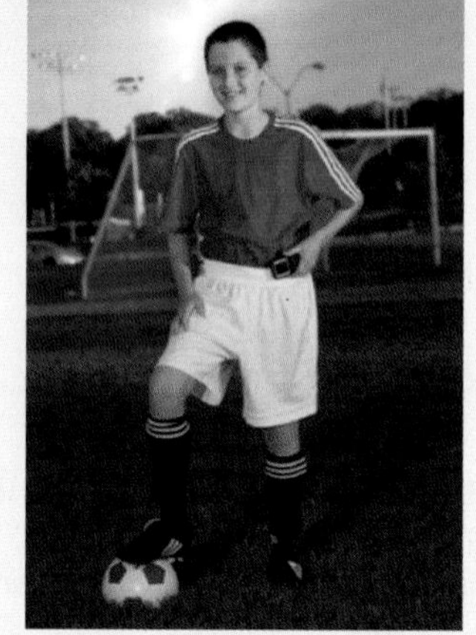

The following first-person narrative describes the reality of living with a particular medical condition—type 1 diabetes in a teenager. In each of the subsequent chapters, you'll find other first-person accounts of diseases and procedures that will make your study of medical terminology more relevant to real-life situations.

Jake Sheldon has type 1 diabetes, which was diagnosed when he was 8 years old. The following narrative was written by his mother, Ruthellen Sheldon, based on his teenage years.

On school days, I wake Jake up at 6:30 AM. He tests his blood sugar by pricking his finger until it bleeds, and then sticks a test strip into the drop of blood. Then he inserts the strip into a small hand-held glucometer and waits 3 to 5 seconds for a reading of his blood sugar. If this is 120 mg/dL or higher, he gives himself insulin 10 to 15 minutes before breakfast. He has an insulin pump, so he types in the amount of carbohydrates he will eat, plus his current blood sugar reading. The pump calculates how much insulin he needs to cover the carbs and any extra insulin he may need to bring down a high blood sugar. If Jake's blood sugar is less than 120 mg/dL when he wakes up, he will wait until he takes his first bite of food to give himself his insulin to avoid hypoglycemia.

Throughout the school day, if his blood sugar is high or low, he visits the nurse. If it's high, he gives himself an insulin bolus, or correction, by pump. If his blood sugar is positive for ketones, he is sent home from school. If his blood sugar is low or less than 70, he eats or drinks some fast-acting sugar (Skittles, Smarties, or Sprite) and waits in the healthroom for his blood sugar to rise so he can return to class.

During the night, his dad and I set an alarm to wake up around 3 hours after bedtime. If his blood sugar is high while he sleeps, we use his pump to give him extra insulin, "a correction." If it is low, we wake him and have him drink Sprite or eat Smarties.

The insulin pump is connected to his body with a small cannula [tube]. It is inserted manually through a needle into his hip region. The needle is then removed and the tiny Teflon cannula remains in his body, delivering fast-acting insulin under the skin. His pump is always connected to him with plastic tubing, and he carries it with him in his pants pocket. When he bathes, he can disconnect the pump, and when he sleeps, he places it on the mattress next to his body.

When Jake is playing sports, he times his meals with the start of the activity so that his blood sugar is around 150 mg/dL. He disconnects his pump during sports, and at halftime he tests his blood sugar. If it is low, he needs to eat. If it is high, he needs to reconnect his pump and administer more insulin.

1

In general, Jake's diabetes doesn't disrupt his life other than for his nighttime checks, wearing an insulin pump, and paying attention to how many carbs he eats. We encourage him to make good nutritional choices and to limit certain foods (doughnuts, Slurpees, candy) to special occasions. He also must carry a glucometer with him at all times and a sugar to take when his blood glucose is low.

Having a child with diabetes forces me to carefully plan the preparation and timing of meals. I always have certain foods and medical supplies in the house, and I also carry snacks and sugar sources wherever I go. My husband and I hope that keeping Jake's blood sugar in tight control will help avoid many of the complications frequently encountered later in life by people with type 1 diabetes.

Throughout high school, Jake took over all diabetes management tasks and managed his diabetes 100 percent independently before his graduation. Moving out of state to college, Jake has had to learn how cafeteria foods, late nights, and new social situations affect his blood sugars. Jake is also learning how to manage ordering and maintaining a vast number of diabetes supplies and prescriptions in his dorm room. Jake will also be transitioning from his pediatric endocrinologist to an adult endocrinologist this year.

Ruthellen Sheldon and her son, Jake, now 18 years old.

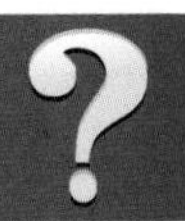

EXERCISES AND ANSWERS

These exercises give you practice writing and understanding the terms presented in the chapter. An important part of your work is to ***check your answers*** *with the Answers to Exercises beginning on page 31.*
Remember the 3 "Rs"—wRite, Review, Repeat—and you will succeed! *Visit the Evolve website for additional games and interactive activities.*

A Using slashes (/), divide the following terms into their component parts and give the meaning for the whole term. The first term is completed as an example.

1. aden/oma *tumor of a gland*
2. arthritis ______________________
3. biopsy ______________________

4. cardiology ____
5. dermal ____
6. cytology ____
7. cystoscope ____
8. cerebral ____
9. cephalic ____
10. adenitis ____

B Complete the following sentences using the medical terms given below.

diagnosis	erythrocyte	hepatitis
electrocardiogram	gynecology	prognosis
electroencephalogram	hematoma	
enteritis	hemoglobin	

1. A mass of blood, or "black-and-blue" mark, is a/an ________________________.
2. A red blood cell is a/an ____.
3. Inflammation of the small intestine is ______________________________.
4. The prediction about the outcome of an illness is a/an ______________________.
5. The record of electricity in the brain is a/an ____________________________.
6. The study of women and women's diseases is __________________________.
7. The record of electricity in the heart is a/an ____________________________.
8. Complete knowledge of a patient's illness on the basis of tests and other information is a/an ____.
9. A protein found in red blood cells is ________________________________.
10. Inflammation of the liver is ______________________________________.

C **Name the tissue or part of the body contained in the following terms and give the meaning of the entire term.**

	Tissue/Body Part	Meaning of Term
1. laparotomy	__________	__________
2. nephrectomy	__________	__________
3. neuritis	__________	__________
4. ophthalmoscope	__________	__________
5. osteotomy	__________	__________
6. renal	__________	__________
7. rhinitis	__________	__________
8. sarcoma	__________	__________

D **Give the meanings of the following terms.**

1. oncologist __________
2. pathologist __________
3. psychosis __________
4. leukocyte __________
5. thrombocyte __________
6. gastritis __________
7. adenoma __________
8. thrombosis __________

E Give the meanings of the following suffixes.

1. -cyte ______
2. -ism ______
3. -ectomy ______
4. -al ______
5. -emia ______
6. -gram ______
7. -algia ______
8. -itis ______
9. -globin ______
10. -ic ______

F Complete the following medical terms to end each sentence.

1. Nerve pain is **neur**______.
2. Presence of large numbers of immature, cancerous white blood cells is a blood condition known as **leuk**______.
3. An x-ray record of a joint is **arthro**______.
4. Study of the kidney is **nephro**______.
5. Tumor of the liver is **hepat**______.
6. Visual examination of the abdomen is **laparo**______.
7. An incision of a joint is called **arthro**______.
8. Abnormal condition of the skin is **dermat**______.
9. Inflammation of the skin is **dermat**______.
10. A specialist in the study of blood is a **hemato**______.

G Give the meanings of the following prefixes.

1. hyper- ____________
2. sub- ____________
3. dys- ____________
4. trans- ____________
5. retro- ____________
6. dia- ____________
7. exo- ____________
8. aut- ____________
9. hypo- ____________
10. endo- ____________
11. peri- ____________
12. pan- ____________
13. epi- ____________
14. a-/an- ____________

H Give the meanings of the following medical terms.

1. autopsy ____________
2. hyperthyroidism ____________
3. anemia ____________
4. dysentery ____________
5. endocrine glands ____________
6. hypoglycemia ____________
7. exocrine glands ____________
8. resection ____________
9. transdermal ____________
10. hyperglycemia ____________

I Complete the following medical terms related to the stomach

1. ____________________gastric Pertaining to **under** the stomach
2. gastr____________________ **Pain** in the stomach
3. gastr____________________ **Inflammation** of the stomach
4. ____________________gastric Pertaining to **across** or **through** the stomach
5. gastr____________________ **Process of visually examining** the stomach
6. ____________________gastric Pertaining to **behind** the stomach
7. gastr____________________ **Study of** the stomach and intestines
8. gastr____________________ **Incision** of the stomach
9. gastr____________________ **Excision** of the stomach
10. gastr____________________ **Instrument to visually examine** the stomach
11. ____________________gastric Pertaining to **above** the stomach

1

J On the line provided, give the meaning of the term in bold

1. An **oncologist** treats abnormal conditions such as sarcomas and carcinomas.

   ____

2. After explaining the diagnosis, Dr. Jones outlined the treatment and assured the patient that the **prognosis** was hopeful. ______________________________

   ____

3. Elderly Mrs. Scott has constant arthralgia in her knees and hips. Her physician prescribes anti-inflammatory drugs and aspirin to treat her **osteoarthritis** but advises that joint replacement may be necessary. ______________________________

   ____

4. A **pathologist** is a medical doctor who performs autopsies and examines biopsy samples. ____

5. **Thrombosis** is a serious condition that may result in blockage of blood vessels.

____

6. **Hyperglycemia** results from lack of insulin (hormone) secretion from the pancreas (endocrine gland near the stomach). Without insulin, sugar cannot enter cells and remains in the blood. ______________________________

7. Schizophrenia is an example of a **psychosis** in which the patient loses touch with reality and displays abnormal behavior. (Delusions and hallucinations may occur.)

____

8. Minimally invasive surgery of the abdomen may be performed using **laparoscopy**. For example, a gallbladder or appendix can be removed with instruments inserted through small incisions. ______________________________

____

9. Clinical signs of **hyperthyroidism** include an enlarged thyroid gland and protruding eyeballs (exophthalmos). ______________________________

____

10. Sally's diagnosis of **dysentery** was made after she returned from a trip to Mexico with abdominal pain, fever, and severe diarrhea (loose, watery stools). ____________

____

11. Mr. Smith died of a **cerebrovascular accident**. Confirmation at autopsy revealed a thrombus blocking one of his cerebral arteries. ______________________________

____

12. **Erythrocytes** contain hemoglobin, which enables them to carry oxygen throughout the body. ______________________________

13. **Leukemia** was confirmed after a bone marrow biopsy and high white blood cell counts. ______________________________

14. Certain types of bleeding or clotting disorders may be caused by reduced numbers of thrombocytes, also known as **platelets**. ______________________________

15. An example of **anemia** is iron deficiency anemia. ______________________________

____

16. **Transdermal** delivery by patch is used for administering drugs such as nicotine, nitroglycerin, and scopolamine (for motion sickness). ______________________________

____

17. When Bill had difficulty urinating (urinary retention), his doctor discovered that his **prostate gland** was enlarged. ______________________________

____

18. To relieve his symptoms related to urinary retention, Bill's urologist performed a **transurethral resection** of his enlarged prostate gland. ______________________________

____

19. Although the small intestine is longer (20 feet) than the large intestine (5 feet), the **diameter** of the large intestine (colon) is greater. ______________________________

____

20. In 2020 millions of people worldwide died in the COVID-19 **pandemic** ______________________________

____

K **In the following medical vignettes, circle the bold term that best completes the meaning of the sentences.**

1. Selma ate a spicy meal at an Indian restaurant. Later that night she experienced (**osteoarthritis, dermatitis, gastroenteritis**). Fortunately the cramping and diarrhea subsided by morning.
2. Christina was feeling very sluggish, both physically and mentally. Her hair seemed coarse, she had noticed weight gain in the past weeks, and she had hot and cold intolerance. Her internist ordered a blood test that revealed low levels of a hormone normally secreted from a gland in the neck. She was referred to a specialist, a/an (**gynecologist, endocrinologist, pathologist**). The physician ordered a blood test that confirmed low levels of the hormone. The diagnosis of (**hypothyroidism, hyperthyroidism, psychosis**) was thus made, and proper treatment prescribed.
3. Dr. Fischer examined the lump in Bruno's thigh. An imaging technique using magnetic waves and radio signals (MRI scan) revealed a suspicious mass in the soft connective tissue of the thigh. Suspecting a cancerous mass of flesh tissue, or (**hematoma, carcinoma, sarcoma**), Dr. Fischer ordered a/an (**prognosis, biopsy, autopsy**) of the mass.
4. On her seventh birthday, Susie fell down during her birthday party. Her mother noticed bruises on Susie's knees and elbows that seemed to "come up overnight." Her pediatrician ordered a blood test, which demonstrated a decreased platelet count and an elevated (**leukocyte, erythrocyte, thrombocyte**) count at 40,000 cells. Susie was referred to a/an (**dermatologist, nephrologist, oncologist**), who made a diagnosis of (**hepatitis, anemia, leukemia**).
5. When Mr. Saluto collapsed and died while eating dinner, the family requested a/an (**laparotomy, gastroscopy, autopsy**) to determine the cause of death. The (**hematologist, pathologist, gastroenterologist**) discovered that Mr. Saluto had died of a (**cardiovascular accident, dysentery, cerebrovascular accident**), otherwise known as a stroke.

ANSWERS TO EXERCISES

1. Tumor of a gland
2. Inflammation of a joint
3. Process of viewing living tissue under a microscope
4. Study of (process of study of) the heart
5. Pertaining to the skin
6. Study of (process of study of) cells
7. Instrument to visually examine the urinary bladder
8. Pertaining to the cerebrum (largest part of the brain)
9. Pertaining to the head
10. Inflammation of a gland

B

1. hematoma
2. erythrocyte
3. enteritis
4. prognosis
5. electroencephalogram
6. gynecology
7. electrocardiogram
8. diagnosis
9. hemoglobin
10. hepatitis

1. abdomen: incision of the abdomen (this is also called exploratory surgery)
2. kidney: excision (removal, resection) of the kidney
3. nerve: inflammation of a nerve
4. eye: instrument to visually examine the eye
5. bone: incision (to cut into, section) of a bone
6. kidney: pertaining to the kidney
7. nose: inflammation of the nose
8. flesh tissue: tumor (cancerous or malignant) of flesh tissue

1. Specialist in the study of tumors (cancerous or malignant tumors)
2. Specialist in the study of disease (examines biopsy samples and performs autopsies)
3. Abnormal condition of the mind
4. White blood cell
5. Clotting cell or platelet
6. Inflammation of the stomach
7. Tumor of a gland (this is a benign or harmless tumor). An adenocarcinoma is a malignant tumor (CARCIN/O means cancerous).
8. Abnormal condition of clotting (occurring in a blood vessel)

1. cell
2. condition, process
3. process of cutting out, excision, resection, removal
4. pertaining to
5. condition of blood (blood condition)
6. record
7. pain; condition of pain
8. inflammation
9. protein
10. pertaining to

1. neuralgia
2. leukemia
3. arthrogram
4. nephrology
5. hepatoma or hepatocellular carcinoma
6. laparoscopy
7. arthrotomy
8. dermatosis
9. dermatitis
10. hematologist

1. excessive, above, more than normal
2. under, below
3. abnormal, bad, difficult, painful
4. across, through
5. behind, back
6. complete, through
7. out, outside
8. self
9. below, deficient, less than normal
10. within, in, inner
11. surrounding
12. all
13. above, upon, on
14. no, not

H

1. Examination of a body to determine the cause of death
2. Excessive activity of the thyroid gland
3. Deficiency of hemoglobin or numbers of red blood cells; literally, "no" (AN-) "blood" (-EMIA)
4. Condition of painful intestines; marked by inflammation, abdominal pain, and frequent and bloody stools and often caused by bacteria
5. Organs that produce (secrete) hormones directly into the bloodstream
6. Blood condition of decreased sugar (lower-than-normal levels)
7. Organs that produce (secrete) chemicals to the outside of the body (through tubes or ducts)
8. Removal (excision) of an organ or structure
9. Pertaining to through the skin
10. Blood condition of increased sugar (higher than normal levels)

I

1. subgastric or hypogastric
2. gastralgia
3. gastritis
4. transgastric
5. gastroscopy
6. retrogastric
7. gastroenterology
8. gastrotomy
9. gastrectomy
10. gastroscope
11. epigastric

J

1. Specialist in the study (and treatment) of tumors
2. Prediction of the outcome of an illness or treatment
3. Inflammation of bones and joints (including degeneration of joints)
4. Specialist in the study of disease
5. Abnormal condition of clotting (clot formation)
6. Blood condition of increased sugar (high blood sugar)
7. Abnormal condition of the mind
8. Visual examination of the abdomen
9. Condition of increased secretion of hormone from the thyroid gland
10. Condition of painful intestines
11. Stroke; trauma to blood vessels of the brain (cerebrum)
12. Red blood cells
13. Increase in cancerous (malignant) white blood cells in blood and bone marrow
14. Clotting cells
15. Deficiency of hemoglobin and/or decrease in number of red blood cells; results in reduced oxygen to cells
16. Pertaining to through the skin
17. Gland in males located in front of the urinary bladder (the prostate is an exocrine gland that secretes fluid to combine with sperm cells during ejaculation)
18. Removal of portions of the prostate gland through the urethra (procedure is called TURP)
19. Measurement of the width across a circle
20. Outbreak of a disease that has spread to all people (pan = all) throughout countries, continents, and even the whole world.

1. gastroenteritis
2. endocrinologist, hypothyroidism
3. sarcoma, biopsy
4. leukocyte, oncologist, leukemia
5. autopsy, pathologist, cerebrovascular accident

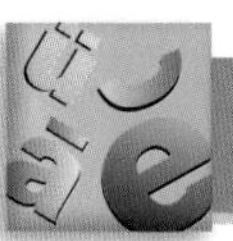

PRONUNCIATION OF TERMS

The terms that you have learned in this chapter are presented here with their pronunciations. The capitalized letters in **BOLDFACE** *indicate the accented syllable. Pronounce each word out loud; then write the meaning in the space provided. All meanings of terms are found in the* ***Mini-Dictionary*** *beginning on page 363, and on the audio section of the Evolve site. After you write all of the meanings, it is a good idea to cover the Term column and write each term from its meaning.*

Term	Pronunciation	Meaning
adenitis	ad-eh-**NI**-tis	____________________
adenoma	ah-deh-**NO**-mah	____________________
anemia	ah-**NE**-me-ah	____________________
arthralgia	ar-**THRAL**-jah	____________________
arthritis	ar-**THRI**-tis	____________________
arthrogram	**AR**-thro-gram	____________________
arthroscope	**AR**-thro-skope	____________________
arthroscopy	ar-**THROS**-ko-pe	____________________
autopsy	**AW**-top-se	____________________
biology	bi-**OL**-o-je	____________________
biopsy	**BI**-op-se	____________________
carcinoma	kar-sih-**NO**-mah	____________________
cardiac	**KAR**-de-ak	____________________
cardiology	kar-de-**OL**-o-je	____________________
cephalic	seh-**FAL**-ik	____________________
cerebral	seh-**RE**-bral	____________________
cerebrovascular accident	seh-re-bro-**VAS**-ku-lar **AK**-sih-dent	____________________
cystoscope	**SIS**-to-skope	____________________

cystoscopy	sis-**TOS**-ko-pe	______
cytology	si-**TOL**-o-je	______
dermal	**DER**-mal	______
dermatitis	der-mah-**TI**-tis	______
dermatosis	der-mah-**TO**-sis	______
diagnosis	di-ag-**NO**-sis	______
diameter	di-**AM**-eh-ter	______
dysentery	**DIS**-en-teh-re	______
electrocardiogram	e-lek-tro-**KAR**-de-o-gram	______
electroencephalogram	e-lek-tro-en-**SEF**-ah-lo-gram	______
endocardium	en-do-**KAR**-de-um	______
endocrine glands	**EN**-do-krin glanz	______
endocrinology	en-do-krih-**NOL**-o-je	______
enteritis	en-teh-**RI**-tis	______
epigastric	eh-pih-**GAS**-trik	______
erythrocyte	eh-**RITH**-ro-site	______
exocrine glands	**EK**-so-krin glanz	______
gastrectomy	gas-**TREK**-to-me	______
gastric	**GAS**-trik	______
gastritis	gas-**TRI**-tis	______
gastroenteritis	gas-tro-en-teh-**RI**-tis	______
gastroenterology	gas-tro-en-ter-**OL**-o-je	______
gastroscope	**GAS**-tro-skope	______
gastroscopy	gas-**TROS**-ko-pe	______

gastrotomy	gas-**TROT**-o-me	______
gynecologist	gi-neh-**KOL**-o-jist	______
gynecology	gi-neh-**KOL**-o-je	______
hematoma	he-mah-**TO**-mah	______
hemoglobin	**HE**-mo-glo-bin	______
hepatitis	hep-ah-**TI**-tis	______
hepatoma	hep-ah-**TO**-mah	______
hyperglycemia	hi-per-gli-**SE**-me-ah	______
hyperthyroidism	hi-per-**THI**-royd-izm	______
hypoglycemia	hi-po-gli-**SE**-me-ah	______
hypothyroidism	hi-po-**THI**-royd-izm	______
laparoscope	**LAP**-ah-ro-skope	______
laparoscopy	lap-ah-**ROS**-ko-pe	______
laparotomy	lap-ah-**ROT**-o-me	______
leukemia	loo-**KE**-me-ah	______
leukocyte	**LOO**-ko-site	______
leukocytosis	loo-ko-si-**TO**-sis	______
nephrectomy	neh-**FREK**-to-me	______
nephrology	neh-**FROL**-o-je	______
nephrosis	neh-**FRO**-sis	______
neural	**NU**-ral	______
neuralgia	nu-**RAL**-jah	______
neuritis	nu-**RI**-tis	______
neurology	nu-**ROL**-o-je	______

neurotomy	nu-**ROT**-o-me	______________________
oncologist	ong-**KOL**-o-jist	______________________
ophthalmoscope	of-**THAL**-mo-skope	______________________
osteitis	os-te-**I**-tis	______________________
osteoarthritis	os-te-o-ar-**THRI**-tis	______________________
pandemic	pan-**DEM**-ik	______________________
pathologist	pah-**THOL**-o-jist	______________________
pericardium	peh-rih-**KAR**-de-um	______________________
platelet	**PLAYT**-let	______________________
prognosis	prog-**NO**-sis	______________________
prostate gland	**PROS**-tayt gland	______________________
psychosis	si-**KO**-sis	______________________
renal	**RE**-nal	______________________
resection	re-**SEK**-shun	______________________
retrogastric	reh-tro-**GAS**-trik	______________________
rhinitis	ri-**NI**-tis	______________________
rhinotomy	ri-**NOT**-o-me	______________________
sarcoma	sar-**KO**-mah	______________________
subgastric	sub-**GAS**-trik	______________________
subhepatic	sub-heh-**PAT**-ik	______________________
thrombocyte	**THROM**-bo-site	______________________
thrombosis	throm-**BO**-sis	______________________
transdermal	tranz-**DER**-mal	______________________
transgastric	tranz-**GAS**-trik	______________________
transurethral	tranz-u-**RE**-thral	______________________

1

PRACTICAL APPLICATIONS

MEDICAL CONDITIONS AND SPECIALISTS

Match the following physician specialists with the condition each would treat.

cardiologist	gastroenterologist	neurologist	urologist
dermatologist	gynecologist	oncologist	
endocrinologist	hematologist	ophthalmologist	

1. Cerebrovascular accident ____________________
2. Skin cancer ____________________
3. Dysentery ____________________
4. Anemia ____________________
5. Lung cancer ____________________
6. Prostate gland enlargement ____________________
7. Hyperglycemia ____________________
8. Cataract (clouding of the lens of the eye) ____________________
9. Heart attack ____________________
10. Abnormal bleeding of the uterus from the vagina ____________________

WHAT'S YOUR DIAGNOSIS?

Case Study

This 7 year-old boy presents with fever, sore throat, runny nose, and persistent fatigue [feeling of being tired all the time]. Physical examination reveals multiple bruises [contusions] of his lower extremities and arms, an erythematous [red] pharynx [throat] with white plaques on the tonsils, and pale gums, lips, and nail beds. CBC [complete blood count] was performed. Increasing fever prompted immediate admission to the children's ward of the hospital.

During the course of admission, the patient's pharyngitis was monitored and subsided. Tonsillitis was ruled out. Fatigue and contusions on his arms and legs were noted and addressed with the parents while taking his social history. A lab hematologist reviewed the high WBC [white blood cell] count, and a WBC differential [percentages of the various types of these cells] shows immature cells. A bone marrow biopsy confirms the diagnosis of WBC malignancy.

Using the information presented in this case study, what's your diagnosis?

A. Hyperthyroidism
B. Leukemia
C. Fever
D. Contusions—arms/legs
E. Leukocytosis

CASE STUDY
A COVID-19 Case

The patient is a 56-year-old African-American man who was well except for hypertension (high blood pressure) and prediabetes hyperglycemia, which was managed by a low-sugar diet. He complains of onset of pharyngitis (inflamation of the throat with pain), fever of 102 degrees, and cough with severe fatigue (tiredness). These symptoms continued for 5 days and were accompanied by night sweats related to the fever. A COVID-19 test was positive. He had a recent loss of appetite but did not complain of loss of smell or taste as many other COVID-19 patients often experience.

After 5 days his fever returned to normal with gradual return of energy over the next week. His family, due to careful attention to restriction of contact (masks, handwashing, isolation) did not contract the virus. He is fully recovere and fortunately did not require hospitalization for lung disease (pneumonia) or respiratory (breathing) distress.

At the time of this patient's illness, in March 2020, there were no established agents to combat the coronavirus and no vaccine available.

1

ANSWERS TO PRACTICAL APPLICATIONS

MEDICAL CONDITIONS AND SPECIALISTS

1. neurologist
2. dermatologist
3. gastroenterologist
4. hematologist
5. oncologist
6. urologist
7. endocrinologist
8. ophthalmologist
9. cardiologist
10. gynecologist

WHAT'S YOUR DIAGNOSIS?

Answer: B. Leukemia

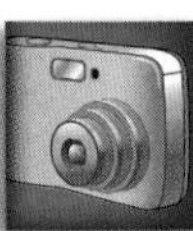

PICTURE SHOW

Answer the questions that follow each image. Answers are found on page 43.

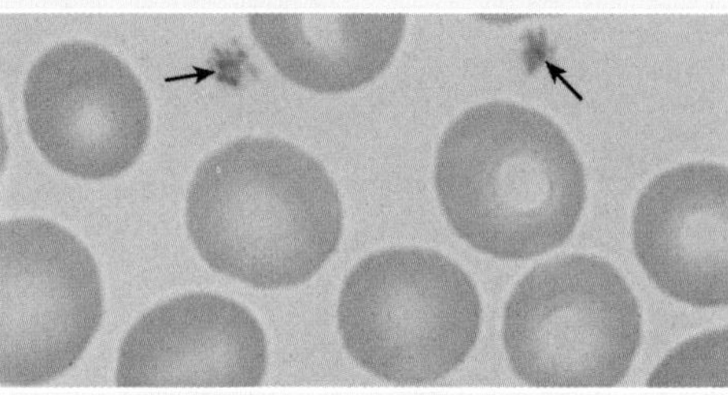

Blood smear.

1. The arrows in this photo of a blood smear are pointing to cells that are necessary in blood clotting. These cells are:
   a. leukocytes
   b. thrombosis
   c. platelets
   d. erythrocytes
2. The other blood cells in the photo contain a protein that helps the cell carry oxygen. These cells are:
   a. leukocytes
   b. thrombosis
   c. platelets
   d. erythrocytes
3. The protein contained in the cells is:
   a. hemoglobin
   b. anemia
   c. sarcoma
   d. carcinoma

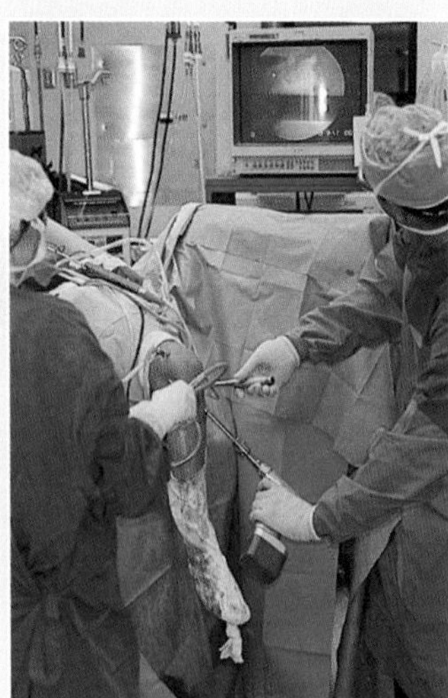

1. The image shows a minimally invasive procedure used to visually examine the knee. This procedure is:
   a. laparotomy
   b. arthroscopy
   c. laparoscopy
   d. arthrectomy

C

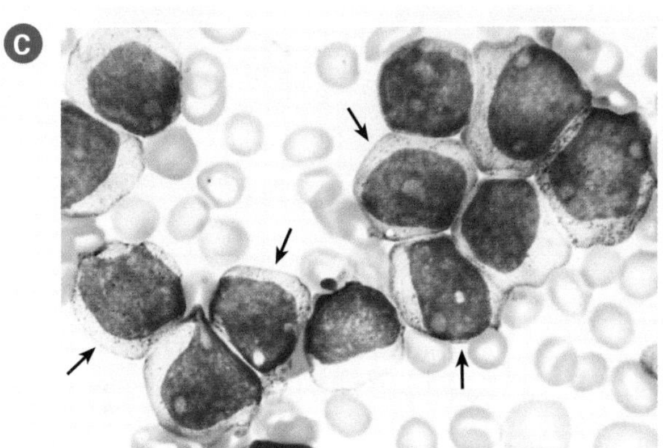

Blood smear.

1. In this blood smear, the arrows point to an increased number of large, immature cells (that would normally fight infection). These cells are:
   a. hepatocytes
   b. erythrocytes
   c. thrombocytes
   d. leukocytes

2. The name of the abnormal condition in which these cells predominate is:
   a. iron deficiency anemia
   b. sickle cell anemia
   c. leukemia
   d. hyperglycemia

D

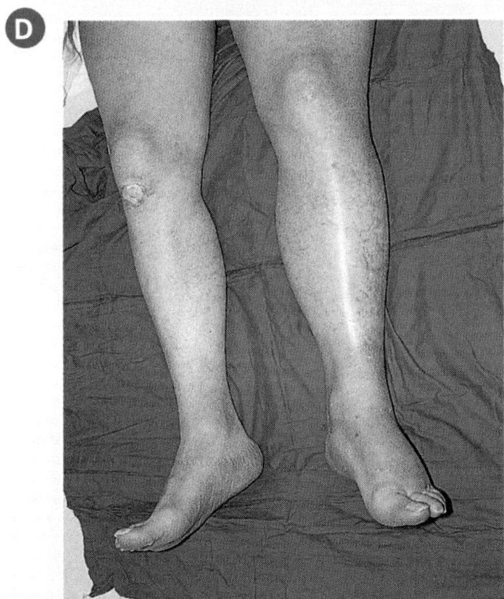

1. Notice that the left leg of the patient is swollen (edema), resulting from blood flow that is slow and sluggish. Fluid seeps out of tiny vessels into tissue spaces. The abnormal condition often associated with this problem is caused by a blood clot in a blood vessel. The condition is called:
   a. hyperglycemia
   b. deep vein thrombosis
   c. cerebrovascular accident
   d. hematoma

E

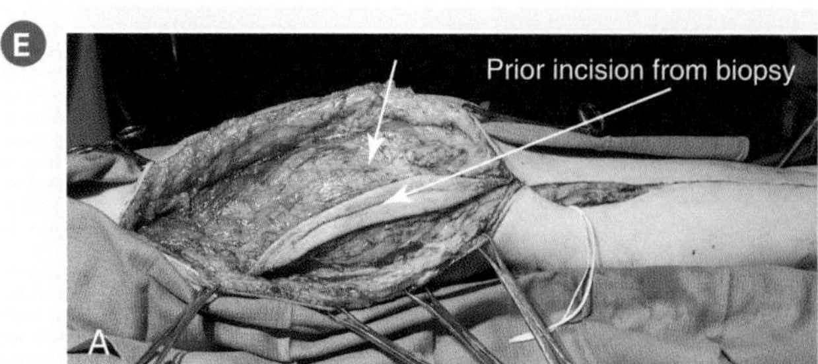

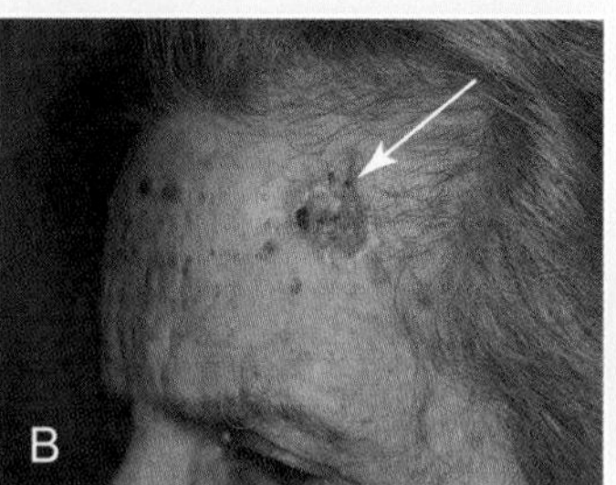

1. The lesion pictured in *A* is a/an:
   a. hepatoma
   b. sarcoma of muscle
   c. adenoma
   d. basal cell carcinoma

2. The lesion pictured in *B* is a/an:
   a. hepatoma
   b. sarcoma of muscle
   c. gastric adenocarcinoma
   d. basal cell carcinoma

F

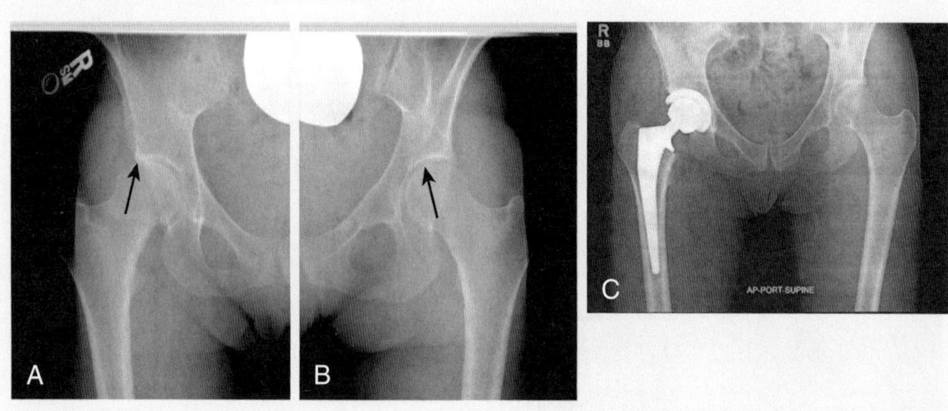

1. The image in *A* shows degeneration of the hip (pelvic) joint with narrowed joint spaces (see arrow). The image in *B* shows a normal hip for comparison (see arrow). The patient with the hip changes has arthralgia, stiffness, and joint tenderness. Your diagnosis?
   a. osteoarthritis
   b. gastroenteritis
   c. hyperthyroidism
   d. osteogenic sarcoma

NOTE: The image in C shows a **THR (total hip replacement)** as treatment for this condition.

ANSWERS TO PICTURE SHOW

A 1. c 2. d 3. a

B 1. b

C 1. d 2. c

D 1. b

E 1. b 2. d

F 1. a

REVIEW

*Here is your chance to test your understanding of the **combining forms, suffixes,** and **prefixes** that you have studied in this chapter. Write the meaning of each term in the space provided and **check** your answers with the Answers to Review section on page 46. All of the meanings for word parts are found in **Glossary of Word Parts** beginning on page 399. **Remember the 3 "Rs"—wRite, Repeat, Review.***

1

COMBINING FORMS

Combining Form	Meaning	Combining Form	Meaning
1. aden/o	________	19. gnos/o	________
2. arthr/o	________	20. gynec/o	________
3. bi/o	________	21. hem/o, hemat/o	________
4. carcin/o	________	22. hepat/o	________
5. cardi/o	________	23. lapar/o	________
6. cephal/o	________	24. leuk/o	________
7. cerebr/o	________	25. nephr/o	________
8. crin/o	________	26. neur/o	________
9. cyst/o	________	27. onc/o	________
10. cyt/o	________	28. ophthalm/o	________
11. dem/o	________	29. oste/o	________
12. derm/o, dermat/o	________	30. path/o	________
13. electr/o	________	31. psych/o	________
14. encephal/o	________	32. ren/o	________
15. enter/o	________	33. rhin/o	________
16. erythr/o	________	34. sarc/o	________
17. gastr/o	________	35. thromb/o	________
18. glyc/o	________		

SUFFIXES

Suffix	Meaning	Suffix	Meaning
1. -al	______	11. -logist	______
2. -algia	______	12. -logy	______
3. -cyte	______	13. -oma	______
4. -ectomy	______	14. -opsy	______
5. -emia	______	15. -osis	______
6. -globin	______	16. -scope	______
7. -ia	______	17. -scopy	______
8. -ic	______	18. -sis	______
9. -ism	______	19. -tomy	______
10. -itis	______		

PREFIXES

Prefix	Meaning	Prefix	Meaning
1. a-, an-	______	9. hypo-	______
2. aut-	______	10. pan-	______
3. dia-	______	11. peri-	______
4. dys-	______	12. pro-	______
5. endo-	______	13. re-	______
6. epi-	______	14. retro-	______
7. exo-	______	15. sub-	______
8. hyper-	______	16. trans-	______

ANSWERS TO REVIEW

COMBINING FORMS

1. gland
2. joint
3. life
4. cancer (cancerous)
5. heart
6. head
7. cerebrum
8. secrete
9. urinary bladder
10. cell
11. people
12. skin
13. electricity
14. brain
15. intestines (often small intestine)
16. red
17. stomach
18. sugar
19. knowledge
20. woman, female
21. blood
22. liver
23. abdomen
24. white
25. kidney
26. nerve
27. tumor
28. eye
29. bone
30. disease
31. mind
32. kidney
33. nose
34. flesh
35. clotting

SUFFIXES

1. pertaining to
2. pain (condition of)
3. cell
4. cutting out; removal; excision
5. blood condition
6. protein
7. condition
8. pertaining to
9. condition; process
10. inflammation
11. specialist in the study of
12. study of
13. tumor, mass
14. to view (process of viewing)
15. abnormal condition
16. instrument to visually examine
17. process of visual examination
18. state of
19. cutting into; incision

PREFIXES

1. no, not
2. self
3. complete, through
4. bad, painful, difficult, abnormal
5. within
6. above, upon, on
7. out, outside
8. excessive, more than normal, too much
9. below, less than normal, under
10. all
11. surrounding
12. before
13. back
14. behind
15. below, under
16. across, through

✓ TERMINOLOGY CHECKUP

Before you leave this chapter, here are important concepts that you should thoroughly understand. In your own words, write the answers on the lines provided. Confirm your answers on the next page. Check the box next to each item when you know you've "got" it!

☐ 1. What is the difference between **endocrine glands** and **exocrine glands.** Give an example of each.

____

____

____

☐ 2. What is the difference between a **diagnosis** and a **prognosis?**

____

____

____

☐ 3. What is the difference between a **carcinoma** and a **sarcoma?** Give an example of each.

____

____

____

☐ 4. What is the difference between **anemia, leukemia,** and **leukocytosis?**

____

____

____

☐ 5. What is the difference between **laparotomy** and **laparoscopy?**

____

____

____

ANSWERS TO TERMINOLOGY CHECKUP

1. **Endocrine glands** secrete chemicals called ***hormones within*** the body. Examples are **thyroid, pituitary, and adrenal glands.**
   Exocrine glands secrete chemicals to the ***outside*** of the body through ducts. Examples are **sweat, tear, and salivary glands.**
2. A **diagnosis** is complete knowledge gained after examining and performing tests on a patient.
   A **prognosis** is a prediction made after the diagnosis. It forecasts and describes the likely ***outcome*** of an illness.
3. A **carcinoma** is a cancerous tumor arising from lining cells of internal organs. An example is an **adenocarcinoma.**
   A **sarcoma** is also a cancerous tumor, but arising from bone, cartilage, muscle, or fat (connective tissues). An example is an **osteosarcoma.**
4. **Anemia** is deficiency of red blood cells (erythrocytes) or deficiency in hemoglobin within red blood cells.
   Leukemia is a cancerous condition of high numbers of abnormal white blood cells (leukocytes).
   Leukocytosis is only a slight increase in normal white blood cells as a response to infection.
5. A **laparotomy** is a large ***incision*** of the abdomen to explore or remove organs and tissues.
   A **laparoscopy** is ***visual examination of the abdomen*** using small incisions for insertion of instruments (laparoscope) to view and remove organs and tissues.

CHAPTER 2

Organization of the Body

Chapter Sections

Introduction 50
Body Systems 50
Body Cavities 53
Divisions of the Back 56
Planes of the Body 58
Terminology 61
In Person: CT and MRI 67
Exercises and Answers 68
Pronunciation of Terms 75
Practical Applications 78
Picture Show 80
Review 83
Terminology CheckUp 85

CHAPTER OBJECTIVES

- To name the body systems and their functions
- To identify body cavities and specific organs within them
- To list the divisions of the back
- To identify the three planes of the body
- To analyze, pronounce, and spell new terms
- To apply medical terms in real-life situations

INTRODUCTION

All the parts of your body are composed of individual units called **cells.** Examples are muscle, nerve, epithelial (skin, and lining of internal organs and cavities), and bone cells.

Similar cells grouped together are **tissues.** Groups of muscle cells are muscle tissue, and groups of epithelial cells are epithelial tissue.

Collections of different tissues working together are **organs.** An organ, such as the stomach, has specialized tissues, such as muscle, epithelial, and nerve, that help the organ function.

Groups of organs working together are the **systems** of the body. The digestive system, for example, includes the mouth, throat (pharynx), esophagus, stomach, and intestines, which bring food into the body, break it down, and deliver it to the bloodstream.

Figure 2-1 reviews the differences between cells, tissues, organs, and systems.

BODY SYSTEMS

There are 11 systems of the body, and each plays an important role in the way the body works.

The **circulatory system** (heart, blood, and blood vessels such as arteries, veins, and capillaries) transports blood (containing all types of blood cells) throughout the body. The **lymphatic system** includes lymph vessels and nodes that carry a clear fluid called lymph. Lymph contains white blood cells called lymphocytes that fight against disease and play an important role in immunity.

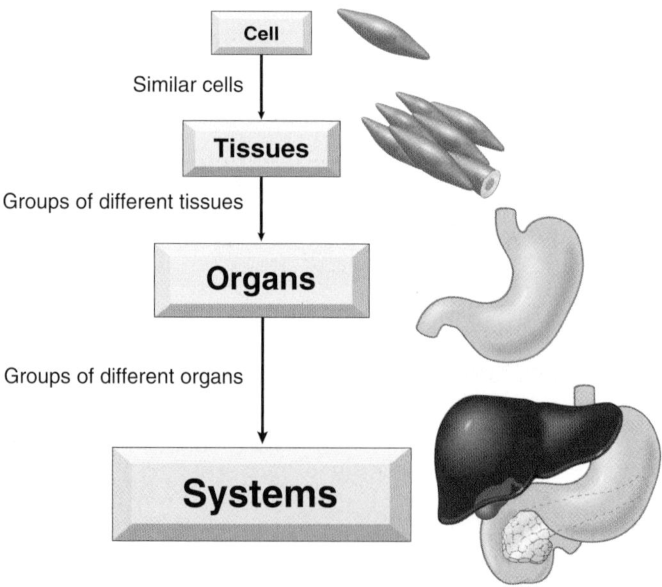

FIGURE 2-1 Cells, tissues, organs, and systems.

The **digestive system** brings food into the body and breaks it down so that it can enter the bloodstream. Food that cannot be broken down is then removed from the body at the end of the system as waste. Organs in the digestive system include the mouth, stomach, and intestines.

The **endocrine system,** composed of glands, sends chemical messengers called hormones into the blood to act on other glands and organs. Examples of endocrine glands are the thyroid gland, adrenal glands, and pituitary gland.

The **female and male reproductive systems** produce the cells (eggs and sperm) that join to form the embryo, which develops in the uterus of a female. Male (testes) and female (ovaries) sex organs produce hormones as well.

The **musculoskeletal system,** including muscles, bones, joints, and other connective tissues such as cartilage, supports the body and allows it to move.

The **nervous system** carries electrical messages to and from the brain and spinal cord.

The **respiratory system** controls breathing, a process by which air enters and leaves the body. Organs of the respiratory system include the trachea (windpipe), bronchial tubes, and lungs.

The **skin and sense organ system,** including the skin and eyes and ears, receives messages from the environment and sends them to the brain. The retina is a layer of sensitive receptor tissue in the back of the eye.

The **urinary system** produces urine and sends it out of the body through the kidneys, ureters, bladder, and urethra.

You can find a table of specific organs/structures and the systems to which they belong on the Evolve site for Chapter 2 in the resources section.

In a separate section of this book, you will find useful information about each body system, with diagrams, terminology, pathology, laboratory tests, and diagnostic and treatment procedures.

At the end of the book, you will find more helpful information. Use these resources as you study:

- **Appendix 1, Body Systems**, page 217
- **Appendix 2, Immunity and COVID-19 Vaccines**, page 297
- **Appendix 3, Diagnostic Tests and Procedures**, page 307
- **Appendix 4, Abbreviations, Acronyms, Symbols, Eponyms & Plurals**, page 329
- **Appendix 5, Quick Drug Reference**, page 349
- **Appendix 6, Health Careers Information**, page 353
- **Mini-Dictionary**, page 363
- **Glossary of Word Parts**, page 399
- **Glossary of English–Spanish Terms**, page 417

2

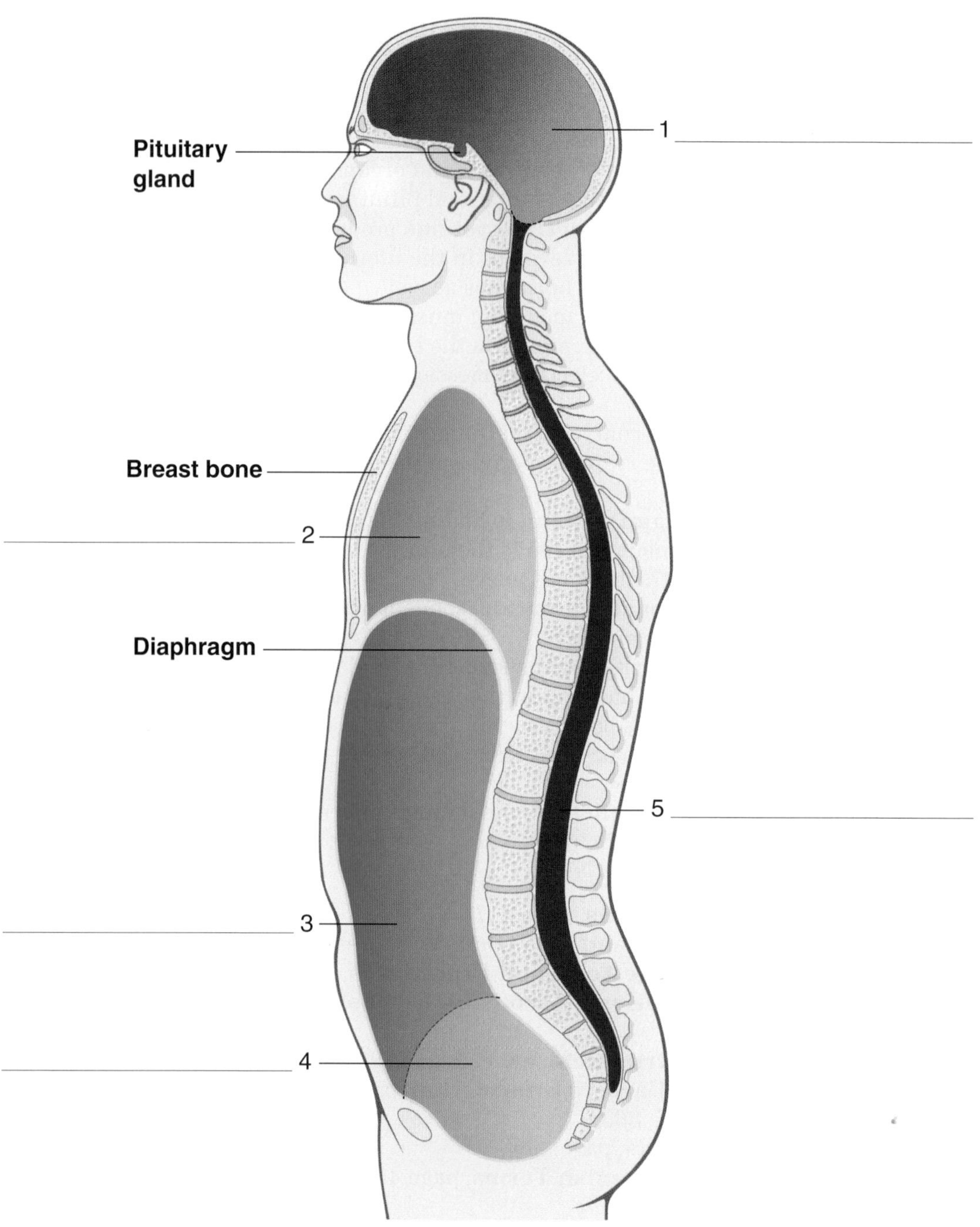

FIGURE 2-2 Body cavities.

BODY CAVITIES

Figure 2-2 shows the five body cavities. A body cavity is a space that contains organs. Label the figure in the spaces provided as you read the following paragraphs.

The **cranial cavity** (1) is located in the head and surrounded by the skull (CRANI/O means skull). The cranial cavity contains the brain and other organs, such as the pituitary gland (an endocrine gland located below the brain).

The **thoracic cavity** (2), also known as the chest cavity (THORAC/O means chest), is surrounded by the breastbone and ribs. The lungs, heart, windpipe (trachea), bronchial tubes (leading from the trachea to the lungs), and other organs are in this cavity.

Figure 2-3 shows a front view of the thoracic cavity. The lungs are each surrounded by a double membrane known as the **pleura.** The space between the pleural membranes is the **pleural cavity.** The large area between the lungs (yellow in Figure 2-3) is the **mediastinum.** The heart, esophagus (food tube), trachea, and bronchial tubes are organs within the mediastinum.

In Figure 2-2, the **abdominal cavity** (3) is the space below the thoracic cavity. The **diaphragm** is the muscle that separates the abdominal and thoracic cavities. Organs in the abdomen include the stomach, liver, gallbladder, and small and large intestines.

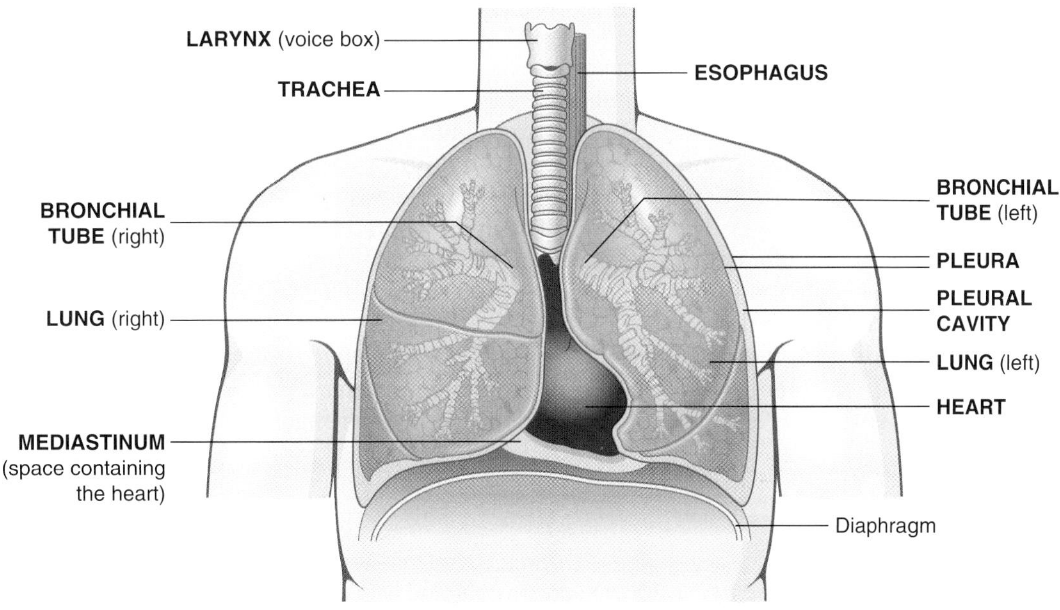

FIGURE 2-3 Thoracic cavity.

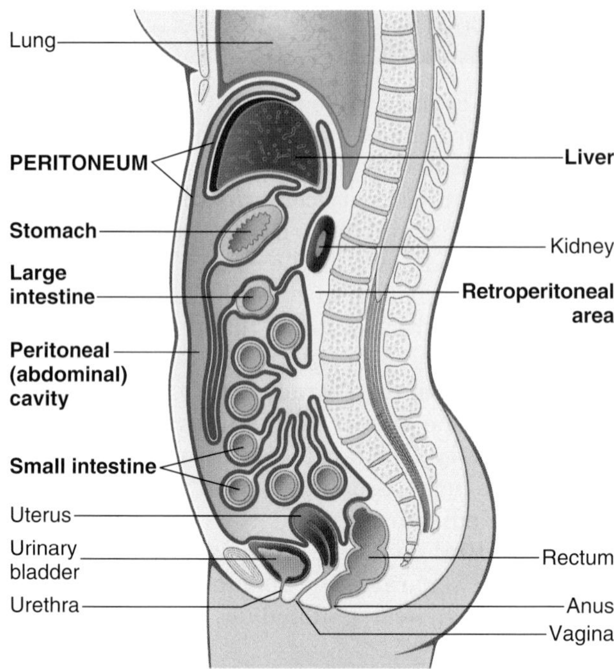

FIGURE 2-4 The **peritoneum** (side view) is a double membrane surrounding the organs in the abdomen (including the liver, stomach, and small and large intestines). The **peritoneal cavity** is the space between the peritoneal membranes. The **retroperitoneal area** is behind the peritoneum. The kidneys are in the retroperitoneal cavity.

2

The organs in the abdomen are covered by a double membrane called the **peritoneum** (Figure 2-4). The peritoneum attaches the abdominal organs to the abdominal muscles and surrounds each organ to hold it in place.

Turn back to Figure 2-2 and locate the **pelvic cavity** (4), below the abdominal cavity. The pelvic cavity is surrounded by the **pelvis** (bones of the hip). The major organs located within the pelvic cavity are the urinary bladder, ureters (tubes from the kidneys to the bladder), urethra (tube from the bladder to the outside of the body), rectum, and anus, and the uterus (muscular organ that nourishes the developing embryo and fetus) in females.

Label the **spinal cavity** (5) on Figure 2-2. This is the space surrounded by the **spinal column** (backbones). The **spinal cord** is the nervous tissue within the spinal cavity. Nerves enter and leave the spinal cord and carry messages to and from all parts of the body.

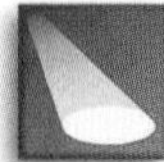

Double membranes

You can visualize the way organs are surrounded by a double membrane by imagining your fist pushing deep into a soft balloon. The balloon is then in two layers folded over your fist, just the way the pleura surrounds the lungs and the peritoneum surrounds the abdominal organs. Double wrapping around organs provides protection and cushioning, as well as a site for attachment to muscles. In the event of inflammation or disease of organs or membranes, fluid may collect in the space between the membranes surrounding the organs. This collection of fluid in the pleural cavity is called a **pleural effusion.** A collection of fluid in the peritoneal cavity is called **ascites** (see pages 64-65).

As a quick review of the terms presented in this section, match the term with its meaning and write it in the space provided.

Term	Meaning
Abdominal cavity	1. Membrane surrounding the lungs ______________
Cranial cavity	2. Space between the lungs, containing the heart
Diaphragm	______________
Mediastinum	3. Bones of the hip ______________
Pelvic cavity	4. Space containing the liver, gallbladder, and stomach; also
Pelvis	called the abdomen ______________
Peritoneum	5. Space within the backbones, containing the spinal cord
Pleura	______________
Spinal cavity	6. Membrane surrounding the organs in the abdomen
Thoracic cavity	______________
	7. Space within the skull, containing the brain
	______________
	8. Space below the abdominal cavity, containing the urinary bladder ______________
	9. Muscle between the thoracic and abdominal cavities
	______________
	10. Entire chest cavity, containing the lungs, heart, trachea, esophagus, and bronchial tubes ______________
	______________

DIVISIONS OF THE BACK

The **spinal column** is a long row of bones from the neck to the tailbone. Each bone in the spinal column is called a **vertebra (backbone)**. Two or more bones are called **vertebrae.**

A piece of flexible connective tissue, called a **disc**, lies between each backbone. The disc, composed of **cartilage**, is a cushion between the bones. If the disc slips or moves out of its place, it can press on the nerves that enter or leave the spinal cord, causing pain. Figure 2-5 shows a side view of vertebrae and discs.

The divisions of the spinal column are pictured in Figure 2-6. Label them according to the following list:

Division	Bones	Abbreviation
1. **Cervical** (neck) region	7 bones	**C1-C7**
2. **Thoracic** (chest) region	12 bones	**T1-T12**
3. **Lumbar** (loin or waist) region	5 bones	**L1-L5**
4. **Sacral** (sacrum or lower back) region	5 fused bones	**S1-S5**
5. **Coccygeal** (coccyx or tailbone) region	4 fused bones	

2

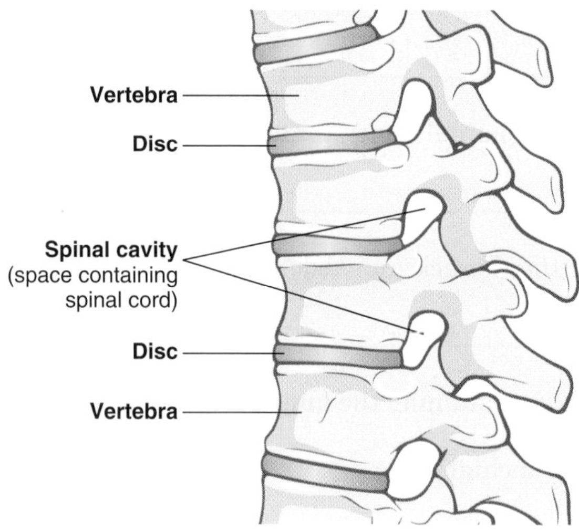

FIGURE 2-5 Vertebrae and discs.

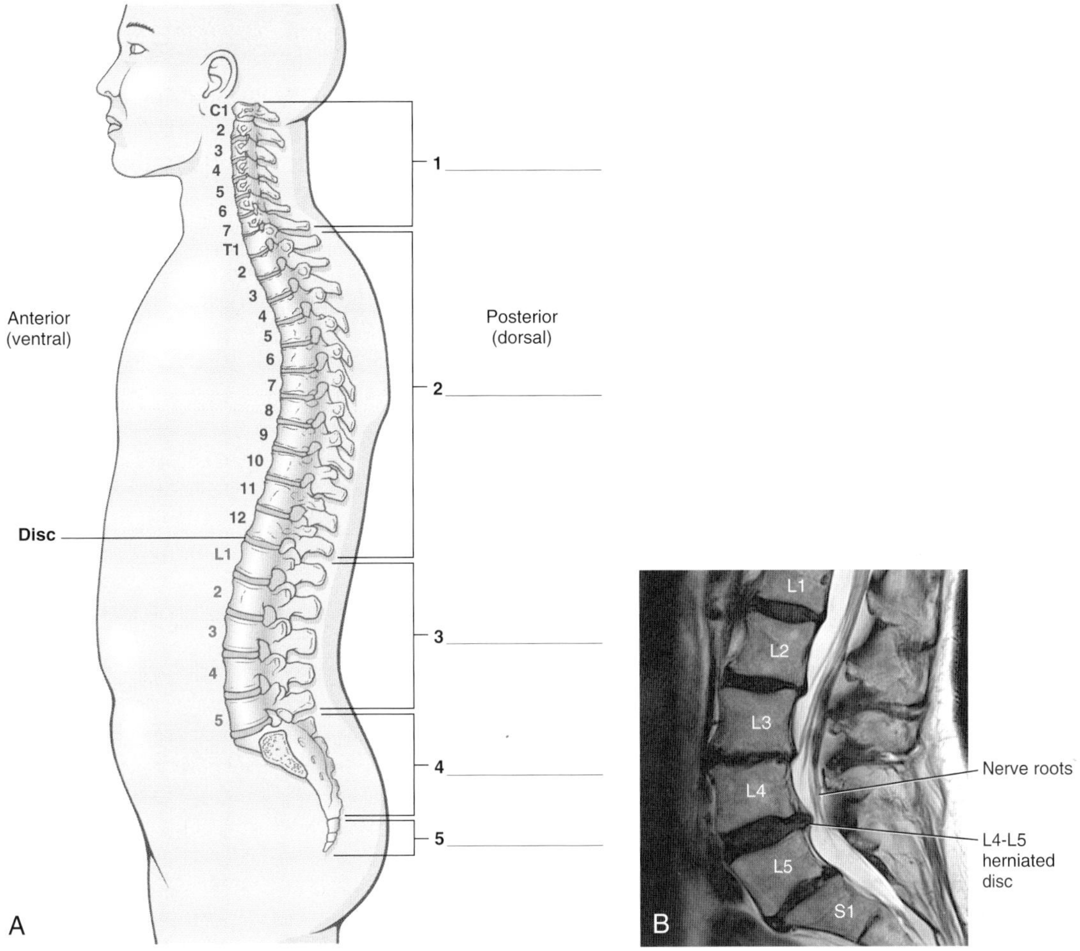

FIGURE 2-6 A, Divisions of the back (spinal column). B, MRI (magnetic resonance imaging) study of a herniated disc at the L4-L5 level of the spinal column.

PLANES OF THE BODY

A plane is an imaginary flat surface. Organs appear in different relationships to one another according to the plane of the body in which they are viewed.

Figure 2-7 shows three planes of the body. Label them as you read the following descriptions:

1. **Frontal (coronal) plane** A vertical plane that divides the body, or body part such as an organ, into front and back portions.

   Anatomically, *anterior* means the front portion and *posterior* means the back portion.

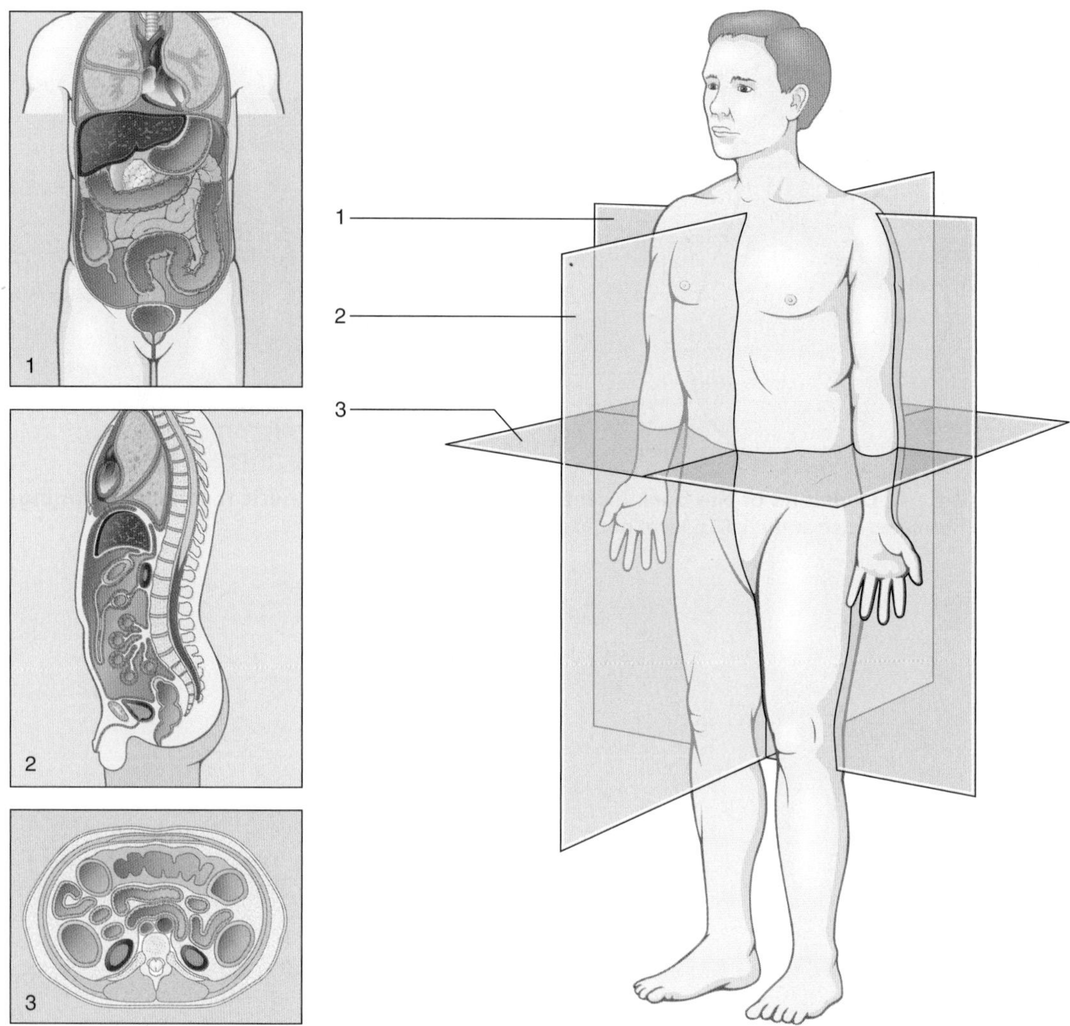

FIGURE 2-7 **Planes of the body.**

2. **Sagittal (lateral) plane**	A vertical plane that divides the body or organ into right and left sides. The **midsagittal plane** divides the body vertically into right and left **halves**.
3. **Transverse (axial) plane**	A horizontal plane that divides the body or organ into upper and lower portions, as in a **cross section.** (Think of cutting a long loaf of French bread into circular sections.)

Knowing the planes of the body is helpful in looking at imaging studies such as x-ray films (radiographs) and computed tomography (CT) scans. See Figure 2-8.

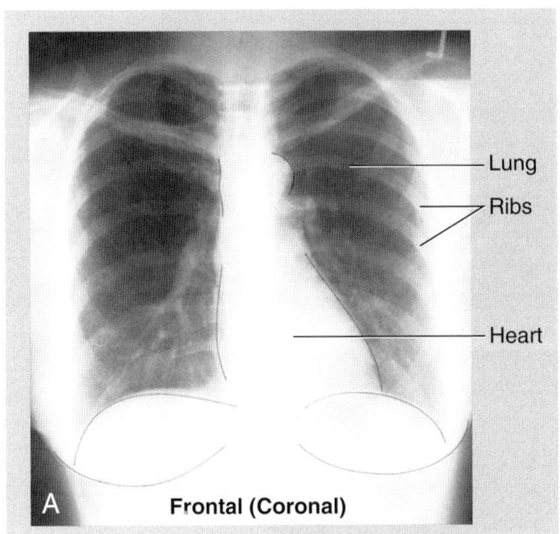

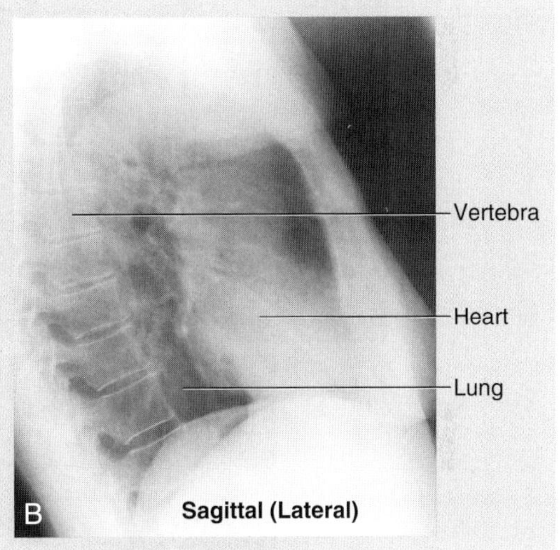

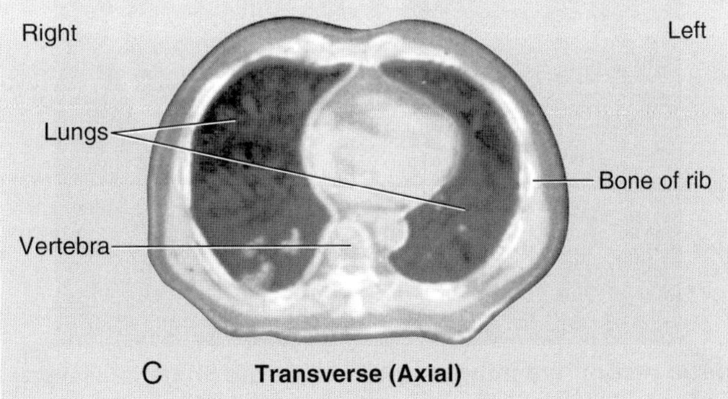

FIGURE 2-8 X-ray views of the chest. A, Frontal (coronal) plane. This radiographic image is an anterior-posterior view of the chest. **B, Sagittal (lateral) plane.** This is a lateral (side) x-ray view of the chest. **C, Transverse (axial) plane.** This computed tomography image is a snapshot of structures at a specific level of the body.

Magnetic resonance imaging (MRI) is another technique for producing images of the body. With **MRI,** magnetic waves instead of x-rays are used to create the images, which show organs and other structures in specialized detail and in all three planes of the body (Figure 2-9). Figure 2-10A shows a patient undergoing MRI. See ***In Person: CT and MRI*** on page 67.

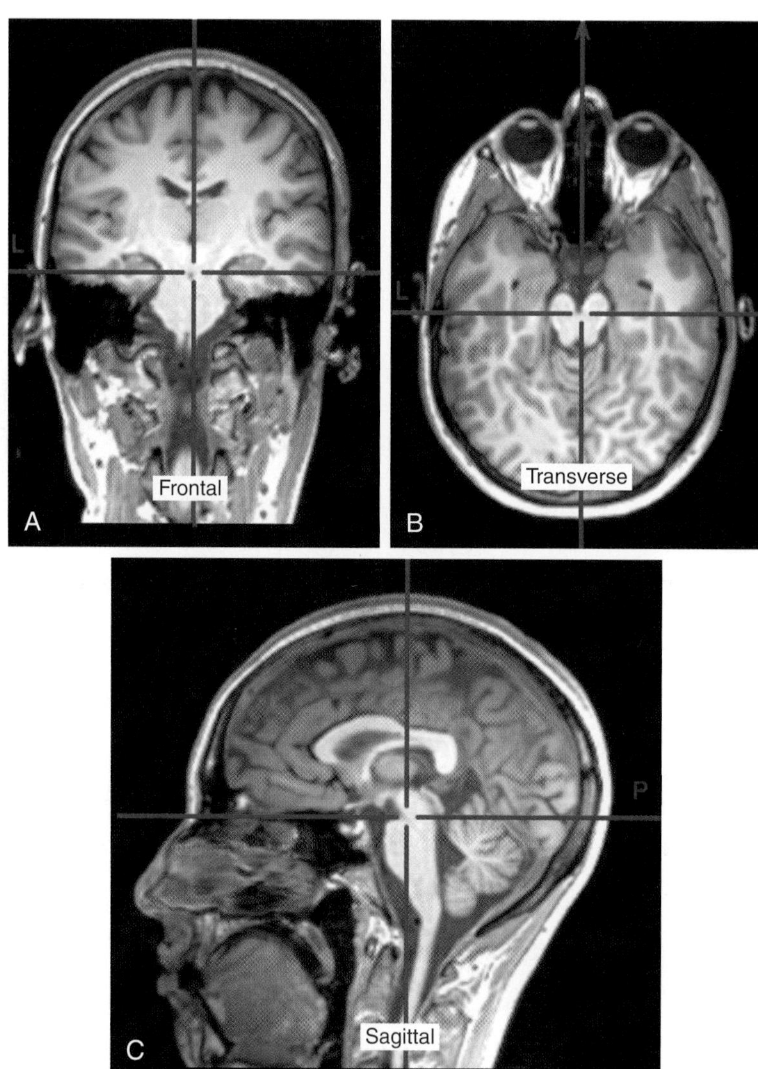

FIGURE 2-9 Magnetic resonance images. Basic views are frontal, transverse, and sagittal. **A, Frontal (coronal) plane** of the head. **B, Transverse (axial) plane** of the head. **C, Sagittal (lateral) plane** showing the head and side of the brain.

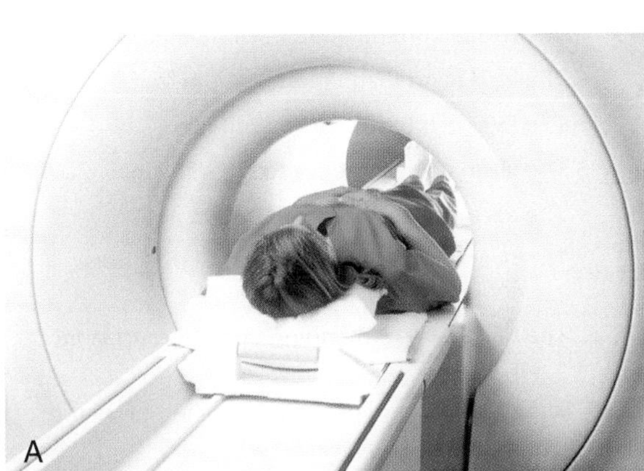

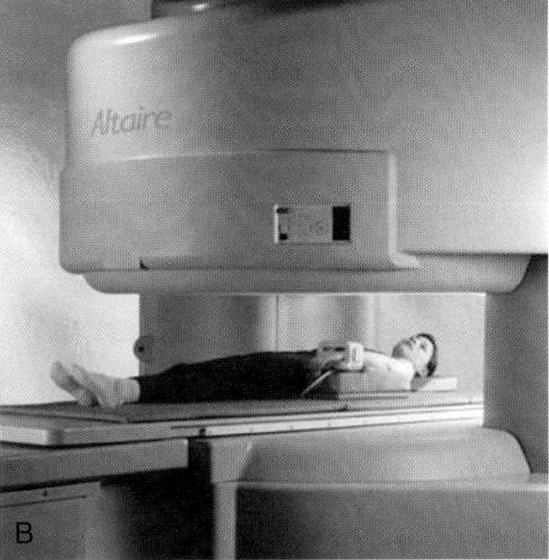

FIGURE 2-10 **A. Patient in an MRI unit surrounded by a superconducting magnet.** Magnetic field changes are picked up by the surrounding machine and processed by a computer to create images. For this examination, the patient must lie very still and have no metal objects on or within the body. **B. Open MRI.** Open MRI machines have a large space to accommodate patients who may experience discomfort or anxiety (claustrophobia) in traditional MRI machines. This design has two flat magnets on the top and bottom areas.

TERMINOLOGY

Write the meanings of the medical terms on the line provided. Check your answers with the ***Mini-Dictionary***, page 363.

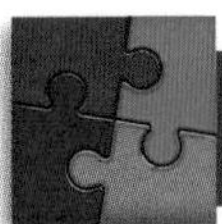

COMBINING FORMS

Combining Form	Meaning	Medical Term	Meaning
abdomin/o	abdomen	abdominal	______________
anter/o	front	anterior *The suffix* -IOR *means pertaining to.* *See Table 2-1 for additional useful positional and directional terms.*	______________
bronch/o	bronchial tubes (leading from the windpipe to the lungs)	bronchoscopy *Pronunciation hint: bron-**KOS**-ko-pe*	______________

TABLE 2-1 POSITIONAL AND DIRECTIONAL TERMS

Position/Direction	Description	Example
Anterior	Front side	The nose is on the anterior of the head.
Posterior	Back side	The heel is on the posterior of the foot.
Inferior	Below	The liver is inferior to the right lung.
Superior	Above	The stomach is superior to the intestines.
Lateral	Side	The ears are lateral to the mouth.
Medial	Middle	The heart is in the medial area of the chest. (mediastinum)
Distal	Far	The distal end of the thigh bone (femur) is at the knee.
Proximal	Near	The proximal end of thigh bone (femur) is at the hip.
Deep	Away from the surface	The stab wound penetrated deep into the skin.
Superficial	On the surface	Superficial veins can be seen on the surface of the skin.
Supine	Facing up	The patient lies supine during an examination of the abdomen.
Prone	Facing down	The backbones are examined with the patient in a prone position.

2

cervic/o neck of the body or neck (cervix) of the uterus

cervical ______________________

You must decide from the context of what you are reading whether ***cervical*** *means pertaining to the neck of the body or pertaining to the uterine cervix (lower portion of the uterus). Figure 2-11 shows the uterus and the cervix.*

chondr/o cartilage (connective tissue attached to bones)

chondroma ______________________

This is a benign tumor.

chondrosarcoma ______________________

This is a malignant tumor. The root SARC, meaning flesh, indicates that the malignant tumor arises from a type of flesh or connective tissue.

coccyg/o coccyx, tailbone

coccygeal ______________________

-EAL *means pertaining to.*

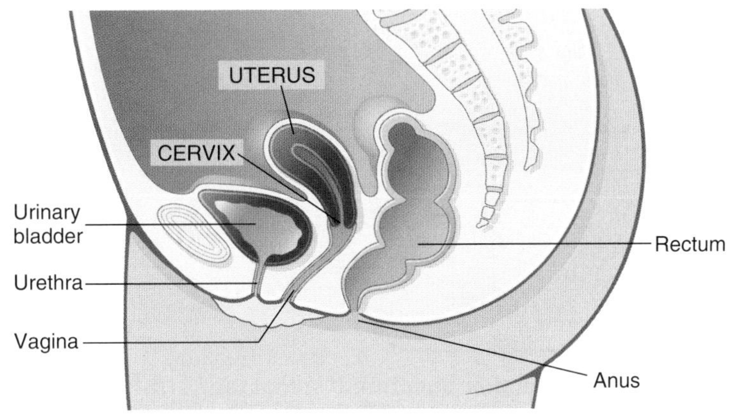

FIGURE 2-11 The uterus and cervix. The cervix is the lower portion of the uterus opening to the vagina.

crani/o	skull	craniotomy ______________________
epitheli/o	skin, surface tissue	epithelial ______________________ *The term **epithelial** was first used to describe the surface (*EPI- *means upon) of the breast nipple (*THELI/O *actually means nipple). More correctly, it describes the cells on the outer layer (surface) of the skin as well as the cells that line internal organs that lead to the outside of the body.*
esophag/o	esophagus (tube from the throat to the stomach)	esophageal ______________________
hepat/o	liver	hepatitis ______________________
lapar/o	abdomen	laparoscopy ______________________
laryng/o	larynx (voice box)	laryngeal ______________________ *The larynx (pronounced* **LAR**-*inks) is found in the upper part of the trachea. See Figure 2-3,* page 53. laryngectomy ______________________
later/o	side	lateral ______________________

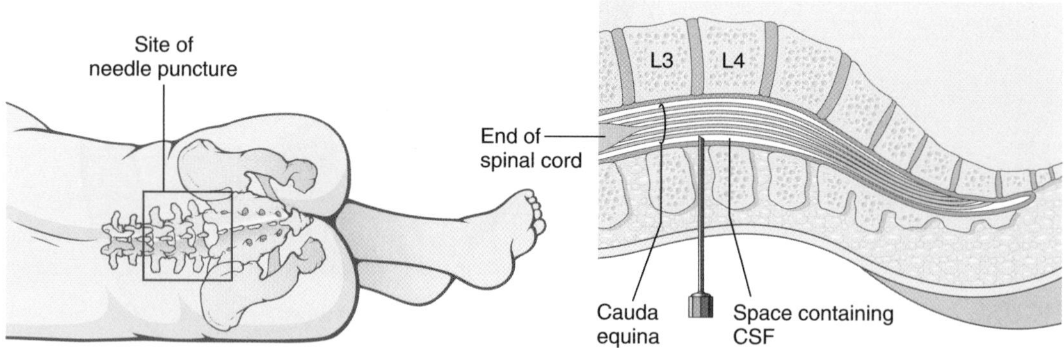

FIGURE 2-12 Lumbar puncture ("spinal tap"). The patient lies on his side with his knees drawn up to the abdomen and the chin brought down to the chest. This position increases the spaces between the vertebrae. The physician inserts a needle between the third and fourth (or fourth and fifth) lumbar vertebrae, and cerebrospinal fluid (CSF) is withdrawn, or medication can be injected.The end of the spinal cord is where the spinal nerves begin to fan out toward the legs. Performing a lumbar puncture below this level avoids injury to the spinal cord.

2

lumb/o	loin (waist)	lumbar ______________ -AR *means pertaining to. A* ***lumbar puncture ("spinal tap")*** *is the placement of a needle within the membranes in the lumbar region of the spinal cord to inject or withdraw fluid. See Figure 2-12.*
lymph/o	lymph (clear fluid in tissue spaces and lymph vessels)	lymphocyte ______________ *Lymphocytes are white blood cells that fight disease. There are two major types of lymphocytes, B cells and T cells. B cells produce disease-fighting proteins called* ***antibodies.***
mediastin/o	mediastinum (space between the lungs)	mediastinal ______________
pelv/o	pelvis (bones of the hip)	pelvic ______________
peritone/o	peritoneum (membrane surrounding the abdominal organs)	peritoneal ______________ *Peritoneal fluid, produced by the peritoneum, lubricates its surfaces to prevent friction. With peritoneal inflammation (peritonitis), fluid may accumulate in the peritoneal cavity. This accumulation of fluid is called* ***ascites*** *(see Figure 2-13).*

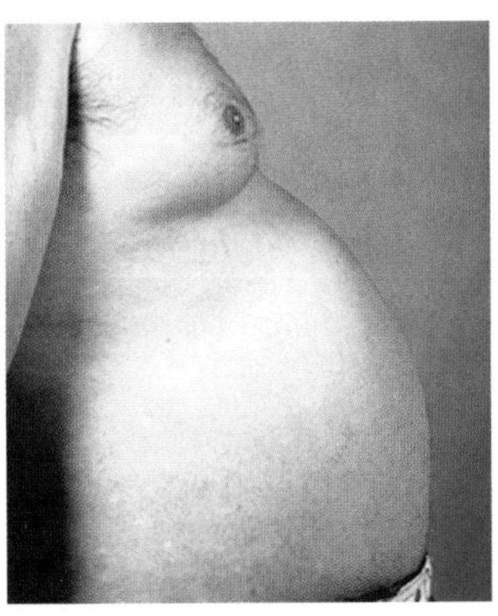

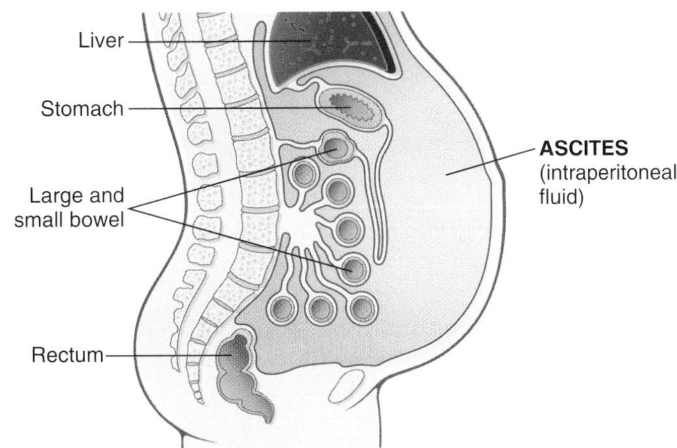

FIGURE 2-13 Ascites. Abnormal intraperitoneal fluid can result from conditions such as liver disease, peritonitis, and ovarian cancer.

pharyng/o	pharynx (throat)	pharyngeal ______ *The pharynx (pronounced* **FAR**-*inks) is the common passageway for food from the mouth and air from the nose. See Figure 2-14.*
pleur/o	pleura	pleuritis ______

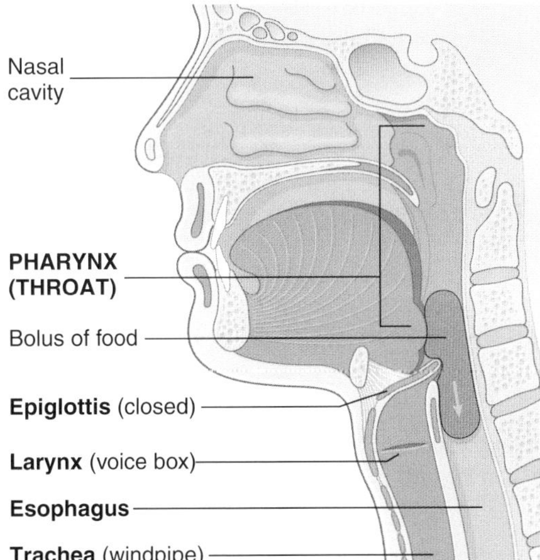

FIGURE 2-14 Pharynx (throat). Notice that the **epiglottis** (a flap of cartilage) closes over the trachea during swallowing so that the bolus (mass) of food travels down the esophagus and not the trachea.

Your Mother Was Right! Don't Talk While You're Eating!

Talking opens the epiglottis so that if you're eating and swallowing while talking, food can accidentally enter the larynx and trachea, causing you to choke.

poster/o	back, behind	posterior ______________ *See Table 2-1 for useful positional and directional terms, on page 62.*
radi/o	x-rays	radiology ______________ *This medical specialty includes x-ray procedures, ultrasonography (images obtained using sound waves), and nuclear medicine (images obtained using radioactive substances).*
sacr/o	sacrum (five fused bones in the lower back)	sacral ______________
spin/o	spine (backbone)	spinal ______________
thorac/o	chest	thoracotomy ______________
		thoracic ______________
trache/o	trachea (windpipe)	tracheotomy ______________ *See Figure 2-15.*
vertebr/o	vertebra (backbone)	vertebral ______________

Don't confuse sacr/o and sarc/o

Notice the difference in spelling! Sacr/o always refers to the sacrum, a part of the back, while sarc/o means flesh and is used in **sarcoma**, a malignant tumor of connective or fleshy tissue of the body.

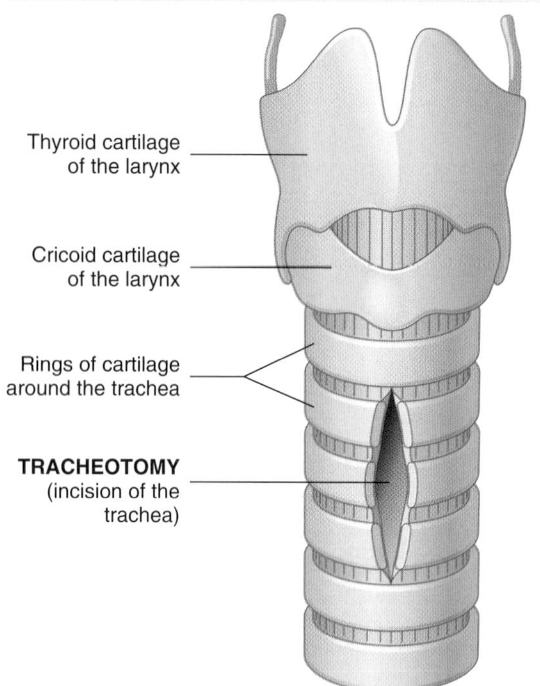

FIGURE 2-15 Tracheotomy. This procedure may be performed to open the trachea below a blockage from a foreign body or tumor. For an emergency procedure, any available instrument, even the barrel of a ballpoint pen, with the inner part removed, can be used to keep the airway open.

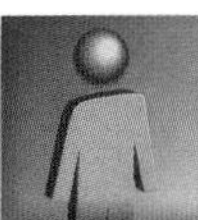

IN PERSON: CT AND MRI

The following first-person narrative provides a detailed look at two common diagnostic procedures—CT and MRI—from the perspective of the patient. It was written by Catherine Ward, a 77-year-old woman with head and neck cancer.

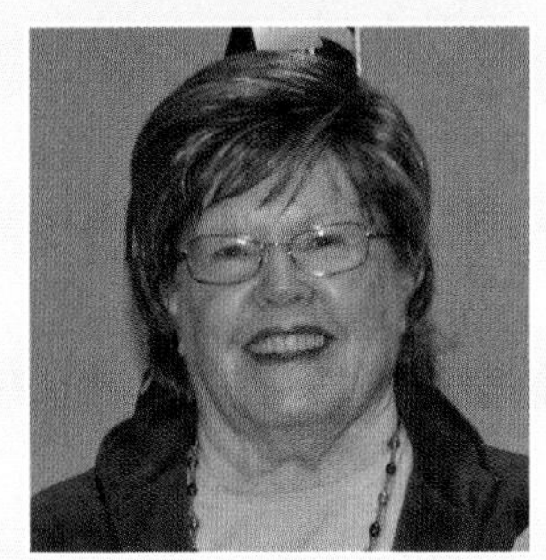

CT—COMPUTED TOMOGRAPHY

Before an upcoming surgical procedure, I was told that I would need to have a CT scan. The doctors wanted to see whether the cancer on my scalp had spread into the bones in my skull. They explained that these images of my head would be in thin "slices," taken as the CT camera rotated around me.

When I arrived in the room, I saw, to my claustrophobic relief, the CT machine was a large, circular hollow tube about 18 inches wide with a narrow table through the center. The technician explained he would add contrast halfway through the procedure through an intravenous (IV) line.

The table was rolled into the machine to a specific spot where a series of pictures were taken. There were several short periods when I was asked to stay as still as possible and hold my breath. The noise was minimal, just soft whirring and clicking. Halfway through the procedure, the contrast was administered into the IV line. Additional pictures were taken, and the test was completed with a minimum of discomfort, much to my grateful surprise.

MRI—MAGNETIC RESONANCE IMAGING

Before yet another surgical procedure, my doctors requested an MRI. They explained that the MRI and CT images are similar but that MRI shows more detail, especially of soft tissue.

The technician asked whether I had any metal (such as a pacemaker or surgical screws) inside or on my body. The magnet used in the MRI machine is so strong that it could cause metal objects to shift, disrupting the imaging process or causing damage to tissue in my body.

The MRI machine is a 6-foot-long round tube, open on both ends. I was rolled inside to the middle of the tube with my head positioned close to the inner sides of the tube. This was really uncomfortable because of my mild claustrophobia. I took deep breaths to relax myself.

I was still taken aback by just how loud it was inside the tube. Even with the earplugs that were provided, the sound of the machine was extremely loud, just like heavy-duty jackhammers. I used a "relax-substitution" method to calm myself, replacing the jarring MRI pounding with more pleasant sounds.

After the machine took a series of images, I was then rolled out of the machine for addition of the IV contrast, and the process was repeated.

I am still amazed that the doctors could get such detailed information on what was going on inside my body using these two tests.

? EXERCISES AND ANSWERS

Complete these exercises and check your answers. An important part of your success in learning medical terminology is checking your answers carefully with the Answers to Exercises on page 74. Be sure to visit the Evolve website, which has additional information, images, games, videos, and interactive activities.

A Match the following systems of the body with their functions.

circulatory	musculoskeletal	respiratory
digestive	nervous	skin and sense organs
endocrine	reproductive	urinary

1. Produces urine and sends it out of the body ____________________

2. Secretes hormones that are carried by blood to other organs ____________________

3. Supports the body and helps it move ____________________

4. Takes food into the body and breaks it down to be absorbed into the bloodstream

   ____

5. Transports blood containing nutrients, gases, and other substances through the body ____________________

6. Moves air into and out of the body ____________________

7. Produces the cells that unite to form a new baby ____________________

8. Receives messages from the environment and sends them to the brain

   ____

9. Carries electrical messages to and from the brain and spinal cord

   ____

B **Select from the following body systems to match the organ or tissue that is found within the system.**

cardiovascular	digestive	endocrine
female reproductive	lymphatic	male reproductive
musculoskeletal	nervous	respiratory
skin and sense organs	urinary	

1. brain ______________________
2. cartilage ______________________
3. kidney ______________________
4. intestines ______________________
5. heart ______________________
6. bronchial tubes ______________________
7. uterus ______________________
8. retina ______________________
9. adrenal glands ______________________
10. testes ______________________

2

C **Use the following terms to complete the chart below. Give the name of the cavity and an organ that is contained within the cavity.**

abdominal	lungs	stomach
brain	pelvic	thoracic
cranial	spinal	urinary bladder
heart	spinal cord	uterus

	Cavity	**Organ**
1. Space located within the bones of the hip	______	______
2. Space located within the skull	______	______
3. Space located within the chest	______	______
4. Space located within the abdomen	______	______
5. Space located within the backbones	______	______

D Complete the following sentences using the terms listed below.

abdomen (abdominal cavity)	mediastinum	spinal column
diaphragm	pelvis	spinal cord
disc	peritoneum	vertebra
	pleura	

1. The bones of the hip are the ______________________
2. The muscle separating the chest and the abdomen is the ______________________
3. The membrane surrounding the organs in the abdomen is the ______________________
4. The membrane surrounding the lungs is the ______________________
5. The space between the lungs in the chest is the ______________________
6. The space that contains organs such as the stomach, liver, gallbladder, and intestines is the ______________________
7. The backbones are the ______________________
8. The nerves running down the back form the ______________________
9. A single backbone is a ______________________
10. A piece of cartilage between two backbones is a ______________________

2

E Name the five divisions of the spinal column from the neck to the tailbone.

1. c ___ ___ ___ ___ ___ ___ ___
2. t ___ ___ ___ ___ ___ ___ ___
3. l ___ ___ ___ ___ ___
4. s ___ ___ ___ ___ ___
5. c ___ ___ ___ ___ ___ ___ ___ ___

F Match the following terms with their meanings below.

anterior
cartilage
CT scan
frontal (coronal) plane
MRI
posterior
sagittal plane
transverse (axial) plane

1. Pertaining to the back ______
2. Pertaining to the front ______
3. A plane that divides the body into an upper and a lower part ______
4. An imaging study that uses magnetic waves; all three planes of the body are viewed ______
5. A plane that divides the body into right and left parts ______
6. Flexible connective tissue found between bones at joints ______
7. A plane that divides the body into front and back parts ______
8. Series of cross-sectional x-ray images ______

G Give meanings for the following terms.

1. craniotomy ______
2. abdominal ______
3. pelvic ______
4. thoracic ______
5. mediastinal ______
6. epithelial ______
7. tracheotomy ______
8. peritoneal ______
9. hepatitis ______
10. cervical ______
11. lymphocyte ______
12. lateral ______
13. bronchoscopy ______

14. diaphragm ______________________________
15. pleura ______________________________
16. chondrosarcoma ______________________________
17. radiology ______________________________

H Match the following terms with their meanings below.

coccygeal	laparotomy	pleuritis
epithelial	laryngeal	sacral
esophageal	lumbar	thoracotomy
laparoscopy	pharyngeal	vertebral

1. Pertaining to the loin (waist) region below the thoracic vertebrae ______________
2. Pertaining to skin (lining or surface) cells ______________
3. Incision of the abdomen ______________
4. Pertaining to the tube from the throat to stomach ______________
5. Pertaining to the voice box ______________
6. Inflammation of the membrane surrounding the lungs ______________
7. Pertaining to the throat ______________
8. Pertaining to the sacrum ______________
9. Incision of the chest ______________
10. Pertaining to the tailbone ______________
11. Visual examination of the abdomen ______________
12. Pertaining to backbones ______________

2

I Circle the boldface term that best completes the meaning of the sentences in the following medical vignettes.

1. After her car accident, Cathy had severe neck pain. An MRI study revealed a protruding **(diaphragm, disc, uterus)** between C6 and C7. The doctor asked her to wear a **(sacral, cervical, cranial)** collar for several weeks.

2. Mr. Sellar was a heavy smoker all his adult life. He began coughing and losing weight and became very lethargic (tired). His physician suspected a tumor of the **(musculoskeletal, urinary, respiratory)** system. A chest CT scan showed a **(lung, pharyngeal, spinal)** mass. Dr. Baker performed **(laparoscopy, craniotomy, bronchoscopy)** to biopsy the lesion.

3. Grace had never seen a gynecologist. She had pain in her **(cranial, pelvic, thoracic)** cavity and increasing **(abdominal, vertebral, laryngeal)** girth (size). Dr. Hawk suspected a/an **(esophageal, ovarian, mediastinal)** tumor after palpating (examining by touch) a mass.

4. Mr. Cruise was explosed to asbestos while working in the shipyards during World War II. Now many years later, his doctor encouraged him to stop smoking because of a recently discovered link between asbestos, smoking, and the occurrence of mesothelioma (malignant tumor of cells of the pleura or the membrane surrounding the lungs). A routine chest x-ray film had shown thickening of the **(esophagus, pleura, trachea)** on both sides of Mr. Cruise's **(abdominal, spinal, thoracic)** cavity.

5. Kelly complained of headaches, together with nausea, disturbances of vision, and loss of coordination in her movements. Also, she had generalized weakness and stiffness on one side of her body. Dr. Brown suspected a tumor of the central **(circulatory, digestive, nervous)** system. Treatment involved a **(thoracotomy, craniotomy, laryngectomy)** to remove the lesion (mass) in her brain.

6. Mr. Smith experienced increasing weakness and loss of movement in his right arm and right leg. He saw his family doctor, who immediately referred him to a **(neurologist, cardiologist, rheumatologist).** This specialist examined him and sent him to **(pathology, hematology, radiology)** for x-ray imaging. (Results are shown in Figure 2-16.) This image is a/an **(MRI study, CT scan, AP film).** The imaging clearly showed a large white region in the brain, indicating an area of dead tissue. Mr. Smith's doctor informed him that he had had a stroke, which is also known as a **(pituitary gland tumor, myocardial infarction, CVA or cerebrovascular accident).**

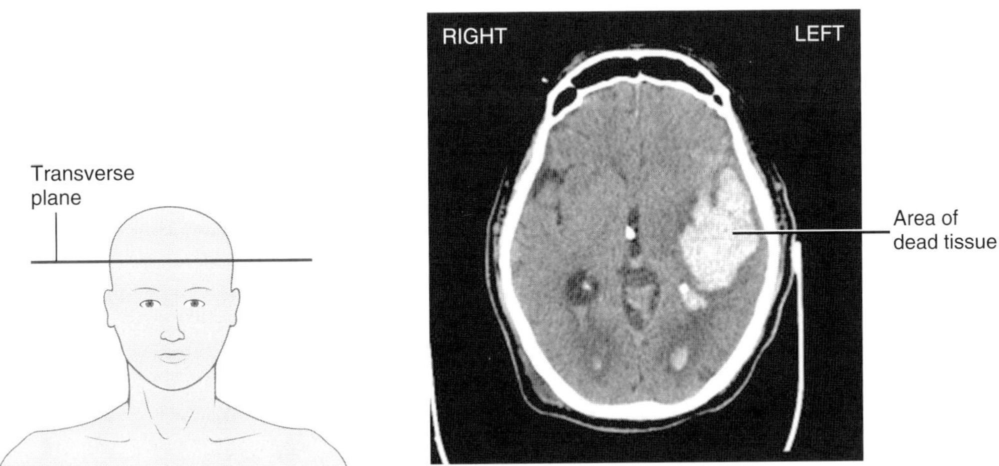

FIGURE 2-16 Cross-sectional x-ray image of Mr. Smith's head.

2

ANSWERS TO EXERCISES

A

1. urinary
2. endocrine
3. musculoskeletal
4. digestive
5. circulatory
6. respiratory
7. reproductive
8. skin and sense organs
9. nervous

B

1. nervous
2. musculoskeletal
3. urinary
4. digestive
5. cardiovascular
6. respiratory
7. female reproductive
8. skin and sense organs
9. endocrine
10. male reproductive

C

1. pelvic (urinary bladder, uterus)
2. cranial (brain)
3. thoracic (lungs, heart)
4. abdominal (stomach)
5. spinal (spinal cord)

D

1. pelvis
2. diaphragm
3. peritoneum
4. pleura
5. mediastinum
6. abdomen (abdominal cavity)
7. spinal column
8. spinal cord
9. vertebra
10. disc

E

1. cervical
2. thoracic
3. lumbar
4. sacral
5. coccygeal

F

1. posterior
2. anterior
3. transverse (axial) plane
4. MRI
5. sagittal plane
6. cartilage
7. frontal (coronal) plane
8. CT scan

G

1. incision of the skull
2. pertaining to the abdomen
3. pertaining to the pelvis (bones of the hip)
4. pertaining to the chest
5. pertaining to the mediastinum (the space between the lungs)
6. pertaining to skin (lining or surface) cells
7. incision of the trachea (windpipe)
8. pertaining to the peritoneum (the membrane surrounding the organs in the abdomen)
9. inflammation of the liver
10. pertaining to the neck of the body or neck (cervix) of the uterus
11. lymph cell (a type of white blood cell)
12. pertaining to the side
13. visual examination of bronchial tubes using an endoscope
14. muscle separating the abdomen from the chest
15. membrane surrounding the lungs
16. malignant tumor (sarcoma) of cartilage
17. study of x-rays

H

1. lumbar
2. epithelial
3. laparotomy
4. esophageal
5. laryngeal
6. pleuritis
7. pharyngeal
8. sacral
9. thoracotomy
10. coccygeal
11. laparoscopy
12. vertebral

I

1. disc, cervical
2. respiratory, lung, bronchoscopy
3. pelvic, abdominal, ovarian
4. pleura, thoracic
5. nervous, craniotomy
6. neurologist, radiology, CT scan, CVA or cerebrovascular accident

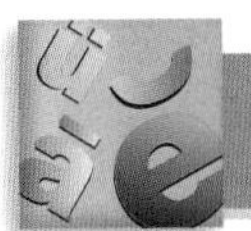

PRONUNCIATION OF TERMS

The terms that you have learned in this chapter are presented here with their pronunciations. The capitalized letters in **BOLDFACE** *represent the accented syllable. Pronounce each word out loud; then write the meaning in the space provided. Meanings of terms are found in the* ***Mini-Dictionary****, beginning on page 363, and on the audio section of the Evolve website.*

Term	Pronunciation	Meaning
abdomen	**AB**-do-men	______
abdominal cavity	ab-**DOM**-in-al **KAV**-ih-te	______
anterior	an-**TE**-re-or	______
bronchial tubes	**BRON**-ke-al toobz	______
bronchoscopy	bron-**KOS**-ko-pe	______
cartilage	**KAR**-tih-lij	______
cervical	**SER**-vih-kal	______
chondroma	kon-**DRO**-mah	______
chondrosarcoma	kon-dro-sar-**KO**-mah	______
circulatory system	**SER**-ku-lah-tor-e **SIS**-tem	______
coccygeal	kok-sih-**JE**-al	______
coccyx	**KOK**-siks	______
cranial cavity	**KRA**-ne-al **KAV**-ih-te	______
craniotomy	kra-ne-**OT**-o-me	______
diaphragm	**DI**-ah-fram	______
digestive system	di-**JES**-tiv **SIS**-tem	______
disc	disk	______
endocrine system	**EN**-do-krin **SIS**-tem	______
epithelial	ep-ih-**THE**-le-al	______

2

esophageal	eh-sof-ah-**JE**-al ________
esophagus	eh-**SOF**-ah-gus ________
female reproductive system	**FE**-male re-pro-**DUK**-tiv **SIS**-tem ________
frontal plane	**FRUN**-tal plane ________
hepatitis	hep-ah-**TI**-tis ________
laparoscopy	lap-ah-**ROS**-ko-pe ________
laparotomy	lap-ah-**ROT**-o-me ________
laryngeal	lah-**RIN**-je-al *or* lah-rin-**JE**-al ________
laryngectomy	lah-rin-**JEK**-to-me ________
larynx	**LAR**-inks ________
lateral	**LAT**-er-al ________
lumbar	**LUM**-bar ________
lymphocyte	**LIMF**-o-site ________
male reproductive system	male re-pro-**DUK**-tiv **SIS**-tem ________
mediastinal	me-de-ah-**STI**-nal ________
mediastinum	me-de-ah-**STI**-num ________
musculoskeletal system	mus-ku-lo-**SKEL**-eh-tal **SIS**-tem ________
nervous system	**NER**-vus **SIS**-tem ________
ovary	**O**-vah-re ________
pelvic cavity	**PEL**-vik **KAV**-ih-te ________
pelvis	**PEL**-vis ________
peritoneal	per-ih-to-**NE**-al ________
peritoneum	per-ih-to-**NE**-um ________
pharyngeal	fah-**RIN**-je-al *or* fah-rin-**JE**-al ________

pharynx	**FAR**-inks ______
pituitary gland	pih-**TOO**-ih-teh-re gland ______
pleura	**PLOO**-rah ______
pleuritis	ploo-**RI**-tis ______
posterior	pos-**TER**-e-or ______
radiology	ra-de-**OL**-o-je ______
respiratory system	**RES**-pir-ah-tor-e **SIS**-tem ______
sacral	**SA**-kral ______
sacrum	**SA**-krum ______
sagittal plane	**SAJ**-ih-tal plane ______
spinal cavity	**SPI**-nal **KAV**-ih-te ______
spinal column	**SPI**-nal **KOL**-um ______
spinal cord	**SPI**-nal kord ______
thoracic cavity	tho-**RAS**-ik **KAV**-ih-te ______
thoracotomy	tho-rah-**KOT**-o-me ______
trachea	**TRAY**-ke-ah ______
tracheotomy	tray-ke-**OT**-o-me ______
transverse plane	trans-**VERS** plane ______
ureter	**YOOR**-eh-ter *or* u-**RE**-ter ______
urethra	u-**RE**-thrah ______
urinary system	**YOOR**-in-air-e **SIS**-tem ______
uterus	**U**-ter-us ______
vertebra	**VER**-teh-brah ______
vertebrae	**VER**-teh-bray ______
vertebral	**VER**-teh-bral ______

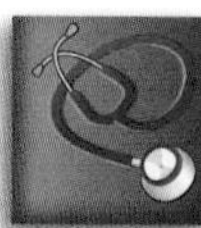

PRACTICAL APPLICATIONS

PROCEDURES

Select one of the procedures listed below to identify the descriptions in the following paragraphs. Answers are found on page 79.

bronchoscopy
craniotomy
laparoscopy
laparotomy
laryngectomy
thoracotomy
tracheotomy

1. A skin incision is made, and muscle is stripped away from the skull. Four or five burr (or bur) holes are drilled into the skull. The bone between the holes is cut using a craniotome (bone saw). The bone flap is turned down or completely removed. After the bone flap is secured, the membrane surrounding the brain is incised and the brain is exposed. This procedure is a ____________________.

2. A major surgical incision is made into the chest for diagnostic or therapeutic purposes. One type of incision is a medial sternotomy (the sternum is the breastbone). A straight incision is made from the upper part of the sternum (suprasternal notch) to the lower end of the sternum (xiphoid process). The sternum must be cut with an electric or air-driven saw. The procedure is done to perform a biopsy or to locate sources of bleeding or injury. It often is performed to remove all or a portion of a lung. This procedure is a ____________________.

3. A needle is inserted below the umbilicus (navel) to inject carbon dioxide (a gas) into the abdomen. The gas distends (expands) the abdomen, permitting better visualization of the organs. A trocar (sharp-pointed instrument used to puncture the wall of a body cavity) within a cannula (tube) is inserted into an incision under the umbilicus. After the cannula is in place in the abdominal cavity, the trocar is removed and an endoscope is inserted through the cannula. The surgeon can then visualize the abdominopelvic cavity and reproductive organs. This procedure is a ____________________.

4. A flexible fiberoptic endoscope is inserted through the mouth and down the throat and trachea to assess the tracheobronchial tree for tumors and obstructions, to obtain biopsy specimens, or to remove secretions and foreign bodies. This procedure is a ____________________.

2

WHAT'S YOUR DIAGNOSIS?

Case Study

A 67-year-old man with a two-pack-a-day h/o (history of) smoking and hypertension (high blood pressure) presents to the ED (emergency department) complaining of hemoptysis (coughing up blood), fatigue, back pain on his right side, polyuria (frequent need to urinate), and headaches. The elevated BP (blood pressure), hemoptysis, and headaches require observation in the ED. The patient is admitted, and diabetes is ruled out as a cause of polyuria. A chest x-ray for hemoptysis reveals a RLL (right lower lobe) mass. Needle biopsy confirms malignancy. The patient agrees to have a lobectomy performed. He is counseled on his tobacco use during recovery, and he agrees to begin therapy for tobacco cessation.

Using the information presented in this case study, what's your diagnosis?

A. Lung cancer—lower lobe
B. Hemoptysis
C. Polyuria
D. Headache
E. Hypertension

ANSWERS TO PRACTICAL APPLICATIONS

PROCEDURES

1. craniotomy
2. thoracotomy
3. laparoscopy
4. bronchoscopy

WHAT'S YOUR DIAGNOSIS?

Answer: A. Lung cancer—lower lobe

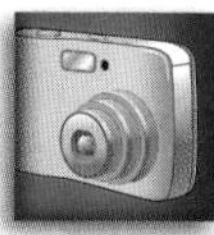

PICTURE SHOW

Answer the questions that follow each image. Answers are found on page 82.

A

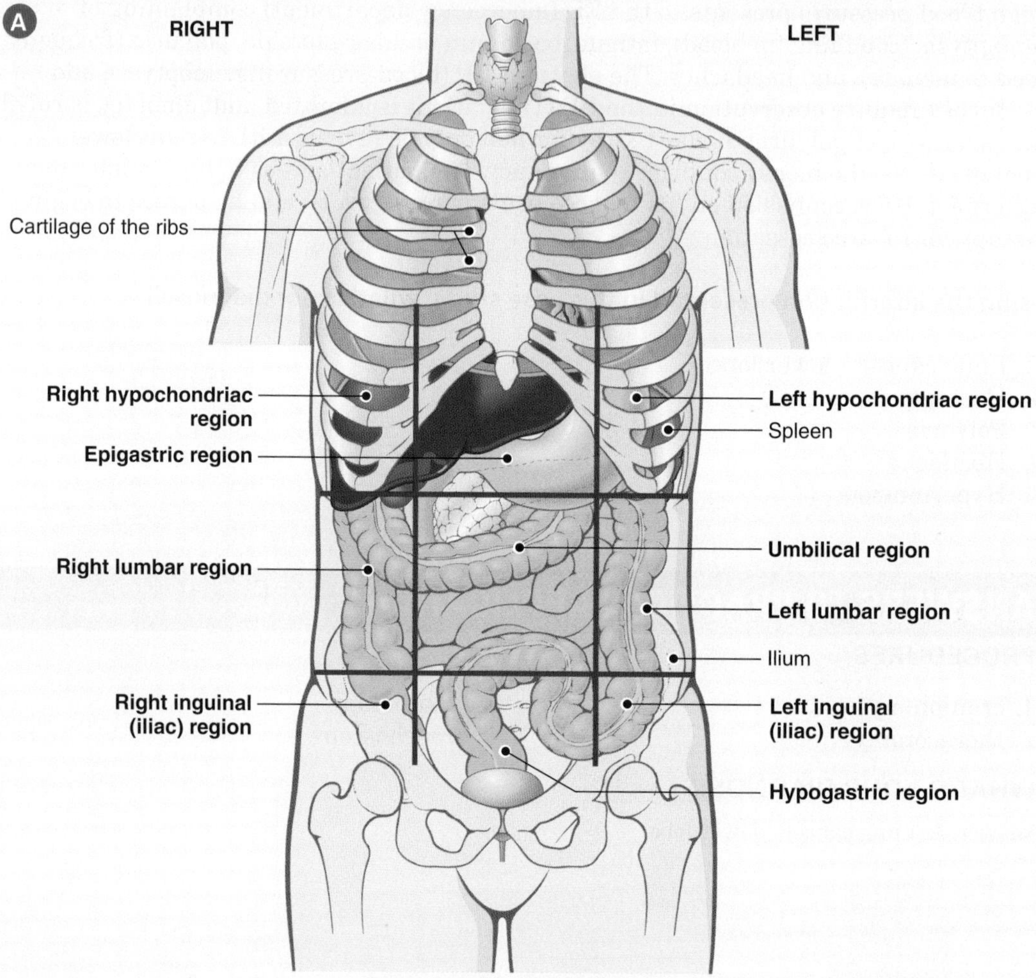

RIGHT

LEFT

Cartilage of the ribs

Right hypochondriac region

Epigastric region

Left hypochondriac region

Spleen

Right lumbar region

Umbilical region

Left lumbar region

Ilium

Right inguinal (iliac) region

Left inguinal (iliac) region

Hypogastric region

Abdominopelvic regions.

1. Which abdominopelvic regions are the middle lateral regions?
   a. epigastric
   b. lumbar (right and left)
   c. hypochondriac (right and left)
   d. inguinal (right and left)

2. Which abdominopelvic region lies above the stomach?
   a. epigastric
   b. inguinal (right and left)
   c. umbilical
   d. hypogastric

3. Which abdominopelvic regions lie under the cartilage of the ribs?
   a. hypogastric
   b. hypochondriac (right and left)
   c. umbilical
   d. inguinal (right and left)

4. Which lateral abdominopelvic regions are in the area of the groin (depression between the thigh and the trunk of the body)?
   a. umbilical
   b. hypochondriac (right and left)
   c. lumbar (right and left)
   d. inguinal (right and left)

B

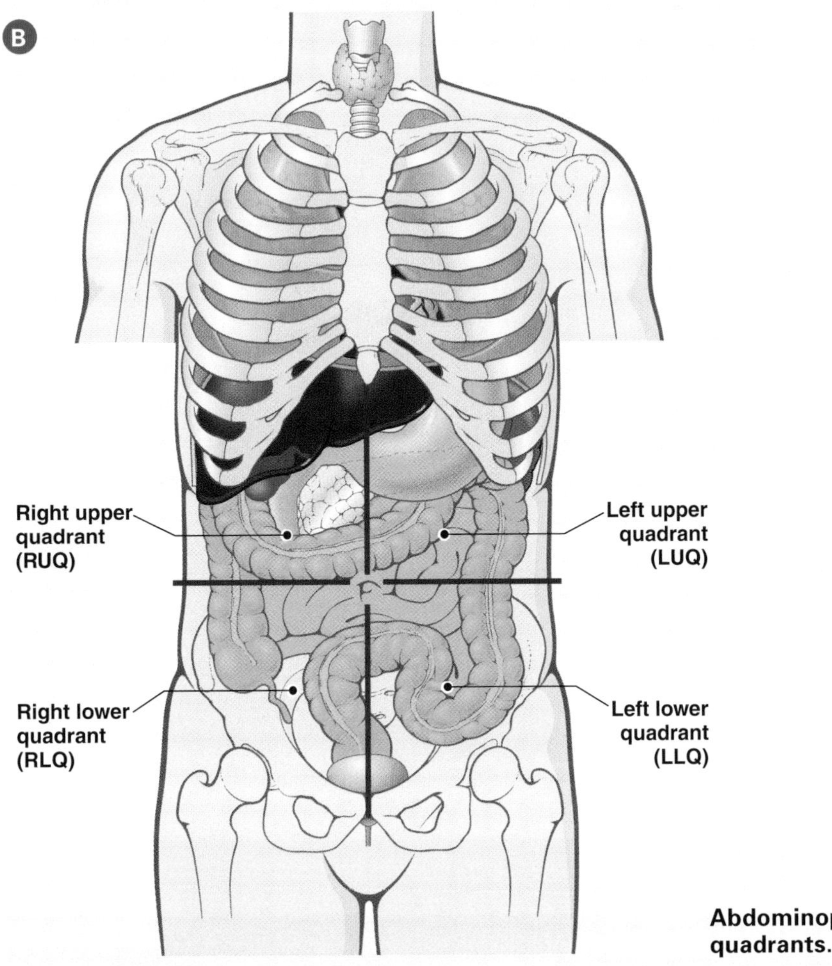

Abdominopelvic quadrants.

1. A large organ in the RUQ is the:
   a. stomach
   b. lung
   c. heart
   d. liver

2. The spleen is located in which quadrant?
   a. LUQ
   b. RUQ
   c. RLQ
   d. LLQ

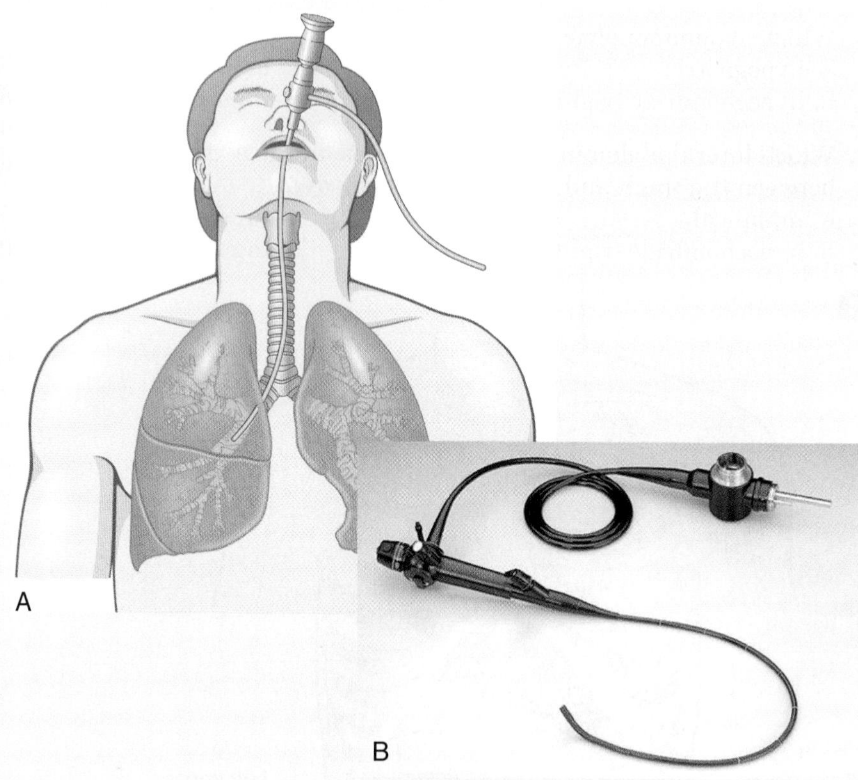

1. In the procedure shown, an endoscope (pictured in *B*) is inserted into the mouth to visualize tubes leading to the lungs. This procedure is:
   a. laryngoscopy
   b. laparoscopy
   c. mediastinoscopy
   d. esophagoscopy
   e. bronchoscopy

2. The instrument is a/an:
   a. mediastinoscope
   b. laparoscope
   c. bronchoscope
   d. esophagoscope
   e. laryngoscope

ANSWERS TO PICTURE SHOW

A 1. b 2. a 3. b 4. d

B 1. d 2. a

C 1. e. This procedure is used for removing material (sputum) from the bronchial tubes, obtaining a biopsy specimen, or removing foreign bodies.

2. c. This flexible bronchoscope permits passage of various instruments to obtain specimens from airways and lungs.

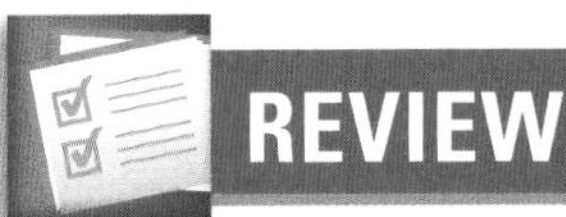

REVIEW

*Write the meanings of the following combining forms and suffixes in the spaces provided. Check your answers with the Answers to Review on page 84. Meanings for word parts also are listed in the **Glossary of Word Parts** beginning on page 399.*
Remember: The key to success is wRite, Repeat, Review!

COMBINING FORMS

Combining Form	Meaning
1. abdomin/o	______
2. anter/o	______
3. bronch/o	______
4. cervic/o	______
5. chondr/o	______
6. coccyg/o	______
7. crani/o	______
8. epitheli/o	______
9. esophag/o	______
10. hepat/o	______
11. lapar/o	______
12. laryng/o	______
13. later/o	______
14. lumb/o	______

Combining Form	Meaning
15. lymph/o	______
16. mediastin/o	______
17. pelv/o	______
18. peritone/o	______
19. pharyng/o	______
20. pleur/o	______
21. poster/o	______
22. radi/o	______
23. sacr/o	______
24. spin/o	______
25. thorac/o	______
26. trache/o	______
27. vertebr/o	______

SUFFIXES

Suffix **Meaning**

1. -ac ____________________
2. -al ____________________
3. -ar ____________________
4. -cyte ____________________
5. -eal ____________________
6. -ectomy ____________________
7. -ic ____________________
8. -itis ____________________
9. -logy ____________________
10. -oma ____________________
11. -scopy ____________________
12. -tomy ____________________

ANSWERS TO REVIEW

COMBINING FORMS

1. abdomen
2. front
3. bronchial tubes
4. neck
5. cartilage
6. tailbone
7. skull
8. skin
9. esophagus
10. liver
11. abdomen
12. voice box
13. side
14. loin, waist region
15. lymph
16. mediastinum
17. bones of the hip region
18. peritoneum
19. throat
20. pleura
21. back, behind
22. x-rays
23. sacrum
24. backbone
25. chest
26. windpipe
27. backbone

SUFFIXES

1. pertaining to
2. pertaining to
3. pertaining to
4. cell
5. pertaining to
6. cutting out, removal, excision, resection
7. pertaining to
8. inflammation
9. study of
10. tumor, mass
11. process of visual examination
12. cutting into, incision, to cut into

✓ TERMINOLOGY CHECKUP

Before you leave this chapter, here are important concepts that you should thoroughly understand. In your own words, write the answers on the lines provided. Confirm your answers on the next page. Check the box next to each item when you know you've "got" it!

☐ 1. Give the locations for the following double membranes: **pleura, peritoneum**, and **pericardium**.

____

____

____

☐ 2. What is the difference between the following parts of the body: **pharynx, larynx, trachea**, and **esophagus**?

____

____

____

☐ 3. Explain the difference between three planes of the body: **frontal (coronal) plane**, **sagittal (lateral) plane,** and **transverse (axial) plane.**

____

____

____

☐ 4. Where is the **mediastinum**? Name organs located in the mediastinum.

____

____

____

☐ 5. What is the difference between the **spinal column** and the **spinal cord**? Name the sections of the spinal column and the spinal cord.

____

____

____

ANSWERS TO TERMINOLOGY CHECKUP

1. The **pleura** is a double membrane surrounding the lungs.
   The **peritoneum** is a double membrane surrounding the abdominal organs.
   The **pericardium** is a double membrane surrounding the heart. In a later chapter, you will learn about the ***meninges***, three membranes surrounding the brain and spinal cord.

2. The **pharynx** is the **throat** (common passageway for air and food).
   The **larynx** is the **voice box** (containing vocal cords and located in the upper portion of the trachea).
   The **trachea** is the **windpipe** (tube that carries air into the bronchial tubes and lungs).
   The **esophagus** is the **food tube** (behind the trachea and carrying food to the stomach).

3. The **frontal (coronal) plane** divides the body into front and back (anterior/posterior) portions.
   The **sagittal (lateral) plane** divides the body into right and left sides.
   The **transverse (axial) plane** divides the body into upper and lower portions (cross sections). Visualizing organs in all three planes is possible with CT and MRI.

4. The **mediastinum** is the central region in the chest. It is the **space between the lungs.** Organs in the mediastinum are the **heart**, **large blood vessels** (aorta and venae cavae), **trachea, bronchial tubes,** and **lymph nodes.**

5. The **spinal cord** is a **bundle of nerves** extending from the base of the brain down the back of the body. It is within the spinal cavity. The **spinal column** is a **series of bones** surrounding spinal cavity and the spinal cord. Sections of the spinal cord and the spinal column are **cervical, thoracic, lumbar, sacral,** and **coccygeal.**

CHAPTER 3

Suffixes

Chapter Sections

Introduction 88
Combining Forms 88
Suffixes and Terminology 89
In Person: Gallbladder Stones 108
Exercises and Answers 109
Pronunciation of Terms 117
Practical Applications 120
Picture Show 122
Review 126
Terminology CheckUp 129

CHAPTER OBJECTIVES

- To identify and define useful diagnostic and procedural suffixes
- To analyze, spell, and pronounce medical terms that contain diagnostic and procedural suffixes
- To apply medical terms in real-life situations

INTRODUCTION

This chapter reviews the suffixes that you have learned in the first two chapters and also introduces new suffixes and medical terms. The combining forms used in the chapter are listed below. Refer to this list as you write the meanings of the terms in the Suffixes and Terminology section that follows (beginning on page 89). Be faithful about completing all of the Exercises (page 109), and remember to check your answers on pages 115 and 116! These exercises will help you spell terms correctly and understand their meanings. Test yourself by completing the Pronunciation of Terms on pages 117 to 119 and Review (pages 126 and 127).

Remember the 3 "Rs"—wRite, Review, Repeat—and you will succeed!

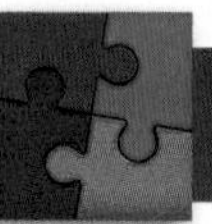

COMBINING FORMS

Combining Form	Meaning
aden/o	gland
amni/o	amnion (sac of fluid surrounding the embryo)
angi/o	vessel (usually a blood vessel)
arteri/o	artery
arthr/o	joint
ather/o	plaque (a yellow fatty material)
axill/o	armpit (underarm)
bronch/o	bronchial tube
bronchi/o	bronchial tube
carcin/o	cancerous
cardi/o	heart
chem/o	drug; also chemical
cholecyst/o	gallbladder
chron/o	time
col/o	colon (large intestine or bowel)
coron/o	heart; crown
crani/o	skull
cry/o	cold
cyst/o	urinary bladder; also a sac of fluid or a cyst
electr/o	electricity
encephal/o	brain
erythr/o	red
esophag/o	esophagus (tube leading from the throat to the stomach)
hem/o	blood
hemat/o	blood
hepat/o	liver
hyster/o	uterus
inguin/o	groin (area in which the thigh meets the trunk of the body)
isch/o	to hold back
lapar/o	abdomen (abdominal wall)

laryng/o	voice box (larynx)
leuk/o	white
mamm/o	breast (use with -ARY, -GRAPHY, -GRAM, and -PLASTY)
mast/o	breast (use with -ECTOMY and -ITIS)
men/o	menses (menstruation); month
mening/o	meninges (membranes around the brain and spinal cord)
my/o	muscle
myel/o	spinal cord (nervous tissue connected to the brain). MYEL/O can also mean bone marrow (soft, inner part of bones, where blood cells are made)
necr/o	death (of cells)
nephr/o	kidney (use with all suffixes except -AL and -GRAM)
neur/o	nerve
oophor/o	ovary
oste/o	bone
ot/o	ear
pelv/o	hip area
peritone/o	peritoneum (membrane surrounding organs in the abdomen)
phleb/o	vein
pneumon/o	lung
pulmon/o	lung
radi/o	x-rays
ren/o	kidney (use with -AL and -GRAM)
rhin/o	nose
salping/o	fallopian (uterine) tube
sarc/o	flesh
septic/o	pertaining to infection
thorac/o	chest
tonsill/o	tonsil
trache/o	windpipe; trachea
ur/o	urine or urea (a waste material); urinary tract
vascul/o	blood vessel

3

SUFFIXES AND TERMINOLOGY

Suffixes are divided into two groups: those that describe **diagnoses** and those that describe **procedures.**

DIAGNOSTIC SUFFIXES

Diagnostic suffixes describe disease conditions or their symptoms. Use the list of combining forms in the previous section to write the meaning of each term. You will find it helpful to check the meanings of the terms with the ***Mini-Dictionary***, beginning on page 363.

Noun Suffix	Meaning	Terminology	Meaning
-algia	condition of pain, pain	arthralgia	______________
		otalgia	______________
		myalgia	______________
		neuralgia	______________
-emia	blood condition	leukemia *Increase in numbers of leukocytes; cells are malignant (cancerous).*	______________
		septicemia *Blood infections result when pathogens enter the blood from a wound.*	______________
		ischemia *Figure 3-1 illustrates ischemia of heart muscle caused by blockage of a coronary (heart) artery.*	______________

3

Septicemia and bacteremia

Bacteremia is bacterial invasion of the blood with or without symptoms. **Septicemia** (sepsis), however, is a more serious bacteremia that moves rapidly and may be life-threatening.

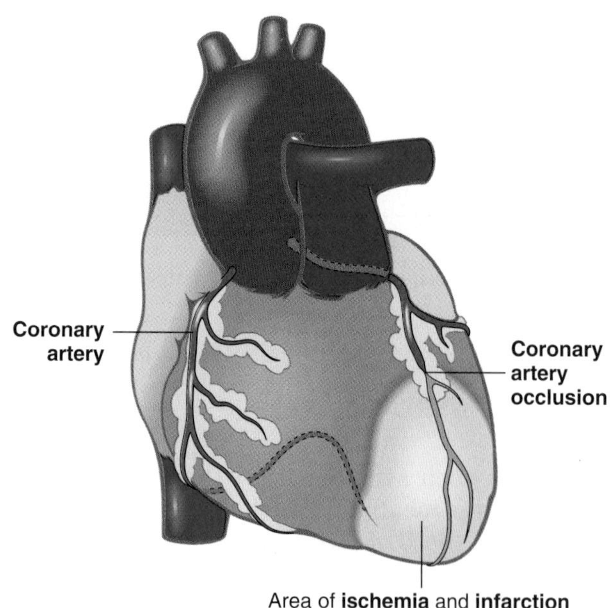

FIGURE 3-1 Ischemia of heart muscle. Blood is held back from an area of the heart muscle by an occlusion (blockage) of a coronary (heart) artery. The muscle then loses its supply of oxygen and nutrition and, if the condition persists, dies. **The death of the affected part of the heart muscle is a myocardial infarction (heart attack).**

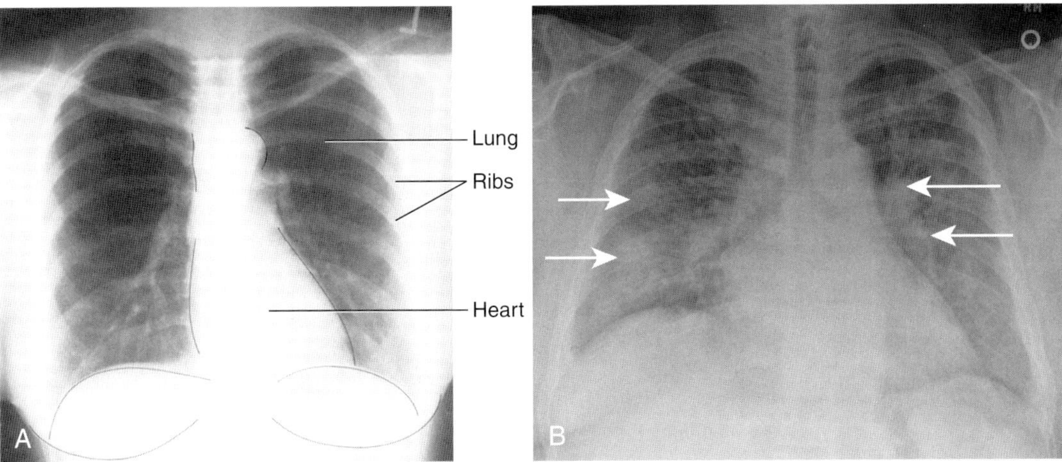

FIGURE 3-2 **A, Chest x-ray** showing **normal lungs. B,** Chest x-ray showing **pneumonia from coronavirus infection**. Notice the bilateral (both sides) "patchy" infiltrates (cells and fluid) as shown with arrows.

		uremia ________________ *Uremia occurs when the kidneys fail to function and urea (a waste material) accumulates in the blood.*
-ia	condition	pneumonia ________________ *The lung is inflamed, causing fluid and material to collect in the air sacs of the lung. Pneumonia is a serious and potentially fatal complication of infection with coronavirus. See Figure 3-2. Oxygen therapy may needed to help breathing and some patients are placed on a ventilator (assisted breathing device) to survive.*
-itis	inflammation	bronchitis ________________ *Bronchial tubes are inflamed, with hypersecretion of mucus.* esophagitis ________________ laryngitis ________________ meningitis ________________ *The meninges are membranes that surround and protect the brain and spinal cord. See Figure 3-3.* cystitis ________________ phlebitis ________________ colitis ________________ *Table 3-1 lists other common inflammatory conditions with their meanings.*

3

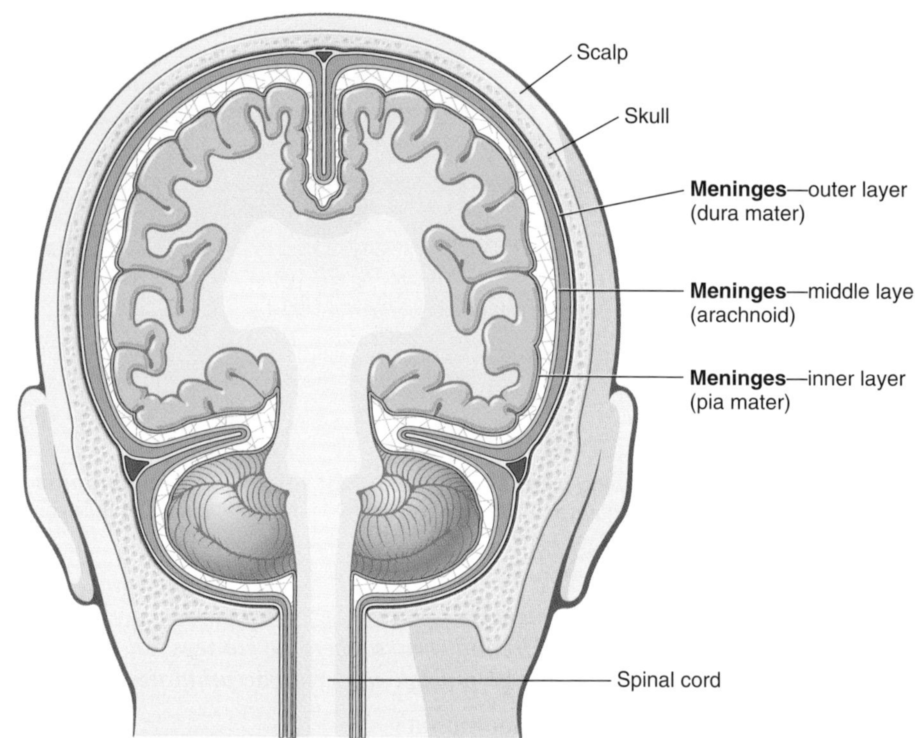

FIGURE 3-3 **Meninges** (frontal view) are the membranes surrounding the brain and spinal cord.

TABLE 3-1	INFLAMMATIONS
appendicitis	Inflammation of the appendix (hangs from the colon in the lower right abdomen)
bursitis	Inflammation of a small sac of fluid (bursa) near a joint
cellulitis	Inflammation of soft tissue under the skin
dermatitis	Inflammation of the skin
endocarditis	Inflammation of the inner lining of the heart (endocardium)
epiglottitis	Inflammation of the epiglottis (cartilage at the upper part of the windpipe)
gastritis	Inflammation of the stomach
hepatitis	Inflammation of the liver
myositis	Inflammation of muscle (MYOS/O means muscle)
nephritis	Inflammation of the kidney
osteomyelitis	Inflammation of bone and bone marrow
otitis	Inflammation of the ear
peritonitis	Inflammation of the peritoneum
pharyngitis	Inflammation of the throat
thrombophlebitis	Inflammation of a vein with formation of clots

-megaly	enlargement	cardiomegaly ______________________
		hepatomegaly ______________________
-oma	tumor, mass	adenoma ______________________ *This is a benign (noncancerous) tumor.*
		adenocarcinoma ______________________ *Carcinomas are malignant (cancerous) tumors of epithelial (skin or lining) tissue in the body. Glands and the linings of internal organs are composed of epithelial tissue. See Figure 3-4B.*
		myoma ______________________ *This is a benign tumor. Myomas commonly occur in the uterus and are known as **fibroids.** See Figure 3-5.*
		myosarcoma ______________________ *Sarcomas are malignant tumors of connective (flesh) tissue. Muscle, bone, cartilage, fibrous tissue, and fat are examples of connective tissues. See Table 3-2.*
		myeloma ______________________ MYEL/O *means bone marrow in this term. Also called **multiple myeloma,** this is a malignant tumor of cells in the bone marrow often occurring in other locations. See Table 3-3 for names of other malignant tumors that do not contain the combining forms* CARCIN/O *and* SARC/O.

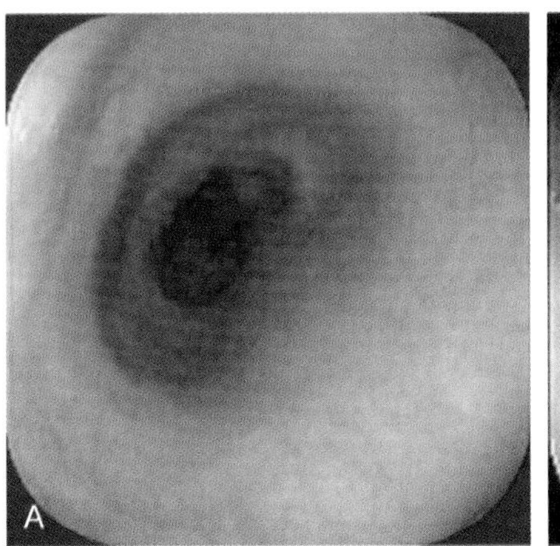

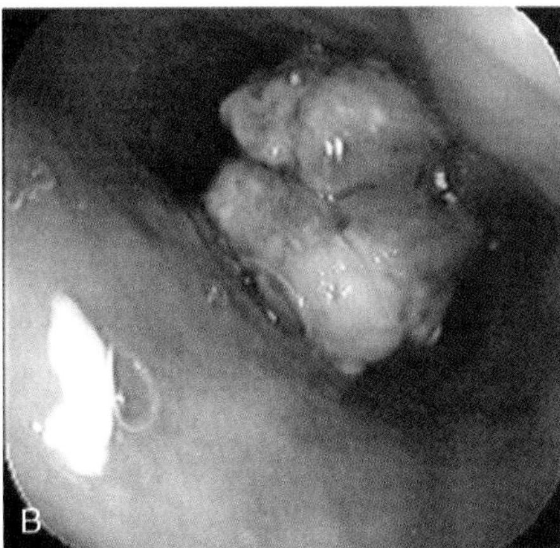

FIGURE 3-4 **A, Normal esophagus. B, Esophageal adenocarcinoma.**

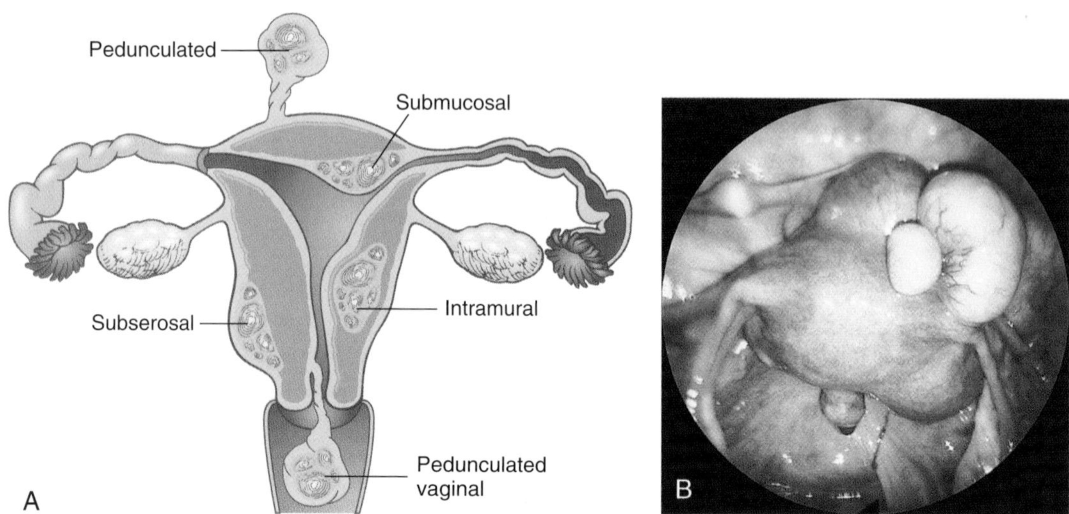

FIGURE 3-5 **A, Location of uterine fibroids (leiomyomas). Pedunculated** growths protrude on stalks. A **subserosal** mass lies under the serosal (outermost) layer of the uterus. A **submucosal** leiomyoma grows under the mucosal (innermost) layer. **Intramural** (mural means wall) masses arise within the muscular uterine wall. **B, Multiple myomas viewed laparoscopically.**

TABLE 3-2	SARCOMAS
chondrosarcoma	Cancer of cartilage tissue (CHONDR/O means cartilage)
fibrosarcoma	Cancer of fibrous tissue (FIBR/O means fibrous tissue)
leiomyosarcoma	Cancer of visceral (attached to internal organs) muscle (LEIOMY/O means visceral or "smooth" muscle)
liposarcoma	Cancer of fatty tissue (LIP/O means fat)
osteogenic sarcoma	Cancer of bone (OSTE/O means bone)
rhabdomyosarcoma	Cancer of skeletal (attached to bones) muscle (RHABDOMY/O means skeletal muscle)

TABLE 3-3	MALIGNANT TUMORS WHOSE NAMES DO NOT CONTAIN THE COMBINING FORMS *CARCIN/O* AND *SARC/O*
hepatoma	Malignant tumor of the liver (commonly called hepatocellular carcinoma)
lymphoma	Malignant tumor of lymph nodes (previously called lymphosarcoma)
melanoma	Malignant tumor of pigmented (MELAN/O means black) cells in the skin
mesothelioma	Malignant tumor of pleural cells (membrane surrounding the lungs)
multiple myeloma	Malignant tumor of bone marrow cells
thymoma	Malignant tumor of the thymus gland (located in the mediastinum)

-osis	condition, abnormal condition	nephrosis ______________________
		necrosis ______________________ *Ischemia may lead to necrosis.* ***Gangrene*** *is type of necrosis.*
		erythrocytosis ______________________ *When* -OSIS *is used with blood cell words, it means a slight increase in number of cells.*
		leukocytosis ______________________
-pathy	disease condition	encephalopathy ______________________ *Pronunciation is* en-sef-ah-**LOP**-*ah-the.* ***Chronic traumatic encephalopathy (CTE)*** *is a serious disease condition of the brain caused by repeated (chronic) high-impact trauma such as in boxing or football.*
		cardiomyopathy ______________________. *Pronunciation is* kar-de-o-mi-**OP**-ah-the
		nephropathy ______________________ *Pronunciation is* neh-**FROP**-ah-the. *Table 3-4 lists other disease conditions.*

3

Leukocytosis versus leukemia

Leukocytosis—slight increase in normal white blood cells (WBCs)—is the body's response to bacterial infection. **Leukemia** is a malignant condition marked by dramatic increase in cancerous WBCs.

Cardiomyopathy and myocardial infarction (MI)

Cardiomyopathy is chronic (ongoing) disease of heart muscle with inflammation and weakness. However, a **myocardial infarction (MI)** is an acute (sudden) condition involving an area of heart muscle that has died as a result of ischemia. An MI is a heart attack.

TABLE 3-4	DISEASE CONDITIONS (*-PATHIES*)
adenopathy	Disease condition of lymph nodes ("glands"); lymphadenopathy
adrenopathy	Disease condition of the adrenal glands
hepatopathy	Disease condition of the liver
myopathy	Disease condition of muscles
neuropathy	Disease condition of nerves
osteopathy	Disease condition of bones
retinopathy	Disease condition of the retina of the eye

-rrhea	flow, discharge	rhinorrhea ______________
		menorrhea ______________ *Normal menstrual flow.*
-rrhage *or* **-rrhagia**	excessive discharge of blood	hemorrhage ______________
		menorrhagia ______________ *Excessive bleeding during menstruation.*
-sclerosis	hardening	arteriosclerosis ______________ ***Atherosclerosis** is the most common type of arteriosclerosis. A fatty plaque (atheroma) collects on the lining of arteries. See Figure 3-6.*
-uria	condition of urine	hematuria ______________ *Bleeding into the urinary tract can cause this sign of kidney disease or of disorders of the urinary and genital tracts.*

All of the following **adjective suffixes** mean *pertaining to* and describe a part of the body, process, or condition. Do not worry about which suffix (-al, -eal, -ar, -ary, or -ic) to use with a particular organ or root. Just identify the suffix as meaning "pertaining to" in each term.

-al *or* **-eal**	pertaining to	peritoneal ______________
		inguinal ______________
		renal ______________
		esophageal ______________
		myocardial ______________ *Don't forget that a heart attack is a **myocardial infarction (MI).** An **infarction** is an area of dead tissue caused by **ischemia** (a condition in which blood supply is held back from a part of the body).*
-ar	pertaining to	vascular ______________ *A **cerebrovascular accident (CVA)** is a stroke.*

Menorrhea and menorrhagia

Menorrhea is the normal discharge of blood and tissue from the lining of the uterus. **Menorrhagia** is abnormally heavy or long menstrual periods. Chronic menorrhagia can result in anemia. Menorrhagia is a common complication of uterine myomas (fibroids).

Hematuria and uremia

Hematuria is blood in the urine, whereas **uremia** is high levels of urea in the blood.

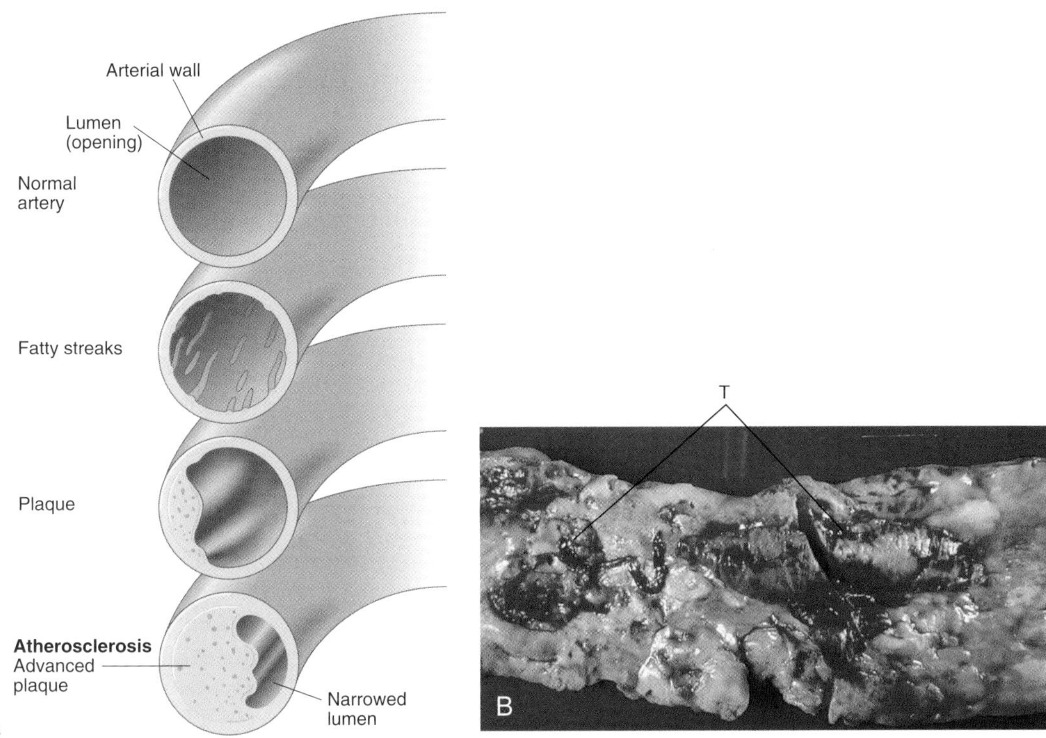

FIGURE 3-6 **Atherosclerosis** (a type of **arteriosclerosis**). **A,** A fatty material (cholesterol) collects in an artery, narrowing it and eventually blocking the flow of blood. **B, Atherosclerotic aorta.** The surface of the aorta is rugged and irregular. Organized thrombi (T) are seen protruding from the inner lining (endothelial) surface.

3

-ary	pertaining to	axillary ______________________
		coronary ______________________ *Coron/o means heart or crown. Coronary arteries are located on the outside of the heart, surrounding it like a crown. They bring oxygen-rich blood to the heart muscle.*
		mammary ______________________
		pulmonary ______________________
-ic	pertaining to	chronic ______________________ ***Chronic** conditions occur over a long period of time, as opposed to **acute** conditions, which are sharp, sudden, and brief.*

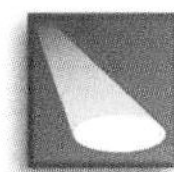

Coronary arteries, atherosclerosis, and myocardial infarction

When the **coronary arteries** are narrowed or blocked by **atherosclerosis**, the heart muscle is deprived of oxygen (ischemia) and may die (necrosis), causing a **myocardial infarction (MI)**. See Figure 3-1.

PROCEDURAL SUFFIXES

The following suffixes describe *procedures* used in patient care.

Suffix	Meaning	Terminology	Meaning
-centesis	puncture to remove fluid	thoracentesis *This term is a shortened form of thoracocentesis. See Figure 3-7.*	______
		amniocentesis *See Figure 3-8.*	______
		arthrocentesis *This procedure is commonly performed on the knee joint to withdraw fluid for diagnosis or treatment.*	______
-ectomy	removal, resection, excision	tonsillectomy *Tonsils and adenoids are lymph tissue in the pharynx (throat). See Figure 3-9A. Lymph is composed of white blood cells that fight infection. Chronic tonsillitis is a an indication for tonsillectomy. See Figure 3-9B.*	______

3

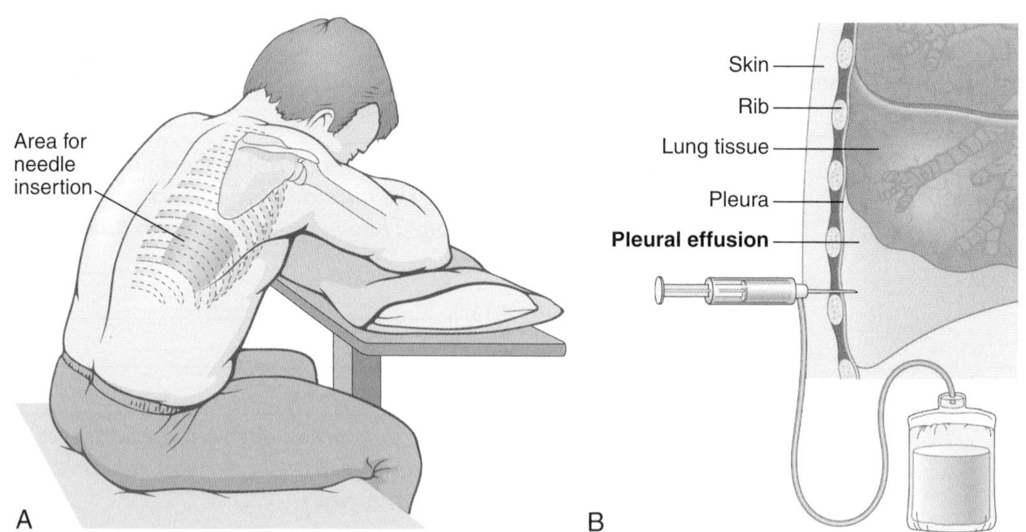

FIGURE 3-7 Technique of thoracentesis. A, The patient is sitting in the correct position for the procedure. **B,** The needle is advanced, and the fluid **(pleural effusion)** is drained.

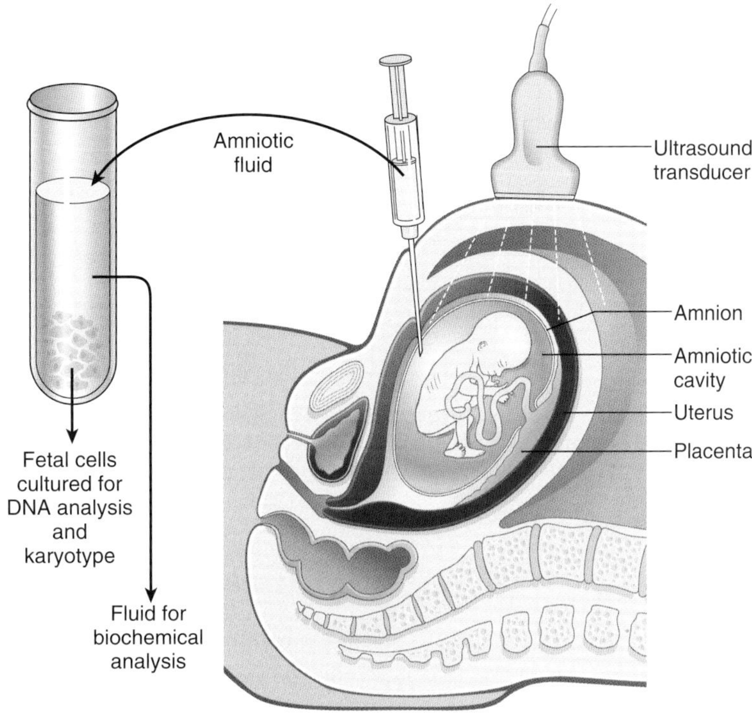

FIGURE 3-8
Amniocentesis. Under ultrasound guidance (imaging based on high-frequency sound waves), the physician inserts a needle through the uterine wall and amnion, into the amniotic cavity. Amniotic fluid, containing fetal cells, is withdrawn and examined for chemicals that indicate fetal defects.

3

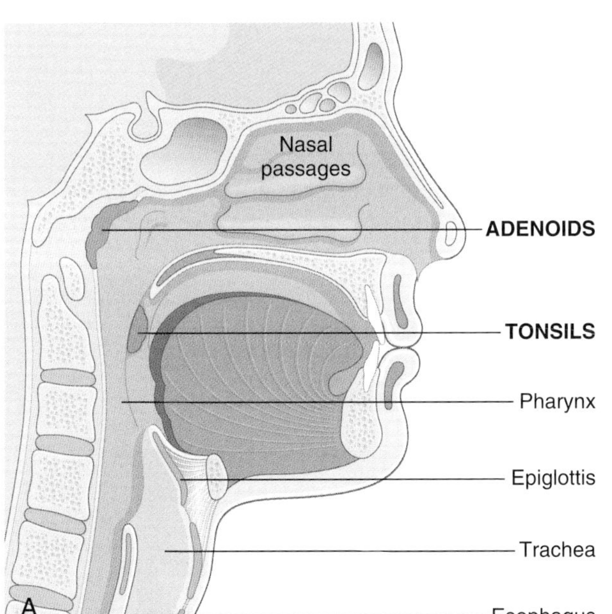

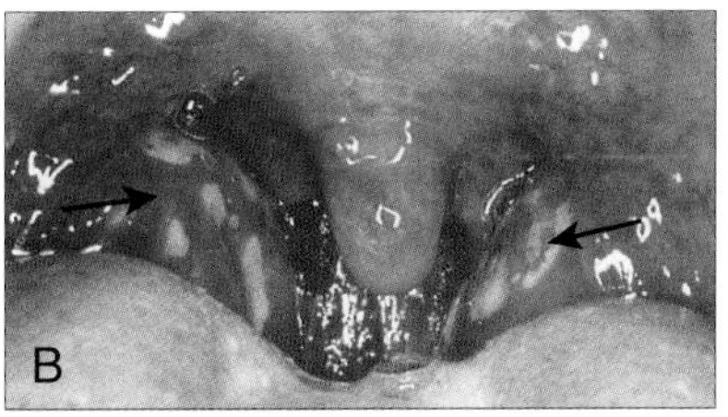

FIGURE 3-9 A. Tonsils and adenoids. B. Tonsillitis. Arrows are pointing to swollen and infected tonsils with intense erythema (redness) and creamy yellow exudates (pus containing leukocytes and bacteria). Removal of chronically infected tonsils and adenoids, called **tonsillectomy and adenoidectomy (T & A)** may be necessary.

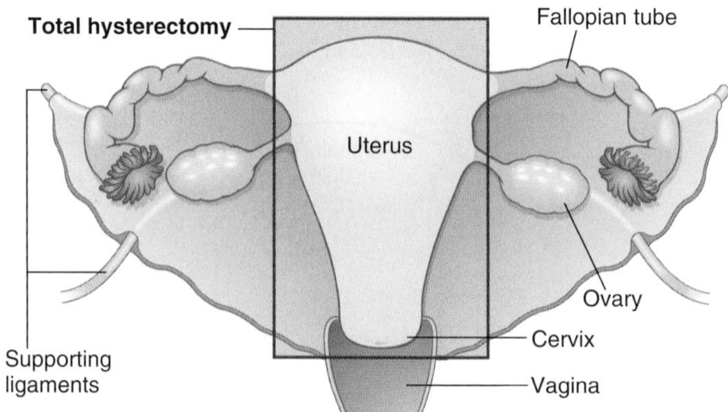

FIGURE 3-10 Total hysterectomy. In a total abdominal hysterectomy (TAH), the uterus is removed through the abdomen. A **TAH-BSO** is a total abdominal hysterectomy with bilateral salpingectomy and oophorectomy. Laparoscopic hysterectomy can be performed as well.

hyster<u>ectomy</u> ______________________________

*In a **total hysterectomy,** the entire uterus, including the cervix, is removed. If only a portion of the uterus is removed, the procedure is a* partial *or **subtotal hysterectomy.** See Figure 3-10.*

oophor<u>ectomy</u> ______________________________

Figure 3-11 shows a laparoscopic oophorectomy.

salping<u>ectomy</u> ______________________________

cholecyst<u>ectomy</u> ______________________________

*See Figure 3-12. Laparoscopic cholecystectomy is performed whenever possible, instead of an open (more invasive) procedure. See **In Person: Gallbladder Stones** on page 108.*

mast<u>ectomy</u> ______________________________

Table 3-5 lists additional resection procedures.

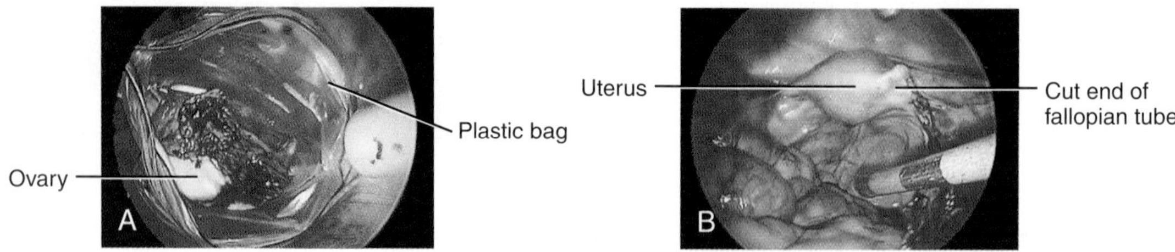

FIGURE 3-11 Laparoscopic oophorectomy. A, Notice the ovary within a plastic bag. The bag was inserted through the laparoscope and then opened, and the ovary was placed inside. **B,** Both are extracted through the laparoscope, leaving the uterus and the cut end of the fallopian tube.

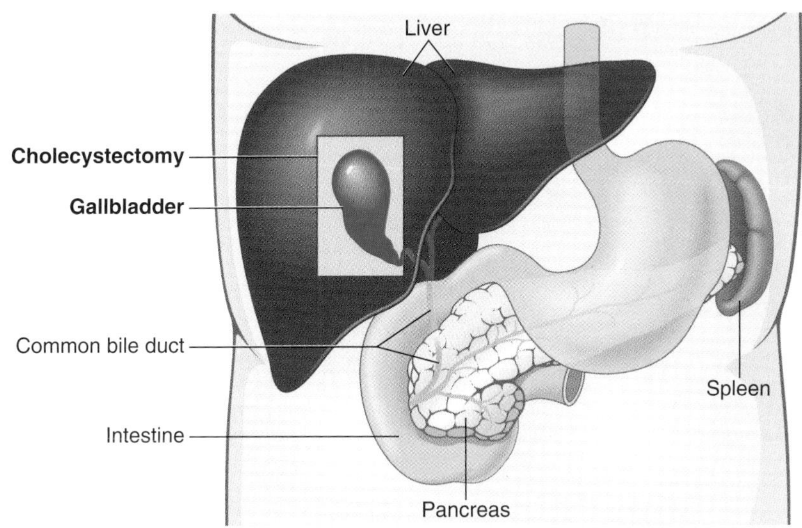

FIGURE 3-12 Cholecystectomy. The liver is lifted up to show the **gallbladder** underneath. The pancreas is a long, thin gland located behind and to the left of the stomach, toward the spleen. The common bile duct carries bile from the liver and gallbladder to the intestine. After cholecystectomy, the liver continues to produce bile and release it, via the common bile duct, into the intestine.

-gram	record	myelogram ________________ MYEL/O *means spinal cord in this term. Contrast material is injected into the membranes around the spinal cord (by lumbar puncture), and then x-ray pictures are taken of the spinal cord. This procedure is performed less frequently now that MRI is available.*
		mammogram ________________ *See Figure 3-13.*

3

TABLE 3-5	RESECTIONS
adenectomy	Excision of a gland
adenoidectomy	Excision of the adenoids
appendectomy	Excision of the appendix
colectomy	Excision of the colon
gastrectomy	Excision of the stomach
laminectomy	Excision of a piece of backbone (lamina) to relieve pressure on nerves from a (herniating) disc
myomectomy	Excision of a muscle tumor (commonly a fibroid of the uterus)
pneumonectomy	Excision of lung tissue: total pneumonectomy (an entire lung) or lobectomy (a single lobe)
prostatectomy	Excision of the prostate gland
splenectomy	Excision of the spleen

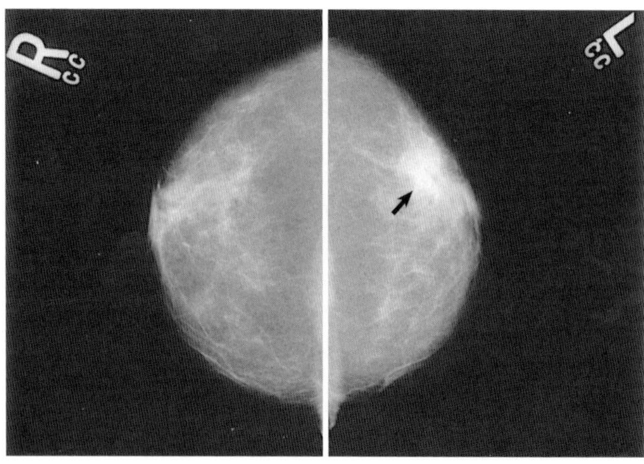

FIGURE 3-13 **Mammograms** from a 63-year-old woman. The right breast is normal, and the left breast contains a carcinoma (breast cancer) (arrow).

-graphy process of recording

electroencephalography ______________________

mammography ______________________

***Tomosynthesis** is a new mammographic technique that shows clearer and more detailed images. See Figure 3-14, A and B.*

angiography ______________________

Contrast material (such as iodine) is injected into an artery or vein, and x-ray images are taken.

3

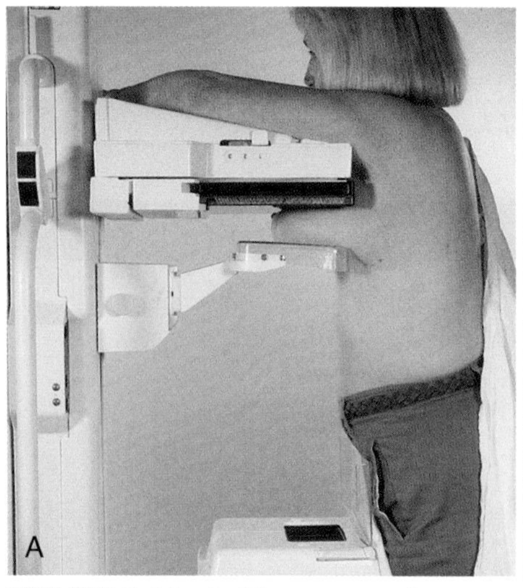

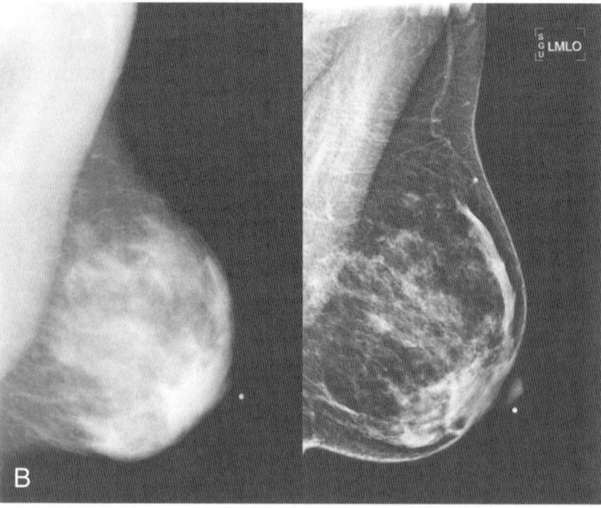

FIGURE 3-14 **A, Mammography**. The breast is compressed, and x-ray images, craniocaudal (top to bottom) and lateral, are taken. **B,** Image on the left is a mammogram and the image on the right is the same anatomy viewed by digital mammography **tomosynthesis**.

-lysis	separation, breakdown, destruction	dia<u>lysis</u> ________________ *Dialysis literally means complete* (DIA-) *separation* (-LYSIS). *In hemodialysis, blood is removed from the body and passes through a kidney machine that separates out waste materials, such as urea, from the blood. Another form of dialysis is* ***peritoneal dialysis.*** *A special fluid is inserted into the peritoneal cavity through a tube in the abdomen. Waste materials (such as urea) seep into the fluid during a period of time. The fluid and wastes are then drained from the peritoneal cavity. See Figure 3-15.*

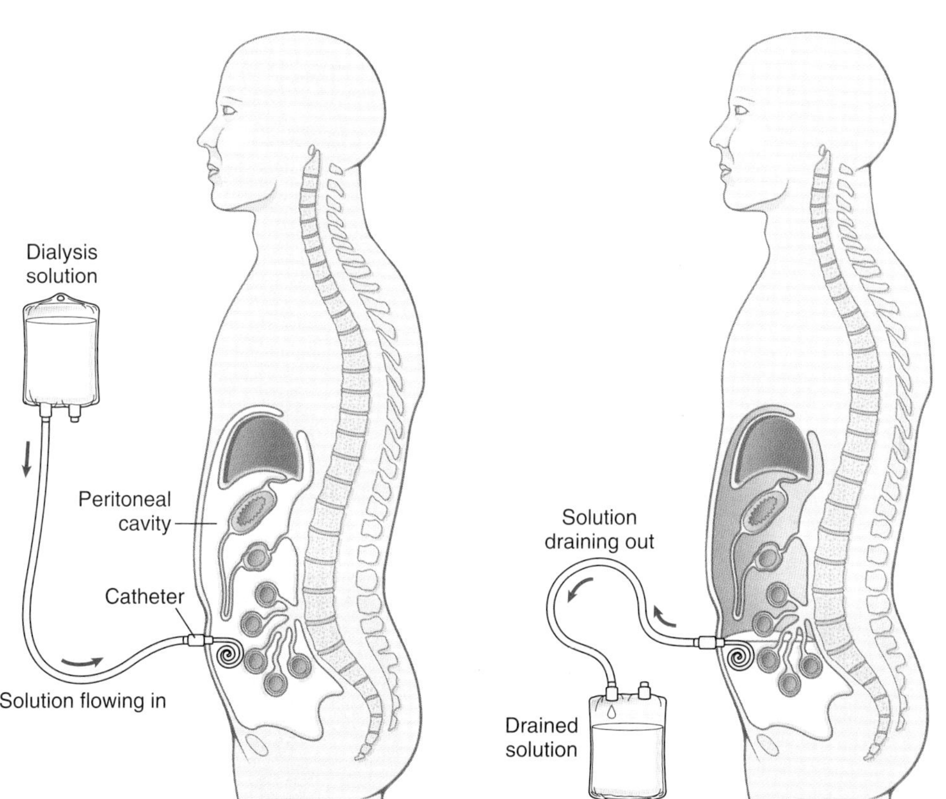

FIGURE 3-15 Peritoneal dialysis. This procedure (or the alternative method of hemodialysis) is necessary when the kidneys are not functioning to remove waste materials (such as urea) from the blood. Without dialysis or kidney transplantation, uremia can result.

3

-plasty	surgical repair or surgical correction	mammoplasty ______________
		rhinoplasty ______________
		angioplasty ______________ *Balloon angioplasty is performed on narrowed, blocked coronary arteries that surround the heart. A wire with a collapsed balloon is placed in a clogged artery. Opening of the balloon widens the vessel, allowing more blood to flow through. A* ***stent*** *(mesh tube) is placed in the artery to hold it open. See Figure 3-16.*
-scopy	process of visual examination	bronchoscopy ______________
		laparoscopy ______________ ***Laparoscopic sleeve gastrectomy*** *is a minimally invasive weight-loss procedure removing about 80% of the stomach through small abdominal incisions. The remaining stomach is a small, tubular sleeve (pouch) that reduces the amount of food consumed and helps decrease appetite.*
		laryngoscopy ______________ *See Figure 3-17.*

3

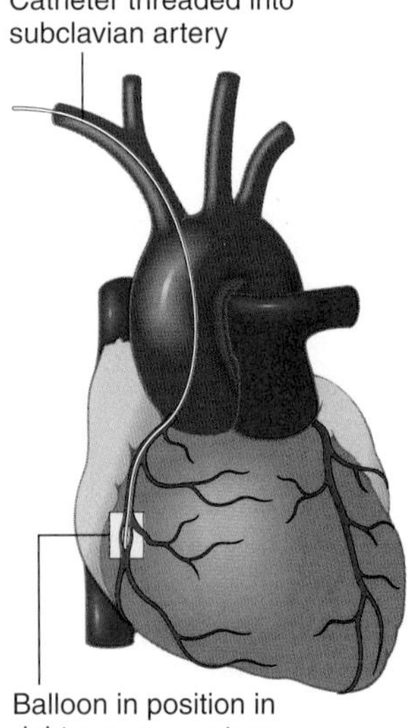

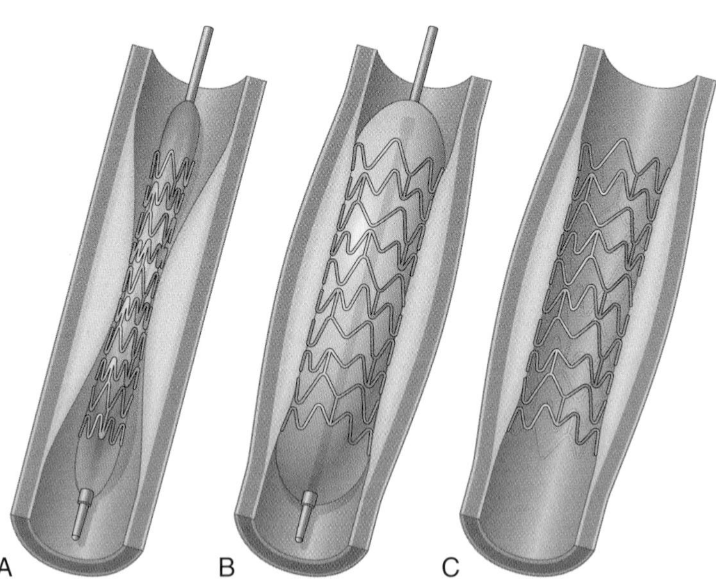

FIGURE 3-16 Angioplasty and placement of an intracoronary artery stent. A, The stent is positioned at the site of the lesion. **B,** The balloon is inflated, expanding the stent. **C,** The balloon is then deflated and removed, and the implanted stent is left in place. Coronary artery stents are stainless steel mesh, tube-like devices that help hold arteries open. Drug-eluting stents release chemicals to dissolve plaque.

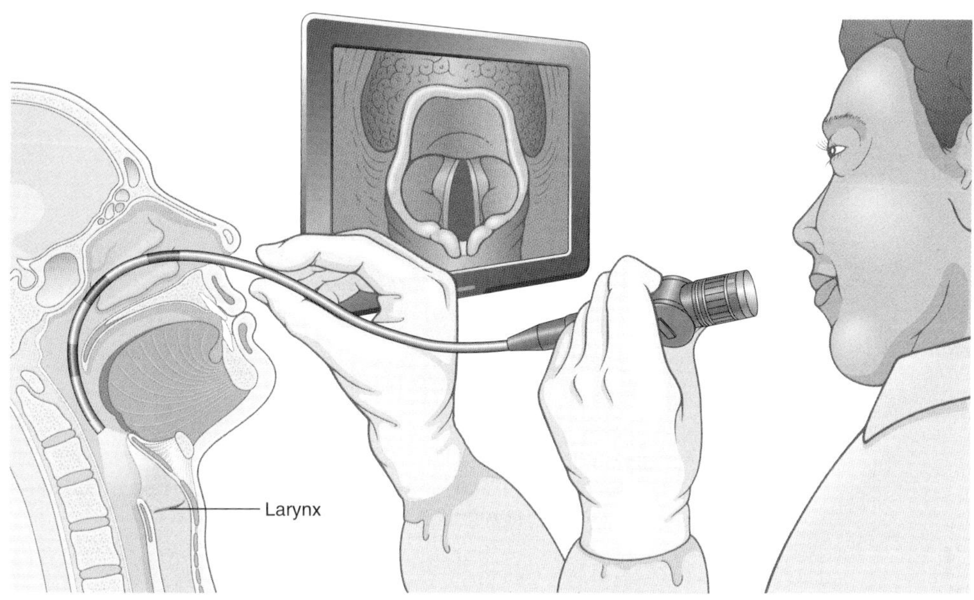

FIGURE 3-17 **Laryngoscopy.**

-stomy opening

colostomy ______________________

A **-STOMY** *procedure is the creation of a permanent or semipermanent opening (stoma) from an organ to the outside of the body. See Figure 3-18. Images of colostomy care are pictured in Figure 3-19. When two tube-like structures are surgically connected* ***within the body****, the new connection is an* ***anastomosis*** *(see Figure 3-20). A* **colocolostomy** *is an anastomosis, a new connection between two previously unconnected portions of the colon.*

tracheostomy ______________________

See Figure 3-21.

-therapy treatment

radiotherapy ______________________

chemotherapy ______________________

cryotherapy ______________________

Skin lesions, such as warts, are removed with cryotherapy. Liquid nitrogen or carbon dioxide snow is applied, and blistering followed by necrosis results.

Radiotherapy versus radiology

Radiotherapy (radiation therapy) is directed by a radiation oncologist, a medical doctor specializing in **treating** cancer using radiation to kill tumor cells. **Radiology** is the specialty of a radiologist, also a medical doctor, who primarily makes a **diagnosis** using x-ray, magnetic wave, and ultrasound techniques.

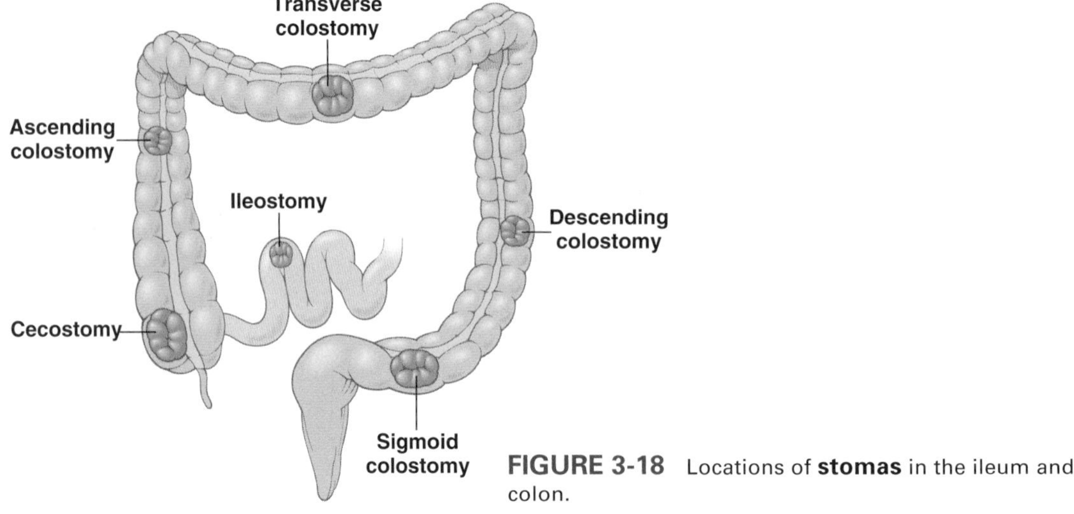

FIGURE 3-18 Locations of **stomas** in the ileum and colon.

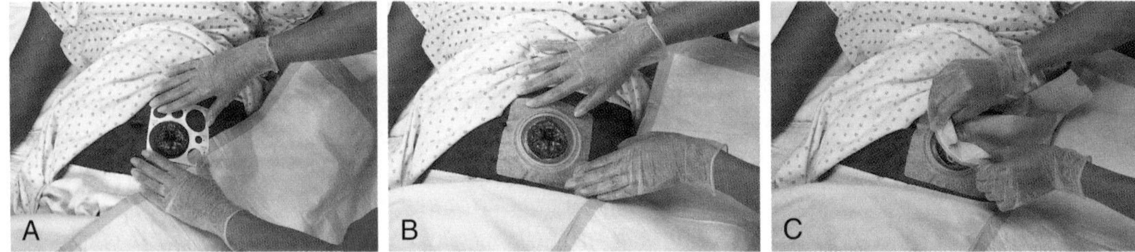

FIGURE 3-19 **Colostomy care.**

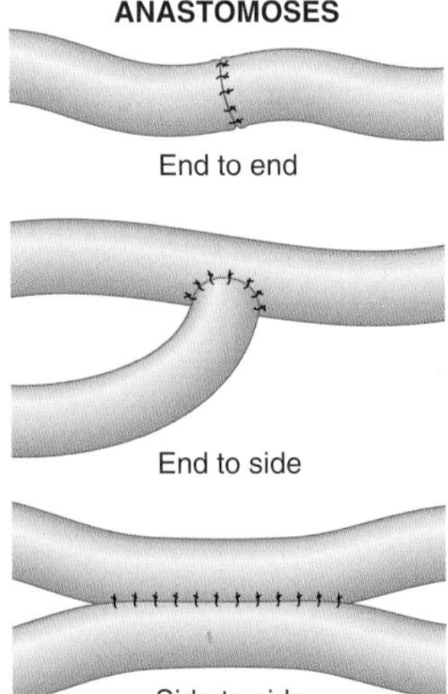

FIGURE 3-20 **Anastomoses** are new surgical connections between previously unconnected tube-like structures.

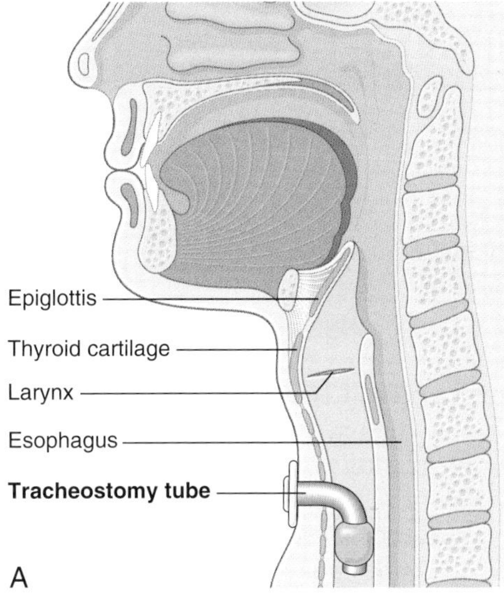

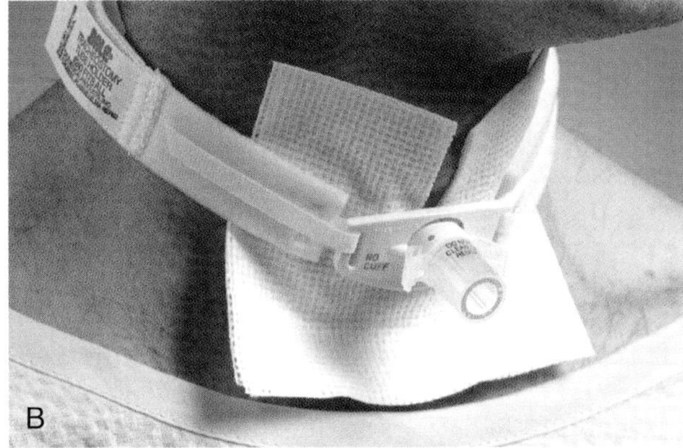

FIGURE 3-21 **A, Tracheostomy** with tube in place. **B, Placement of tracheostomy gauze dressing** and Velcro tracheostomy tube holder after laryngectomy.

-tomy	incision, cutting into	cranio<u>tomy</u> ____________
		laparo<u>tomy</u> ____________
		phlebo<u>tomy</u> ____________ *See Figure 3-22.*

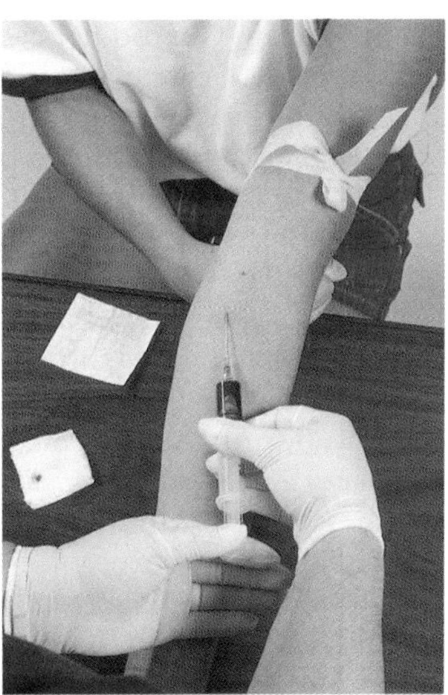

FIGURE 3-22 **Phlebotomy.** After a vein is entered with a needle inserted through the skin, the plunger of the syringe is slowly pulled out to withdraw blood.

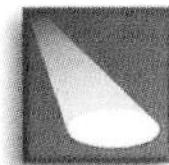

-TOMY versus -STOMY

-TOMY indicates a temporary **incision,** as opposed to -STOMY, which is a permanent or semipermanent **opening.**

3

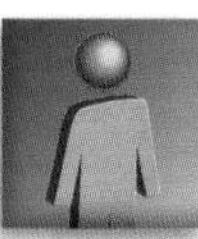

IN PERSON: GALLBLADDER STONES

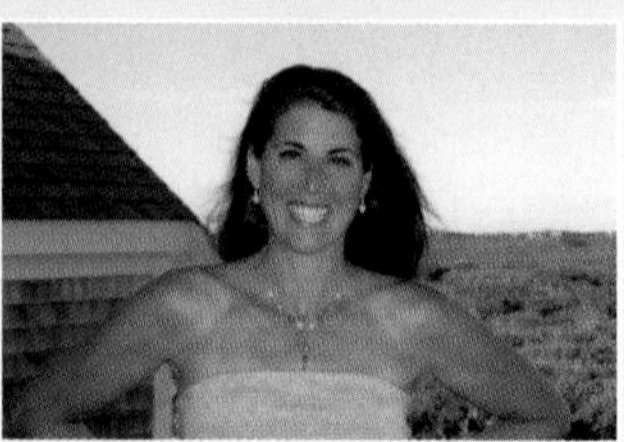

This first-person narrative describes the symptoms and treatment of a 46-year-old woman with gallbladder stones.

Everyone enjoys a little dessert after dinner, but when the ice cream or a creamy tart leads to pain, most would avoid it. I loved sweets, and despite the revenge they took on my waistline, I still would not pass up an ice cream cone—until my gallbladder decided it had had enough. After several late nights spent doubled over in pain, I tried to steer clear of fatty foods but could not resist the temptation of frozen yogurt.

With one hand I pushed my cart through the supermarket; with the other hand I fed myself some delicious low-fat (not nonfat) frozen yogurt. I never dreamed that the attendant at the quick-service window actually gave me soft-serve ice cream. Within 10 minutes of eating the questionable yogurt, I broke out into a sweat; a wave of nausea took me over, and a knifelike pain stabbed me in my right upper quadrant. It hurt even more when I pressed my hand on the area in an attempt to brace the pain.

Several months earlier, after a similar painful episode, I had undergone an ultrasound of my gallbladder, and the surgeon then recommended cholecystectomy. The US showed multiple stones in my gallbladder. Most of the stones were just the right size to lodge in the common bile duct and cause blockage of the outflow of bile that occurs after a fatty meal. When I heard the ultrasound results, I swore off all fatty foods.

I just did not imagine that ice cream masquerading as "low-fat yogurt" would be the straw that broke the camel's back! Soon enough, I abandoned my shopping cart and apologized to the manager of the store for vomiting all over aisle 4. The unrelenting pain did not cease when I vomited—it only intensified. I have no idea how I made it home and into bed. I managed to call my surgeon and arrange for "semiemergent" surgery the next morning.

Dr. Fernandez and his team performed a laparoscopic cholecystectomy and relayed to me as I came out of anesthesia that I no longer had a "bag of marbles" for a gallbladder. I had a gassy, distended feeling in my abdomen over the 2 weeks after surgery (carbon dioxide gas is injected into the abdomen before surgery to allow space between abdominal organs). I felt "tight as a drum" for the first few days, and then day by day it went away. My four tiny incisions healed just fine, and in about 2 weeks I was feeling back to normal. Now I can eat ice cream to my heart's content, only suffering the padding on my waistline, not the stabbing pain just above. Without missing a beat, my liver now delivers the bile into my small intestine right after I eat a fatty meal. The bile emulsifies (breaks down) the fat. I just don't have a storage bag to hold bile in reserve.

I've had an appendectomy, my wisdom teeth removed, and now I gave up my gallbladder! How many more "useless" body parts are there to go?

Elizabeth Chabner is the CEO/founder of Masthead, a company devoted to bringing innovative products to patients with breast cancer. She is a physician, swimmer, cross country skier, and the proud mother of four children ages 18-23.

3

? EXERCISES AND ANSWERS

Complete these exercises and check your answers. An important part of your success in learning medical terminology is checking your answers carefully with the Answers to Exercises beginning on page 115. Visit the Evolve website for additional interactive activities and information.

A Give meanings for the following suffixes.

1. -algia ______________________
2. -emia ______________________
3. -itis ______________________
4. -megaly ______________________
5. -oma ______________________
6. -pathy ______________________
7. -rrhea ______________________
8. -rrhagia ______________________
9. -sclerosis ______________________
10. -uria ______________________

B Give definitions for the following terms:

1. myalgia ______________________
2. septicemia ______________________
3. uremia ______________________
4. phlebitis ______________________
5. cardiomegaly ______________________
6. myosarcoma ______________________
7. nephrosis ______________________
8. encephalopathy ______________________
9. rhinorrhea ______________________
10. menorrhagia ______________________

C Match the following medical terms with their meanings below. Write each term next to its meaning.

adenocarcinoma
cardiomyopathy
esophagitis
hematoma
hepatomegaly
ischemia
leukocytosis
myeloma
otalgia
pneumonia

1. Enlargement of the liver ______________________
2. Pain in the ear ______________________
3. Holding back blood from an organ (depriving it of blood supply) ______________________
4. Abnormal condition of white blood cells (slight increase in normal cells to fight infection) ______________________
5. Abnormal condition of the lung (inflammation and accumulation of material often caused by bacterial infection) ______________________
6. Tumor (malignant) of bone marrow ______________________
7. Inflammation of the tube leading from the throat to the stomach ______________________
8. Disease of heart muscle ______________________
9. Collection or mass of blood ______________________
10. Tumor (cancerous) of glandular tissue ______________________

D Underline the suffix meaning <u>pertaining to</u> in the following terms and give the area or part of the body referred to.

1. esophageal ______________________
2. inguinal ______________________
3. renal ______________________
4. vascular ______________________
5. coronary ______________________
6. pulmonary ______________________
7. axillary ______________________
8. peritoneal ______________________
9. mammary ______________________
10. myocardial ______________________

E Give meanings for the following suffixes related to procedures.

1. -ectomy ________________
2. -gram ________________
3. -centesis ________________
4. -graphy ________________
5. -plasty ________________
6. -lysis ________________
7. -stomy ________________
8. -scopy ________________
9. -tomy ________________
10. -therapy ________________

F Select from the following terms to complete the sentences below.

angiography	colocolostomy	mammogram
angioplasty	colostomy	oophorectomy
bronchoscopy	hysterectomy	phlebotomy
chemotherapy	laryngoscopy	thoracentesis

1. Surgical repair of a blood vessel using a catheter (tube), balloon, and stent is ________________.
2. Treatment using chemicals to destroy malignant cells is ________________.
3. X-ray record of the breast is a/an ________________.
4. Puncture to remove fluid from the chest is ________________.
5. New opening of the large intestine to the outside of the body is a/an ________________.
6. New internal connection (anastomosis) between two parts of the large bowel (intestine) is a/an ________________.
7. Removal of the uterus is a/an ________________.
8. Process of recording x-ray images of blood vessels after injection of contrast is ________________.
9. Visual examination of the voice box is ________________.
10. Incision of a vein to withdraw blood is ________________.

G Write the medical term for the following definitions.

1. Excessive bleeding (discharge of blood) ______
2. Hardening of fatty plaque (in the lining of the arteries) ______
3. Pertaining to time (occurring over a long period of time) ______
4. X-ray record of the spinal cord ______
5. Sharp, sudden, brief ______
6. Treatment using cold temperatures ______
7. Record of electricity in the brain ______
8. Puncture to remove fluid from the membrane surrounding the fetus ______
9. Muscle pain ______
10. Malignant tumor of bone marrow ______
11. Enlargement of the heart ______
12. Abnormal condition of the death of cells ______
13. Disease condition of the kidney ______
14. Incision of the skull ______

H What part of the body is inflamed?

1. neuritis ______
2. arthritis ______
3. salpingitis ______
4. otitis ______
5. hepatitis ______
6. nephritis ______
7. esophagitis ______
8. laryngitis ______
9. encephalitis ______
10. osteitis ______
11. meningitis ______
12. bronchitis ______
13. rhinitis ______
14. peritonitis ______
15. vasculitis ______
16. mastitis ______
17. tonsillitis ______
18. colitis ______
19. pharyngitis ______
20. phlebitis ______

I **Provide the terms for the following procedures.**

1. Excision of the gallbladder ______
2. Excision of the appendix ______
3. Excision of a breast ______
4. Excision of the uterus ______
5. Excision of an ovary ______
6. Excision of the voice box ______
7. Excision of a kidney ______
8. Excision of a gland ______
9. Excision of the large intestine ______
10. Excision of a fallopian tube ______
11. Excision of tonsils ______
12. Incision of the skull ______
13. Incision of the abdomen ______
14. Incision of the chest ______
15. Opening of the windpipe to the outside of the body ______
16. Opening of the colon to the outside of the body ______
17. Puncture to remove fluid from the chest ______
18. Puncture to remove fluid from a joint ______
19. Incision of a vein (needle or catheter is inserted) ______
20. Visual examination of the voice box ______

J Supply the correct medical term for the following:

1. A stroke is a **cerebro**__________ __________ [two words].
2. A heart attack is a **myo**__________ __________ [two words].
3. Use of a machine that filters wastes from the blood is **hemo**__________.
4. Injection of fluid into the abdominal cavity and then withdrawal of that fluid (containing waste material) is **peri**__________ __________ [two words].
5. A benign tumor of muscle is a **my** __________.
6. A malignant tumor of muscle is a **myo** __________.
7. High level of wastes (urea) in the blood is **ur** __________.
8. Blood in the urine is **hemat** __________.
9. High number of malignant (cancerous) white blood cells is **leuk** __________.
10. Slightly elevated number of white blood cells due to an infection in the body is **leuko** __________.
11. Normal discharge of blood during menstruation is **men** __________.
12. Excessive bleeding during menstruation is **men** __________.
13. Hardening of arteries is called **arterio** __________.
14. Use of high-energy rays to treat cancerous tumors is **radio** __________.

K Circle the boldface term that best completes the meaning of the sentences in the following medical vignettes.

1. After routine breast self-examination, Nora felt a small lump in her breast. She consulted her doctor, who scheduled a diagnostic **(mammoplasty, mastectomy, mammogram).** The examination showed a stellate (star-shaped) mass, and a **(biopsy, necropsy, laparoscopy)** revealed an infiltrating ductal carcinoma. Nora decided to have her breast removed **(hysterectomy, mastectomy, salpingectomy),** although her physician gave her the option of having lumpectomy followed by **(cryotherapy, thoracotomy, radiotherapy).**
2. In addition to her surgery, Nora had a sentinel node biopsy of a/an **(inguinal, thoracic, axillary)** lymph node to determine whether the cancer had spread. Injection of contrast revealed the primary (sentinel) lymph node, which was removed and microscopically examined.
3. Victoria had never been comfortable with the bump on her nose. She saw a plastic surgeon, who performed **(mammoplasty, rhinoplasty, angioplasty).**
4. Sylvia had irregular bleeding in between her periods. She was 50 years old and beginning menopause. On pelvic exam, Dr. Hawk felt a large, lobulated uterus. Biopsy revealed a large fibroid, which is a benign (noncancerous) tumor of muscle tissue **(myeloma, myoma, hematoma).** The doctor discussed three surgical options: removal of the fibroid, blockage of blood flow to the fibroid (embolization), or a total abdominal **(gastrectomy, hysterectomy, cholecystectomy).**

5. Sam was experiencing cramps, diarrhea, and a low-grade fever. He was diagnosed with ulcerative **(colitis, meningitis, laryngitis)** and had several bouts of **(uremia, menorrhagia, septicemia)** caused by inflammation and rupture of the bowel wall.
6. Bill felt chest pain every time he climbed a flight of stairs. He went to his doctor, who did a coronary **(myelogram, angiogram, dialysis),** which revealed **(adenocarcinoma, nephrosis, atherosclerosis)** in one of his coronary arteries. The doctor recommended **(angioplasty, thoracentesis, amniocentesis).** This would prevent further **(myosarcoma, ischemia, leukocytosis)** and help Bill avoid a **(peritoneal, vascular, myocardial)** infarction, or heart attack, in the future.

ANSWERS TO EXERCISES

1. condition of pain
2. blood condition
3. inflammation
4. enlargement
5. tumor, mass
6. disease condition
7. flow, discharge
8. excessive discharge of blood
9. hardening
10. condition of urine

B

1. muscle pain
2. blood infection
3. high levels of wastes (urea) in the blood
4. inflammation of a vein
5. enlargement of the heart
6. malignant tumor of muscle
7. abnormal condition of the kidney
8. disease of the brain
9. discharge from the nose
10. excessive bleeding during menstruation.

C

1. hepatomegaly
2. otalgia
3. ischemia
4. leukocytosis
5. pneumonia
6. myeloma (also called multiple myeloma)
7. esophagitis
8. cardiomyopathy
9. hematoma
10. adenocarcinoma

D

1. esophag**eal**—esophagus (tube leading from the throat to the stomach)
2. inguin**al**—groin (area where the thigh meets the trunk of the body)
3. ren**al**—kidney
4. vascul**ar**—blood vessels
5. coron**ary**—heart
6. pulmon**ary**—lungs
7. axill**ary**—armpit (underarm area)
8. periton**eal**—peritoneum (membrane surrounding the abdominal cavity)
9. mamm**ary**—breast
10. myocardi**al**—heart muscle

E

1. removal, excision, resection
2. record
3. puncture to remove fluid
4. process of recording
5. surgical repair
6. separation; breakdown
7. new opening
8. process of visual examination
9. cutting into, incision, section
10. treatment

F

1. angioplasty
2. chemotherapy
3. mammogram
4. thoracentesis
5. colostomy
6. colocolostomy
7. hysterectomy
8. angiography
9. laryngoscopy
10. phlebotomy

3

G

1. hemorrhage
2. atherosclerosis
3. chronic
4. myelogram
5. acute
6. cryotherapy
7. electroencephalogram
8. amniocentesis
9. myalgia
10. myeloma or multiple myeloma
11. cardiomegaly
12. necrosis
13. nephropathy
14. craniotomy

H

1. nerve
2. joint
3. fallopian tubes
4. ear
5. liver
6. kidney
7. esophagus
8. larynx (voice box)
9. brain
10. bone
11. meninges (membranes surrounding the brain and spinal cord)
12. bronchial tubes
13. nose
14. peritoneum
15. blood vessels
16. breast
17. tonsils
18. colon (large intestine)
19. throat (pharynx)
20. veins

I

1. cholecystectomy
2. appendectomy
3. mastectomy
4. hysterectomy
5. oophorectomy
6. laryngectomy
7. nephrectomy
8. adenectomy
9. colectomy
10. salpingectomy
11. tonsillectomy
12. craniotomy
13. laparotomy
14. thoracotomy
15. tracheostomy
16. colostomy
17. thoracentesis
18. arthrocentesis
19. phlebotomy
20. laryngoscopy

3

J

1. cerebro**vascular accident**—clot or hemorrhage in an artery of the brain leads to decreased blood flow (ischemia) to brain tissue and necrosis (death of brain cells).
2. myo**cardial infarction**—ischemia of heart muscle leads to infarction (necrosis of heart muscle cells).
3. hemo**dialysis**—complete separation of waste material from the blood using a machine that receives the patient's blood and after filtration sends the blood back into the patient's body.
4. peri**toneal dialysis**—fluid is introduced into the abdominal cavity and then removed after wastes have passed into the fluid from the peritoneal blood vessels.
5. my**oma**—benign muscle tumors occurring in the uterus are fibroids.
6. myo**sarcoma**—malignant tumors of connective or flesh tissue are sarcomas.
7. ur**emia**—this indicates failure of the kidneys to eliminate nitrogen-containing wastes, such as urea, creatinine, and uric acid, from the bloodstream.
8. hemat**uria**—this indicates bleeding in the urinary tract.
9. leuk**emia**—immature, cancerous white blood cells are produced in excess from the bone marrow or lymph nodes.
10. leuko**cytosis**—normal, mature white blood cells are produced to fight infection.
11. men**orrhea**—lining of the uterus breaks down as a result of changes in hormone levels.
12. men**orrhagia**—long or heavy menstrual periods; often caused by benign muscle tumors or fibroids in the uterus.
13. arterio**sclerosis**—the most common type is atherosclerosis, or the collection of fatty plaques in arteries.
14. radio**therapy**—using high-energy x-rays, gamma rays, and protons to destroy cancerous cells.

K

1. mammogram, biopsy, mastectomy, radiotherapy
2. axillary
3. rhinoplasty
4. myoma, hysterectomy
5. colitis, septicemia
6. angiogram, atherosclerosis, angioplasty, ischemia, myocardial

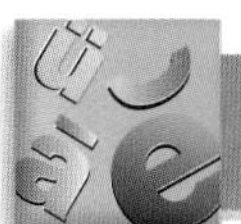

PRONUNCIATION OF TERMS

The terms that you have learned in this chapter are presented here with their pronunciations. The capitalized letters in ***BOLDFACE*** *represent the accented syllable. Pronounce each word out loud; then write the meaning in the space provided. Meanings of all terms can be checked with the* ***Mini-Dictionary*** *beginning on page 363 and on the audio section of the Evolve website*

Term	Pronunciation	Meaning
acute	ah-**KUT**	
adenocarcinoma	ah-deh-no-kar-sih-**NO**-mah	
adenoma	ah-deh-**NO**-mah	
amniocentesis	am-ne-o-sen-**TE**-sis	
anastomosis	ah-nah-sto-**MO**-sis	
angiography	an-je-**OG**-rah-fe	
angioplasty	**AN**-je-o-plas-te	
arteriosclerosis	ar-te-re-o-skleh-**RO**-sis	
arthralgia	ar-**THRAL**-je-ah	
arthropathy	ar-**THROP**-ah-the	
atherosclerosis	ah-theh-ro-skleh-**RO**-sis	
axillary	**AKS**-ih-lair-e	
bronchitis	brong-**KI**-tis	
bronchoscopy	brong-**KOS**-ko-pe	
carcinoma	kar-sih-**NO**-mah	
cardiomegaly	kar-de-o-**MEG**-ah-le	
cardiomyopathy	kar-de-o-mi-**OP**-ah-the	
chemotherapy	ke-mo-**THER**-ah-pe	
cholecystectomy	ko-le-sis-**TEK**-to-me	
chronic	**KRON**-ik	
colitis	ko-**LI**-tis	
colostomy	ko-**LOS**-to-me	

3

colocolostomy	ko-lo-ko-**LOS**-to-me______
coronary	**KOR**-o-nair-e______
craniotomy	kra-ne-**OT**-o-me______
cystitis	sis-**TI**-tis______
dialysis	di-**AL**-ih-sis______
electroencephalography	e-lek-tro-en-sef-ah-**LOG**-rah-fe______
encephalopathy	en-sef-ah-**LOP**-ah-the______
erythrocytosis	eh-rith-ro-si-**TO**-sis______
esophageal	e-sof-ah-**JE**-al______
esophagitis	e-sof-ah-**JI**-tis______
hematuria	he-mah-**TUR**-e-ah______
hemorrhage	**HEM**-o-rij______
hysterectomy	his-teh-**REK**-to-me______
infarction	in-**FARK**-shun______
inguinal	**ING**-gwih-nal______
ischemia	is-**KE**-me-ah______
laparoscopy	lap-ah-**ROS**-ko-pe______
laparotomy	lap-ah-**ROT**-o-me______
laryngitis	lah-rin-**JI**-tis______
laryngoscopy	lah-rin-**GOS**-ko-pe______
leukemia	loo-**KE**-me-ah______
leukocytosis	loo-ko-si-**TO**-sis______
mammogram	**MAM**-o-gram______
mammography	mah-**MOG**-rah-fe______
mammoplasty	**MAM**-o-plas-te______
mastectomy	mas-**TEK**-to-me______
meningitis	men-in-**JI**-tis______
menorrhagia	men-or-**RA**-jah______

3

menorrhea	men-o-**RE**-ah ________
myalgia	mi-**AL**-jah ________
myelogram	**MI**-eh-lo-gram ________
myeloma	mi-eh-**LO**-mah ________
myocardial	mi-o-**KAR**-de-al ________
myoma	mi-**O**-mah ________
myosarcoma	mi-o-sar-**KO**-mah ________
necrosis	neh-**KRO**-sis ________
nephrosis	neh-**FRO**-sis ________
neuralgia	nu-**RAL**-jah ________
oophorectomy	o-of-o-**REK**-to-me *or* oo-for-**EK**-to-me ________
otalgia	o-**TAL**-jah ________
peritoneal	per-rih-to-**NE**-al ________
phlebitis	fleh-**BI**-tis ________
phlebotomy	fleh-**BOT**-o-me ________
pneumonia	noo-**MO**-ne-ah ________
pulmonary	**PUL**-mo-nair-re ________
radiotherapy	ra-de-o-**THAIR**-ah-pe ________
renal	**RE**-nal ________
rhinoplasty	**RI**-no-plas-te ________
rhinorrhea	ri-no-**RE**-ah ________
salpingectomy	sal-pin-**JEK**-to-me ________
septicemia	sep-tih-**SE**-me-ah ________
thoracentesis	tho-rah-sen-**TE**-sis ________
tonsillectomy	ton-sih-**LEK**-to-me ________
tracheostomy	tra-ke-**OS**-to-me ________
uremia	u-**RE**-me-ah ________
vascular	**VAS**-ku-lar ________

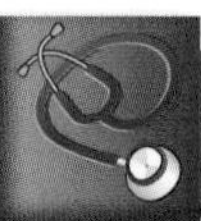

PRACTICAL APPLICATIONS

Answers are given on page 121.

MATCHING

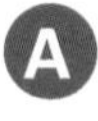

A **Match the procedure in Column I with an abnormal condition (diagnosis) it is associated with in Column II.**

COLUMN I PROCEDURE		COLUMN II ABNORMAL CONDITION (Diagnosis)
1. angioplasty	_____	A. uterine adenocarcinoma
2. mammoplasty	_____	B. ligament tear of the patella (kneecap)
3. cholecystectomy	_____	C. ovarian cyst
4. tonsillectomy	_____	D. blockage of the windpipe
5. dialysis	_____	E. renal failure
6. hysterectomy	_____	F. absence of a breast (postmastectomy)
7. thoracentesis	_____	G. pleural effusion (collection of fluid)
8. oophorectomy	_____	H. coronary atherosclerosis
9. tracheostomy	_____	I. gallbladder calculi (stones)
10. arthroscopy	_____	J. pharyngeal lymph node enlargement

B **Match the sign/symptom (abnormal condition) in Column I with an organ or tissue in Column II.**

COLUMN I SIGN/SYMPTOM (Abnormal Condition)		COLUMN II ORGAN OR TISSUE
1. colitis	_____	A. uterus
2. phlebitis	_____	B. ear
3. menorrhagia	_____	C. bone marrow
4. myocardial ischemia	_____	D. coronary arteries
5. otalgia	_____	E. large bowel
6. uremia	_____	F. membrane surrounding spinal cord and brain
7. meningitis	_____	G. vein
8. leukemia	_____	H. kidney

3

WHAT'S YOUR DIAGNOSIS?

Case Study

A 45-year-old obese woman presents complaining of menorrhagia [heavy periods] with cramping pelvic pain, dizziness when standing, and rapid heart rate. Manual physical examination demonstrates multiple enlarged masses in her uterus. Blood workup reveals low RBCs [red blood cells] and hematocrit [percentage of red blood cells in a volume of blood], normal WBCs and platelets, and slightly elevated blood sugar level. U/S [ultrasound] of the abdomen and pelvis shows multiple fibroids [leiomyomas] of the uterine wall. Patient is admitted to the hospital with recommendation for hysterectomy. During the course of admission she speaks to the resident dietitian about a compulsive eating disorder and agrees to undergo therapy at the hospital's weight loss clinic.

Using the information presented in the case study, what's your diagnosis?

A. Pelvic pain—female
B. Obesity
C. Anemia
D. Menorrhagia
E. Fibroid uterus

ANSWERS TO PRACTICAL APPLICATIONS

MATCHING

A

1. H
2. F
3. I
4. J
5. E
6. A
7. G
8. C
9. D
10. B

B

1. E
2. G
3. A
4. D
5. B
6. H
7. F
8. C

WHAT'S YOUR DIAGNOSIS?

Answer: E. Fibroid uterus

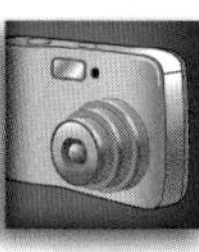

PICTURE SHOW

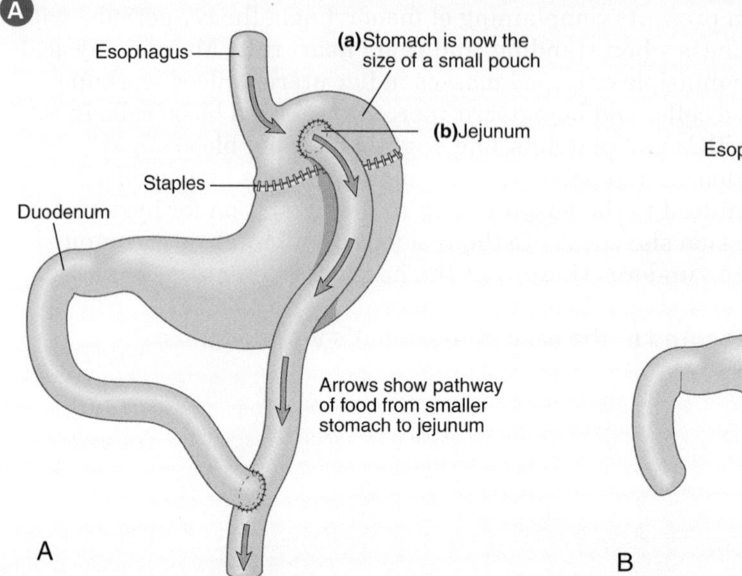

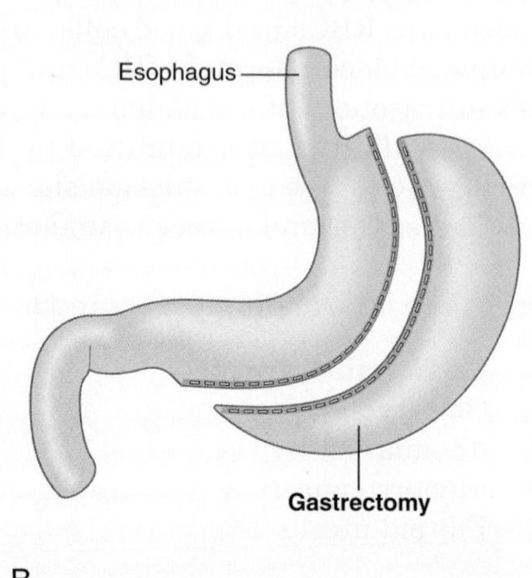

3

1. The drawing in Figure A shows a procedure **(bariatric surgery)*** used to treat extreme obesity. First, the stomach (a) is stapled so that it is reduced to the size of a small pouch. Next, the jejunum (b), which is the second part of the small intestine, is brought up to connect with the smaller stomach. This diverts food so that it has a shorter travel time through the intestine with less time for absorption into the bloodstream. What is the name of this surgical procedure?
   a. esophageal bypass
   b. total gastric resection
   c. gastric bypass
   d. duodenal resection

2. The new connection, or anastomosis, between the stomach and the second part of the small intestine is a:
   a. gastrostomy
   b. jejunostomy
   c. gastroduodenostomy
   d. gastrojejunostomy

3. The drawing in Figure B shows another type of bariatric surgery. It is a simpler procedure that creates a smaller stomach pouch without the complications of more invasive surgery. It is called a/an:
   a. gastric sleeve procedure (sleeve gastrectomy)
   b. duodenal anastomosis
   c. gastroduodenal anastomosis
   d. esophageal pouch procedure

* Bar/o = weight.
-iatric = pertaining to treatment.

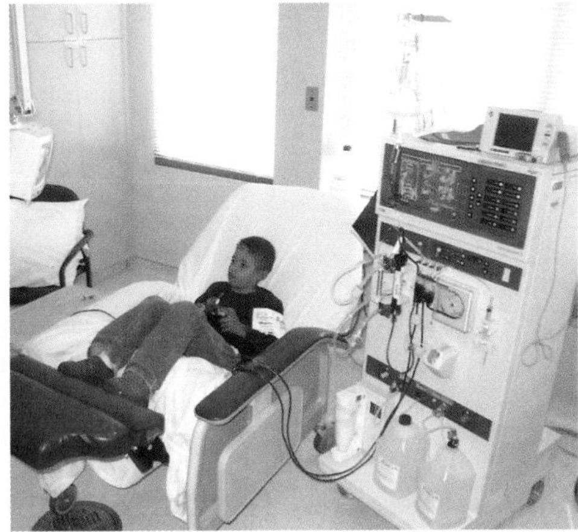

1. In the image shown, blood leaves the patient's body to enter a machine that filters out waste materials. The filtered blood then circulates back to the patient's body. This procedure is:
   a. pericardiocentesis
   b. peritoneal dialysis
   c. hemodialysis
   d. amniocentesis

2. The procedure is a treatment for patients with failure of the:
   a. kidneys
   b. pancreas
   c. liver
   d. all three organs listed

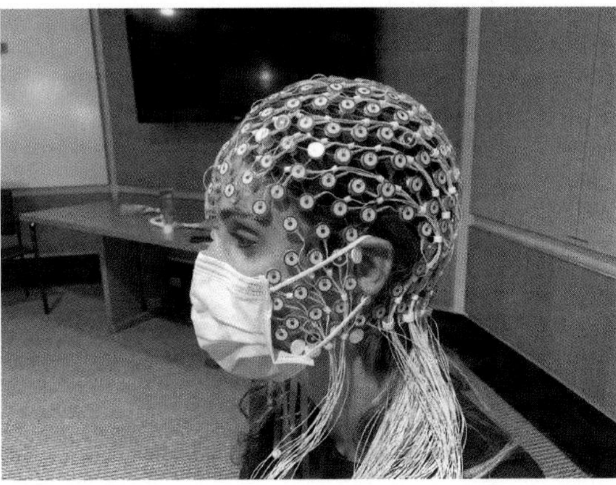

1. This patient is undergoing a procedure that records brain wave activity. It is called:
   a. electrocardiography
   b. electroencephalography
   c. electromyography
   d. electrocraniography

2. It may be used to diagnose:
   a. seizure disorders (epilepsy)
   b. dyspnea
   c. septicemia
   d. atherosclerosis

D

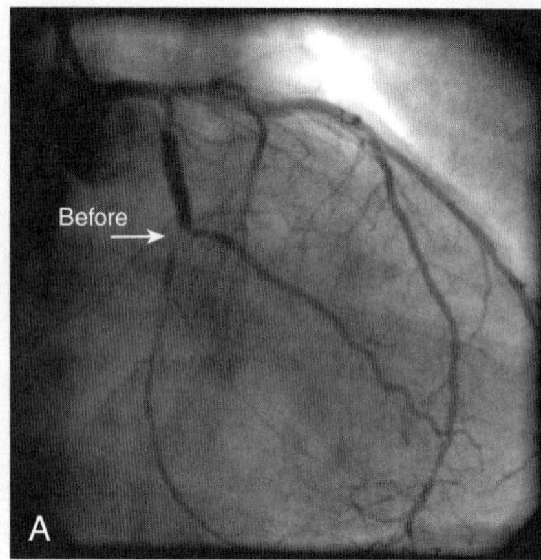

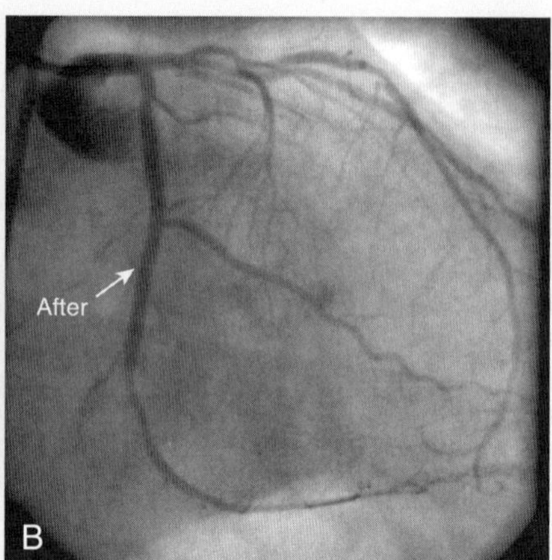

1. The arrow in ***A*** shows a narrowing of a coronary artery, preventing blood flow to the heart muscle. A condition caused by decreased blood flow is called:
   a. nephrosis
   b. uremia
   c. cardiomegaly
   d. ischemia

2. ***B*** shows the coronary artery after stenting. The imaging procedure that is shown is:
   a. electrocardiography
   b. angiography
   c. radiotherapy
   d. mammography

3. The treatment procedure in which coronary arteries are opened using a balloon catheter and stenting is:
   a. rhinoplasty
   b. phlebotomy
   c. angioplasty
   d. thoracentesis

E

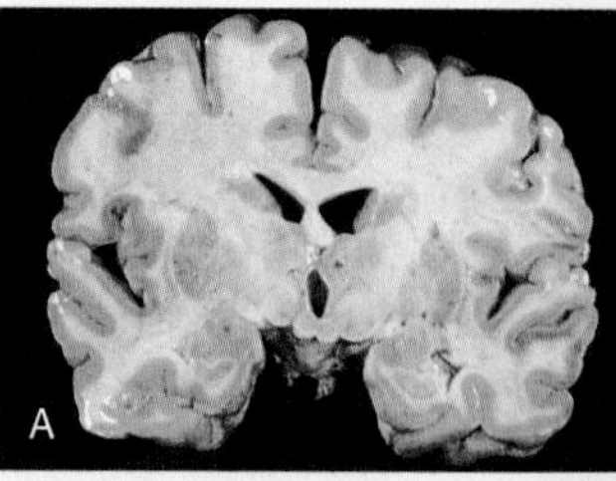

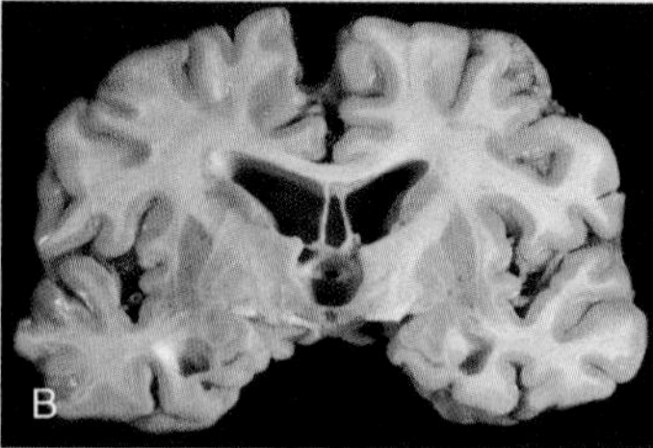

1. These two autopsy images of the brain show a normal brain (A) and the brain of a professional football player who died at age 27 (B). The football player had frequent headaches, difficulty thinking, impulsive behavior, and emotional instability. His brain shows the damaging effects of repeated blows to the head.
   a. arteriosclerosis
   b. chronic traumatic encephalopathy
   c. multiple myeloma
   d. cerebral thrombosis

F

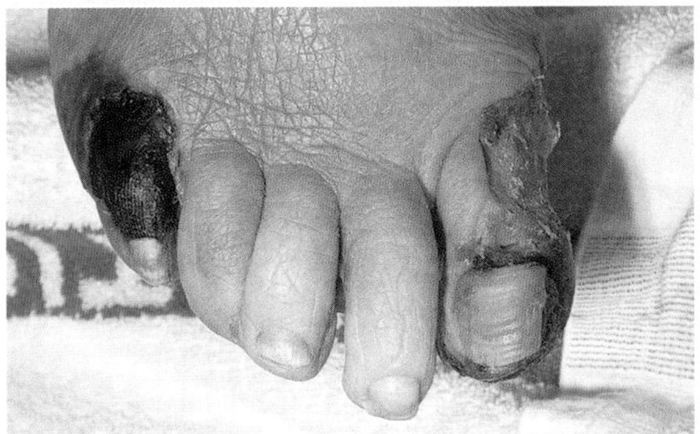

1. The darkened tissue on the toes pictured in the image is called **gangrene**. It is an example of:
   a. dermatitis
   b. necrosis
   c. uremia
   d. hematoma

2. Gangrene may develop as a result of blood vessel injury, frostbite, or conditions such as diabetes and atherosclerosis. It results from:
   a. hematuria
   b. chronic cystitis
   c. ischemia
   d. cardiomyopathy

ANSWERS TO PICTURE SHOW

A 1. c 2. d 3. a

B 1. c 2. a

C 1. b 2. a

D 1. d 2. b 3. c

E 1. b

F 1. b 2. c

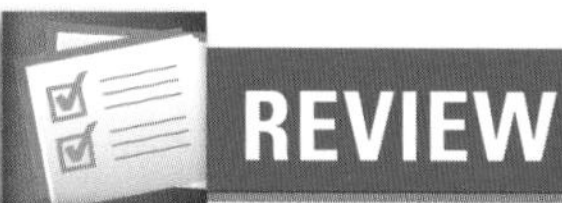

REVIEW

Write the meanings for the following word parts. Remember to check your answers with the Answers to Review section on page 128.

SUFFIXES

Suffix	Meaning	Suffix	Meaning
1. -al	____________	15. -megaly	____________
2. -algia	____________	16. -oma	____________
3. -ar	____________	17. -osis	____________
4. -ary	____________	18. -pathy	____________
5. -centesis	____________	19. -plasty	____________
6. -eal	____________	20. -rrhage	____________
7. -ectomy	____________	21. -rrhagia	____________
8. -emia	____________	22. -rrhea	____________
9. -gram	____________	23. -sclerosis	____________
10. -graphy	____________	24. -scopy	____________
11. -ia	____________	25. -stomy	____________
12. -ic	____________	26. -therapy	____________
13. -itis	____________	27. -tomy	____________
14. -lysis	____________	28. -uria	____________

COMBINING FORMS

Combining Form	Meaning	Combining Form	Meaning
1. aden/o	____________	4. arteri/o	____________
2. amni/o	____________	5. arthr/o	____________
3. angi/o	____________	6. ather/o	____________

3

Combining Form	Meaning

7. axill/o ______________________
8. bronch/o ______________________
9. carcin/o ______________________
10. cardi/o ______________________
11. chem/o ______________________
12. cholecyst/o ______________________
13. chron/o ______________________
14. col/o ______________________
15. coron/o ______________________
16. crani/o ______________________
17. cry/o ______________________
18. cyst/o ______________________
19. encephal/o ______________________
20. erythr/o ______________________
21. esophag/o ______________________
22. hemat/o ______________________
23. hepat/o ______________________
24. hyster/o ______________________
25. inguin/o ______________________
26. isch/o ______________________
27. lapar/o ______________________
28. laryng/o ______________________
29. leuk/o ______________________
30. mamm/o ______________________
31. mast/o ______________________
32. men/o ______________________

Combining Form	Meaning

33. mening/o ______________________
34. my/o ______________________
35. myel/o ______________________
36. necr/o ______________________
37. nephr/o ______________________
38. neur/o ______________________
39. oophor/o ______________________
40. oste/o ______________________
41. ot/o ______________________
42. pelv/o ______________________
43. peritone/o ______________________
44. phleb/o ______________________
45. pneumon/o ______________________
46. pulmon/o ______________________
47. radi/o ______________________
48. ren/o ______________________
49. rhin/o ______________________
50. salping/o ______________________
51. sarc/o ______________________
52. septic/o ______________________
53. thorac/o ______________________
54. tonsill/o ______________________
55. trache/o ______________________
56. ur/o ______________________
57. vascul/o ______________________

ANSWERS TO REVIEW

SUFFIXES

1. pertaining to
2. condition of pain, pain
3. pertaining to
4. pertaining to
5. puncture to remove fluid
6. pertaining to
7. removal, resection, excision
8. blood condition
9. record
10. process of recording
11. condition
12. pertaining to
13. inflammation
14. separation, breakdown, destruction
15. enlargement
16. tumor, mass
17. abnormal condition
18. disease condition
19. surgical repair
20. excessive discharge of blood
21. excessive discharge of blood
22. flow, discharge
23. hardening
24. visual examination
25. opening
26. treatment
27. incision; cutting into
28. urine condition

COMBINING FORMS

1. gland
2. amnion
3. vessel
4. artery
5. joint
6. plaque, collection of fatty material
7. armpit
8. bronchial tubes
9. cancerous
10. heart
11. drug, chemical
12. gallbladder
13. time
14. colon (large intestine)
15. heart
16. skull
17. cold
18. urinary bladder
19. brain
20. red
21. esophagus
22. blood
23. liver
24. uterus
25. groin
26. to hold back
27. abdomen
28. larynx (voice box)
29. white
30. breast
31. breast
32. menstruation
33. meninges
34. muscle
35. spinal cord or bone marrow
36. death
37. kidney
38. nerve
39. ovary
40. bone
41. ear
42. hip area
43. peritoneum
44. vein
45. lung
46. lung
47. x-rays
48. kidney
49. nose
50. fallopian tube
51. flesh
52. pertaining to infection
53. chest
54. tonsil
55. trachea (windpipe)
56. urine, urinary tract
57. blood vessel

✓ TERMINOLOGY CHECKUP

In your own words, write the answers on the lines provided. Confirm your answers and check the box next to each item when you know you've "got" it!

☐ 1. Explain the concept of **ischemia.** How can it lead to **necrosis**? How does this relate to a **myocardial infarction** and a **cerebrovascular accident**?

____

____

____

☐ 2. Explain the difference between the following procedural suffixes: **-tomy, -ectomy,** and **-stomy.** Congratulate yourself if you can explain what a surgeon does in an **anastomosis**!

____

____

____

☐ 3. What is **uremia**? How is it treated? Name two different types of **treatments for uremia.**

____

____

____

☐ 4. What is the difference between the combining forms **my/o** and **myel/o**? Give meanings for the following terms that contain these combining forms: **myoma, myosarcoma, myeloma,** and **myelogram**.

____

____

____

☐ 5. Define the following surgical resections: **cholecystectomy, splenectomy,** and **oophorectomy.**

____

____

____

ANSWERS TO TERMINOLOGY CHECKUP

1. **Ischemia** leads to necrosis because cells are deprived of necessary blood supply (containing oxygen and nutrients). A **myocardial infarction (heart attack)** is when ischemia and necrosis occur in the heart muscle. A **cerebrovascular accident (stroke)** is when ischemia and necrosis occur in the brain.
2. A procedure ending in **-tomy** is an incision or section. A procedure ending in **-ectomy** is an excision or resection. A procedure ending in **-stomy** is the creation of a new opening in an organ to the outside of the body. An **anastomosis** is a new surgical connection between two tubelike structures **within** the body.
3. **Uremia** is a high concentration of waste products (urea, creatinine, and uric acid) in the blood when the kidneys fail to function. It is treated by **dialysis.** Two types of dialysis are **hemodialysis** and **peritoneal dialysis.** A kidney transplant is another treatment for failed kidneys and uremia.
4. **My/o** means muscle. **Myel/o** can mean either bone marrow or spinal cord. **Myoma** is a tumor (benign) of muscle. **Myosarcoma** is a tumor (malignant) of muscle. **Myeloma** is malignant condition originating in bone marrow. **Myelogram** is an x-ray record of the spinal cord.
5. **Cholecystectomy** is removal of a gallbladder. **Splenectomy** is removal of the spleen. **Oophorectomy** is removal of one or both (bilateral) ovaries. In case you are wondering, the body copes very well without these organs. After **cholecystectomy**, without a gallbladder to store bile, the liver secretes bile as needed. After **splenectomy,** without a spleen to produce white blood cells and process worn-out red blood cells, lymph nodes and the liver take over these functions. After **bilateral oophorectomy,** without ovaries to produce eggs and female hormones, adrenal glands produce small amounts of female hormones.

CHAPTER 4

Prefixes

Chapter Sections

Introduction 132
Combining Forms and Suffixes 132
Prefixes and Terminology 134
In Person: Total Knee Replacement (TKR) 151
Exercises and Answers 152
Pronunciation of Terms 162
Practical Applications 165
Picture Show 168
Review 171
Terminology CheckUp 175

CHAPTER OBJECTIVES

- To identify and define common prefixes used in medical terms
- To analyze, spell, and pronounce medical terms that contain prefixes
- To apply medical terms in real-life situations

INTRODUCTION

This chapter reviews the prefixes you studied in Chapter 1 and introduces new prefixes. The list of Combining Forms and Suffixes that follows will help you understand the terminology presented beginning on page 134. Remember to complete all exercises and check your answers. The Pronunciation of Terms and Review are opportunities to test your understanding of all terminology in this chapter.

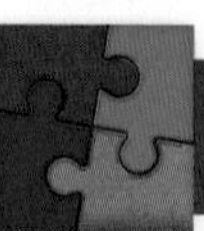

COMBINING FORMS AND SUFFIXES

Combining Form	Meaning
abdomin/o	abdomen
an/o	anus (opening of the digestive tract to the outside of the body)
bi/o	life
cardi/o	heart
carp/o	carpals (wrist bones)
cis/o	to cut
cost/o	ribs
crani/o	skull
cutane/o	skin
dur/o	dura mater (outermost meningeal membrane surrounding the brain and spinal cord)
gen/o	to produce, to begin
glyc/o	sugar
hemat/o	blood
later/o	side
men/o	menses (monthly discharge of blood from the lining of the uterus)
nat/i	birth
neur/o	nerve
norm/o	rule, order
oste/o	bone
ox/o	oxygen
peritone/o	peritoneum (membrane surrounding the organs in the abdomen)
plas/o	formation, growth, development
ren/o	kidney
scapul/o	scapula (shoulder blade)
son/o	sound
thyroid/o	thyroid gland
top/o	to put, place, position
troph/o	development, nourishment
urethr/o	urethra (tube leading from the bladder to the outside of the body)
uter/o	uterus
ven/o	vein
vertebr/o	vertebra (backbone)

4

Suffix	Meaning
-al	pertaining to
-ation	process, condition
-cision	process of cutting
-crine	secretion
-dipsia	thirst
-emia	blood condition
-gen	to produce
-graphy	process of recording
-ia	condition
-ic	pertaining to
-ine	pertaining to
-ism	condition, process
-lapse	to fall, slide
-lysis	loosening, breakdown, separation, destruction
-meter	to measure
-mission	to send
-mortem	death
-oma	tumor, mass
-ous	pertaining to
-partum	birth
-pathy	disease condition
-phagia	eating
-phasia	speech
-plasia	formation (condition)
-plasm	formation (tissue)
-plegia	paralysis
-pnea	breathing
-ptom	a happening
-rrhea	flow, discharge
-scopy	process of visual examination
-section	to cut
-stasis	to stand, place, stop, control
-tension	pressure
-thesis	to put, place (state of putting or placing)
-tic	pertaining to
-trophy	nourishment; development
-um	structure
-uria	urine condition
-y	process, condition

4

PREFIXES AND TERMINOLOGY

Prefix	Meaning	Terminology	Meaning
a-, an-	no, not, without	apnea ______ *In this term, the root (PNE, meaning breathing) is embedded in the suffix (-PNEA). Sleep apnea occurs when breathing stops suddenly during sleep.*	
		aphasia ______ *A stroke affecting the language area of the brain can produce this condition.*	
		atrophy ______ *Disuse of a muscle can result in muscular atrophy. Muscles shrink as cells decrease in size.*	
		anemia ______ *Anemia is a condition in which there is a lower-than-normal number of red blood cells or a decrease in hemoglobin within the cells. Table 4-1 lists different forms of anemia.*	
		amenorrhea ______	
ab-	away from	abnormal ______	
ad-	toward, near	adrenal glands ______ *See Figure 4-1.*	

4

TABLE 4-1	ANEMIAS
aplastic anemia	Bone marrow fails to produce red blood cells (erythrocytes), white blood cells (leukocytes), and clotting cells (platelets).
hemolytic anemia	Red blood cells are destroyed (-LYTIC), and bone marrow cannot compensate for their loss. This condition can be hereditary or acquired (after infection or chemotherapy) or can occur when the immune system acts against normal red blood cells (autoimmune condition).
iron deficiency anemia	Low iron levels lead to low hemoglobin concentration or deficiency of red blood cells.
pernicious anemia	Mucous membranes of the stomach fail to produce a substance (intrinsic factor) necessary for the absorption of vitamin B_{12} and the proper formation of red blood cells. Pernicious means harmful.
sickle cell anemia	Erythrocytes assume an abnormal crescent or sickle shape; this "sickling" is due to the inheritance of an abnormal type of hemoglobin. The sickle-shaped cells clump together, causing clots that block blood vessels.

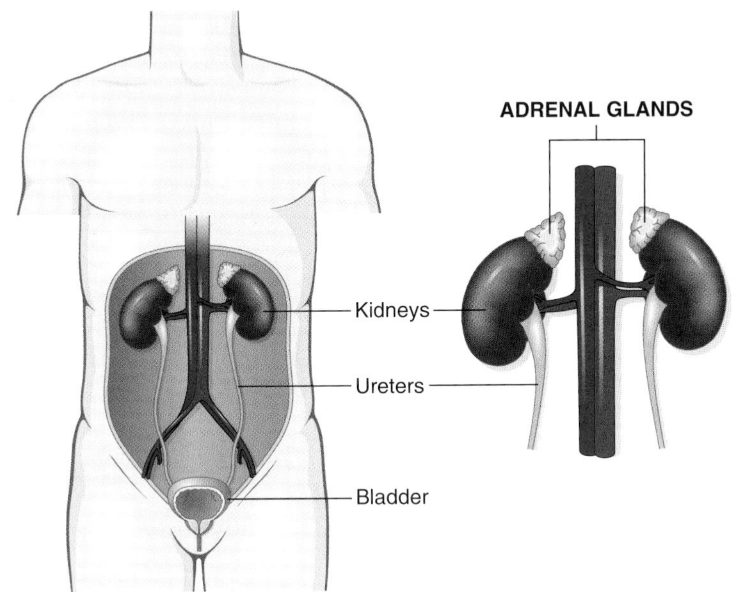

FIGURE 4-1 Adrenal glands. These two endocrine glands are above each kidney.

4

ana-	up, apart	analysis ______________________
ante-	before, forward	antepartum ______________________
anti-	against	antibody ______________________ *Protein made by white blood cells—literally, a "body" working "against" foreign substances.* antigen ______________________ *Antigens are foreign substances, such as bacteria and viruses. When antigens enter the body, they stimulate white blood cells to produce antibodies that act against the antigens.*

Analysis of urine

A **urinalysis** (urine + analysis) is the separation of urine to determine its components. The following chart shows typical urinalysis findings:

Test	**Normal**	**Abnormal**
1. Color	light yellow	red (hematuria)
2. Clarity	clear	cloudy (infection)
3. pH (chemical nature)	slightly acidic	alkaline (infection)
4. Protein	very slight	proteinuria (renal disease)
5. Sugar	none	glycosuria (diabetes mellitus)

antibiotic ______

*Antibiotics are produced **outside** the body by microorganisms and primitive plants called molds. Examples are amoxicillin and erythromycin. As antibacterial medications, they are taken by mouth or through intravenous injection, or applied topically to be absorbed through the skin.*

Don't confuse antibiotics with antibodies.

Remember that **antibiotics are medicines** dispensed by pharmacies to fight against antigens such as bacteria, while **antibodies are proteins** (immunoglobulins) made ***inside*** the body by white blood cells called lymphocytes (B cells).

bi-	two, both	bilateral ______
brady-	slow	bradycardia ______
con-	with, together	congenital ______ *A congenital anomaly is an irregularity (anomaly) present at birth. Examples are webbed fingers and toes and heart defects. See Figure 4-2.*

4

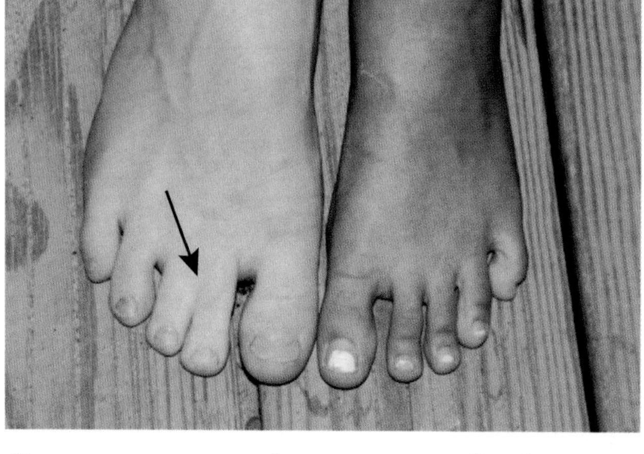

FIGURE 4-2 Webbed toes. The foot on the left (pale) shows "webbing" of the toes (syndactyly). On the right, another person's foot (darker) has normal toes.

dia-	complete through	diarrhea ______ *Feces (stools) are loose and watery. Normal water reabsorption through the walls of the colon is impaired. One serious cause of chronic diarrhea is bacterial infection such as C. difficile. Severe diarrhea can be life-threatening, but can be treated with a fecal transplant.*

What is a fecal transplant?

A fecal transplant is a procedure in which feces are taken from a healthy donor and transferred to the colon of a patient with a serious bacterial infection. The fecal transplant is introduced via colonoscopy or in pill form. Symptoms improve within days of fecal transplant but usually need several weeks to become permanent.

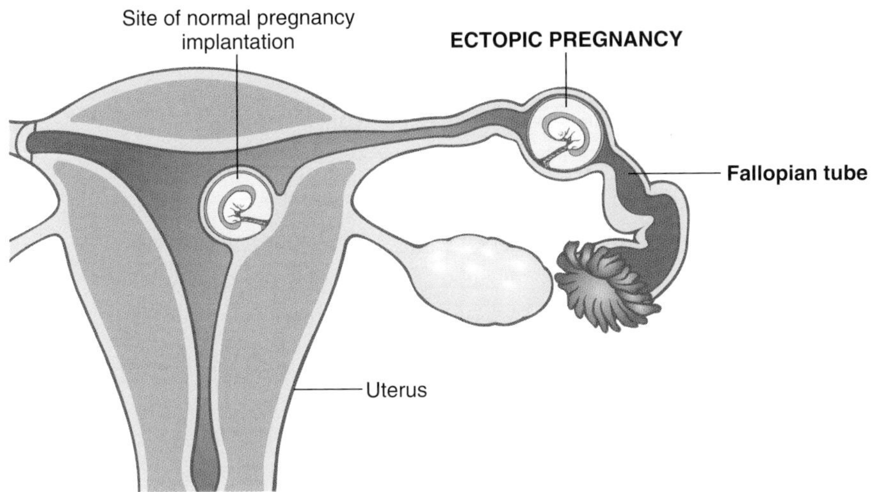

FIGURE 4-3 Ectopic pregnancy. The fallopian tube (ectopic tubal pregnancy) is the most common site for ectopic pregnancies (95%), but they can also occur on the ovary or on the surface of the peritoneum. Normal implantation takes place on the inner lining (endometrium) of the uterus.

dys-	bad, painful, difficult, abnormal	dys pnea ________
		dys phagia ________
		dysplasia ________
		dys menorrhea ________
		dys uria ________ *Dysuria is often a symptom of a urinary tract infection (UTI).*
ec-	out, outside	ec topic pregnancy ________ *Figure 4-3 shows an ectopic tubal pregnancy.*

-Plasia, -phagia, and -phasia

Don't confuse these very different suffixes: **-plasia (PLAY**-zhah) means formation, **-phagia (FAY**-jah) means eating or swallowing, and **-phasia (FAY**-ze-ah) means speech.

TABLE 4-2	TYPES OF ENDOSCOPY PROCEDURES
arthroscopy	Visual examination of a joint
bronchoscopy	Visual examination of the bronchial tubes
colonoscopy	Visual examination of the colon (large intestine)
cystoscopy	Visual examination of the urinary bladder
esophagogastroscopy	Visual examination of the esophagus and stomach
hysteroscopy	Visual examination of the uterus
laparoscopy	Visual examination of the abdomen
laryngoscopy	Visual examination of the larynx (voice box)
mediastinoscopy	Visual examination of the mediastinum
sigmoidoscopy	Visual examination of the sigmoid colon (the lower, S-shaped part of the large intestine)

endo- within, in, inner

endoscopy ______________________

Table 4-2 lists types of endoscopy procedures.

endocrine glands ______________________

The adrenal glands are endocrine glands. Table 4-3 lists the major endocrine glands and the hormones that they secrete.

4

TABLE 4-3 MAJOR ENDOCRINE GLANDS AND SELECTED HORMONES

GLAND	HORMONES
adrenal glands	Adrenaline (epinephrine)
ovaries	Estrogen Progesterone
pancreas	Insulin
parathyroid glands	Parathyroid hormone (PTH)
pituitary gland	Adrenocorticotropic hormone (ACTH) Follicle-stimulating hormone (FSH) Growth hormone (GH) Thyroid-stimulating hormone (TSH)
testes	Testosterone
thyroid gland	Thyroxine (T4)

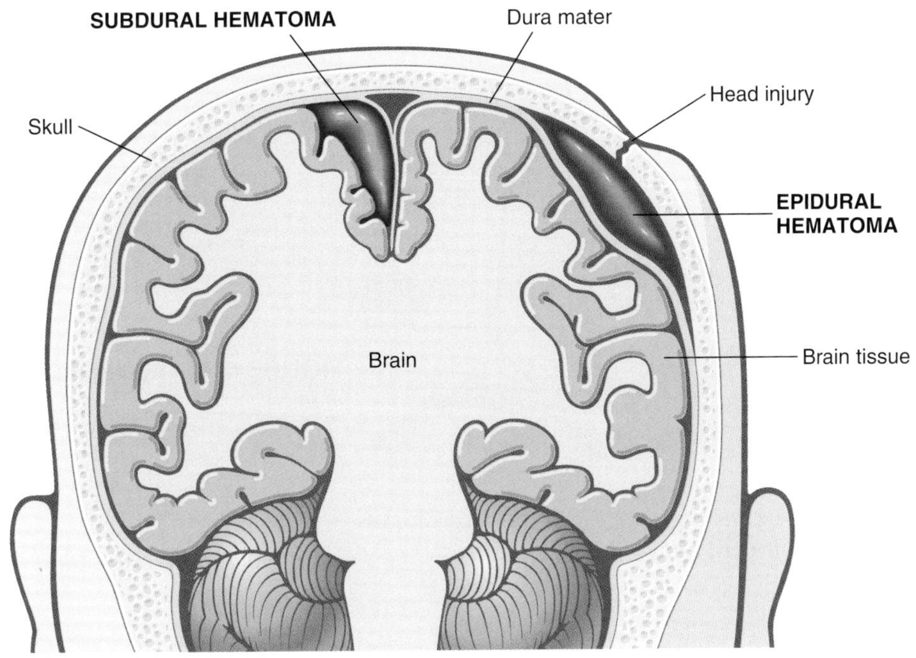

FIGURE 4-4 Epidural and subdural hematomas. The dura mater is the outermost of the three meninges (membranes) around the brain and spinal cord.

epi-	above, upon	epidural hematoma ______________ *Figure 4-4 illustrates epidural and subdural hematomas.*
		epidermis ______________ *The three layers of the skin, from outermost to innermost, are the epidermis, dermis, and subcutaneous layer. See* Appendix 1, Body Systems, *page 217.*
ex-	out	excision ______________
extra-	outside of	extrahepatic ______________
hemi-	half	hemigastrectomy ______________
		hemiplegia ______________ *One side of the body is paralyzed; usually caused by a cerebrovascular accident or brain lesion, such as a tumor. The resulting paralysis occurs on the side opposite the brain disorder.*

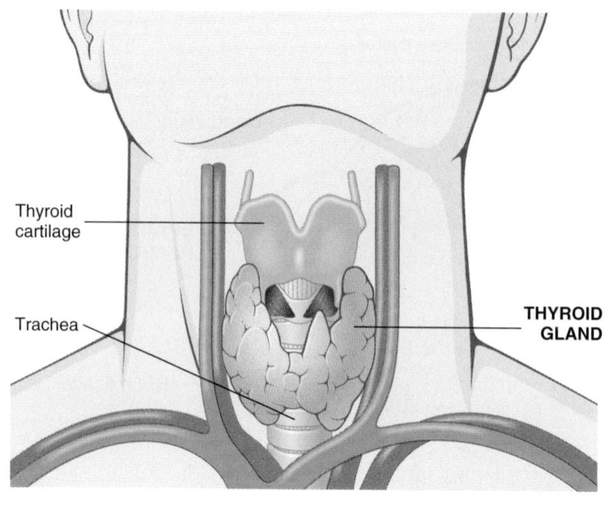

FIGURE 4-5 **Thyroid gland**, located in the front of the trachea in the neck. The thyroid gland produces too much hormone in hyperthyroidism.

4

hyper-	excessive, too much, above	hyperthyroidism ______________ *Figure 4-5 shows position of the thyroid gland in the neck.*
		hyperplasia ______________ *Cells increase in number. The prostate gland is enlarged in benign prostatic hyperplasia (BPH).*
		hypertrophy ______________ *Cells increase in size, not in number. The opposite of hypertrophy is* ***atrophy*** *(cells shrink in size). See Figure 4-6.*
		hypertension ______________ *Risk factors that contribute to high blood pressure are increasing age, smoking, obesity, heredity, and a stressful lifestyle.*
		hyperglycemia ______________ *May also be a sign of* ***diabetes mellitus.*** *Insulin either is not secreted or is improperly utilized so that sugar accumulates in the bloodstream and spills over into the urine (glycosuria).*

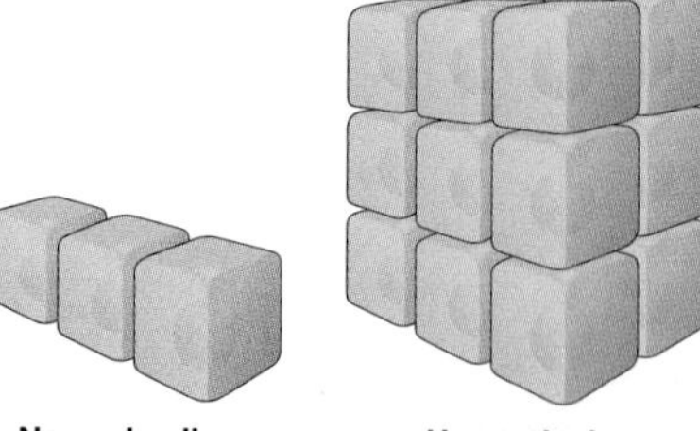

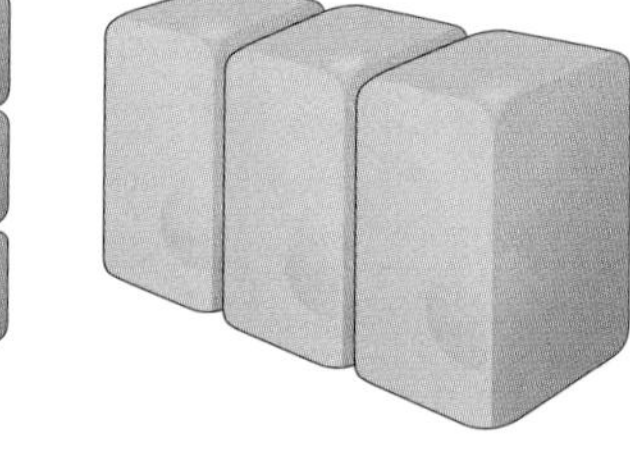

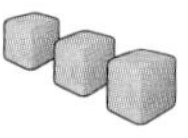

FIGURE 4-6 Differences between **normal cells, hyperplasia, hypertrophy,** and **atrophy.**

hypo-	deficient, too little, below	hypoglycemia ______________________ *Overproduction of insulin or an overdose (from outside the body—exogenously) of insulin can lead to hypoglycemia, as glucose is removed from the blood at an increased rate.* hypoxia ______________________
in-	in, into	incision ______________________
inter-	between	intervertebral ______________________ *An intervertebral disc lies between any two vertebrae.*
intra-	within	intrauterine ______________________ intravenous ______________________ *The abbreviation for intravenous is IV. See Figure 4-7.*

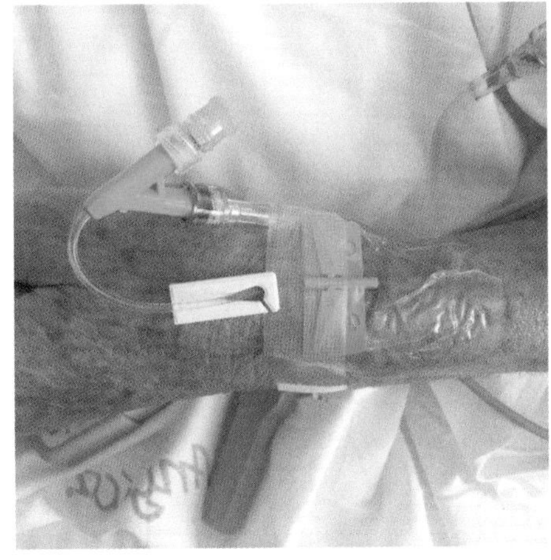

FIGURE 4-7 Intravenous setup for anesthesia administration.

Hypoxia and COVID-19

Hypoxia occurs in COVID-19 patients when the coronavirus damages lung tissue, causing blood oxygen levels to fall (hypoxemia). A **pulse oximeter** is a small device that measures oxygen levels in your blood. Small beams of light pass through the finger, measuring the changes of light absorption in oxygen-rich and oxygen-poor blood. Normal results range from 95%–100%. Values under 90% are considered low, and patients require oxygen treatment.

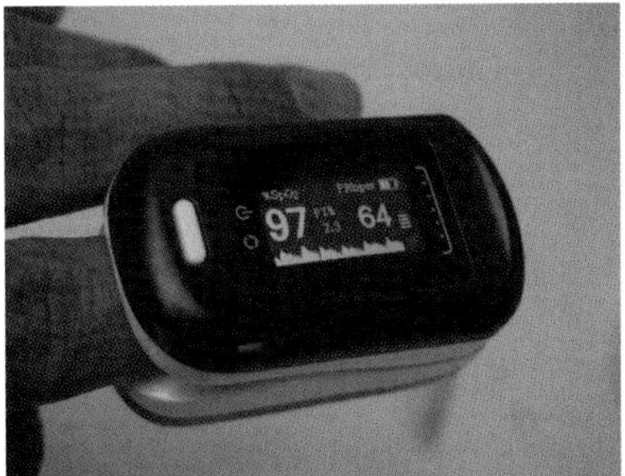

Pulse oximeter

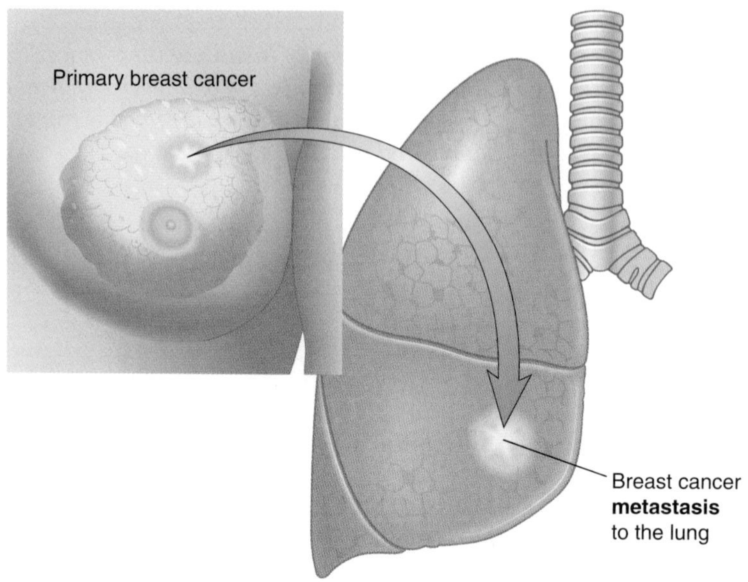

FIGURE 4-8 Metastasis. Note the difference between a primary breast cancer and breast cancer that has metastasized to the lung.

4

mal- bad

malignant ____________________

meta- change, beyond

metastasis ____________________

This term literally means a "change of place; -STASIS means place. It is the spread of a cancerous tumor from its original place to a secondary location in the body. See Figure 4-8.

metacarpals ____________________

The carpal bones are the wrist bones, and the metacarpals are the hand bones, which are ***beyond*** *the wrist. See the x-ray images of the hands in Figure 4-9.*

Malignant versus benign

The root IGN comes from the Latin *ignis,* meaning "fire." A malignant tumor is a cancerous growth that spreads like a "wildfire" from its original location to other organs. A benign tumor (BEN- means "good") is a noncancerous growth that does not spread.

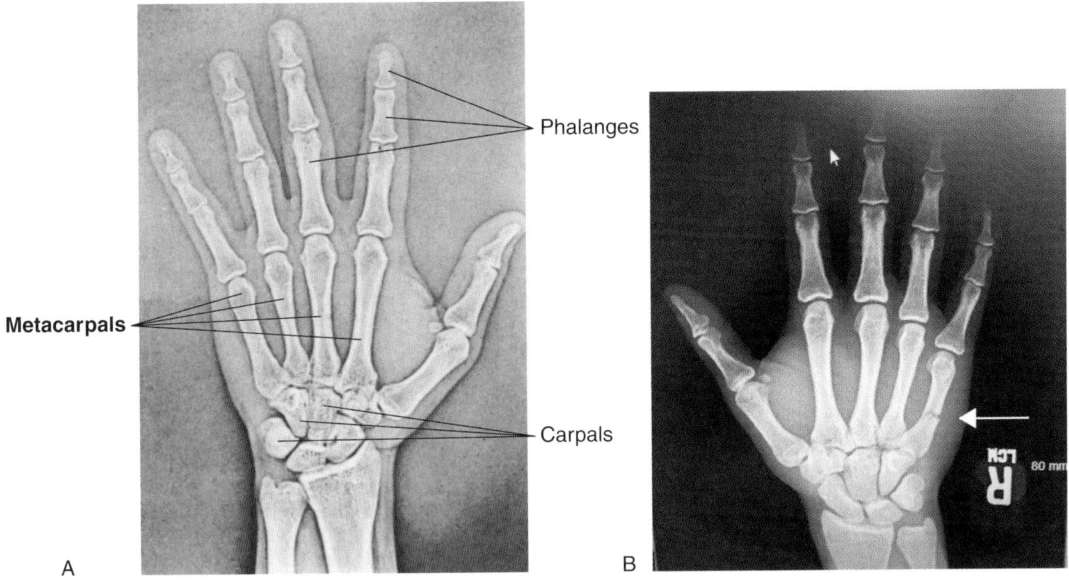

FIGURE 4-9 Metacarpals. **A,** This x-ray image of a normal hand shows metacarpals, carpals (wrist bones), and phalanges (finger bones). **B,** Notice the metacarpal fracture (see arrow).

4

neo- new

neoplasm ______________________

neoplastic ______________________

neonatal ______________________

Neonates (see Figure 4-10) who are born prematurely are often cared for in the ***neonatal intensive care unit (NICU).***

Intensive care units

Note the pronunciations and meanings of hospital intensive care units:

MICU (**MIK**-u)	medical intensive care unit
MSICU (**M-SIK**-u)	medical/surgical intensive care unit
NICU (**NIK**-u)	neonatal intensive care unit
PACU (**PAK**-u)	post anesthesia care unit
PICU (**PIK**-u)	pediatric or psychiatric intensive care unit
SICU (**SIK**-u)	surgical intensive care unit

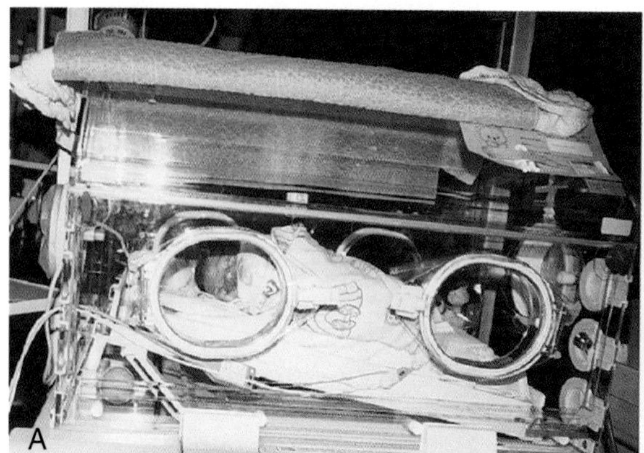

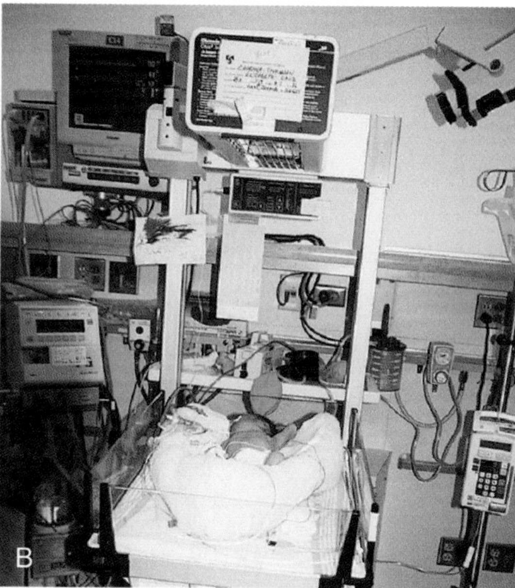

FIGURE 4-10 Neonates in the neonatal intensive care unit (NICU). A, Benjamin Oliver Chabner, born May 22, 2001, at 32 weeks (8 weeks premature). **B,** Samuel August "Gus" Thompson, born August 13, 2001, at 36 weeks. Gus needed an endotracheal tube through which he received surfactant, a substance necessary to inflate his lungs. Both children are healthy and a delight to their grandmother. See the dedication page for current photos!

para- beside, near, along the side of

parathyroid glands ______________________________

Figure 4-11 shows the position of the parathyroid glands on the back side of the thyroid gland. The parathyroid glands are endocrine glands that regulate the amount of calcium in bones and in the blood.

paralysis ______________________________

This term came from the Greek paralytikos, *meaning "one whose side was loose or weak," as after a stroke. Now it means a loss of movement in any part of the body caused by a break in the connection between nerve and muscle.*

paraplegia ______________________________

-PLEGIA *means paralysis, and this term originally meant paralysis of any limb or side of the body. Since the nineteenth century, however, it has indicated paralysis of the lower half of the body.*

peri- surrounding

periosteum ______________________________

perianal ______________________________

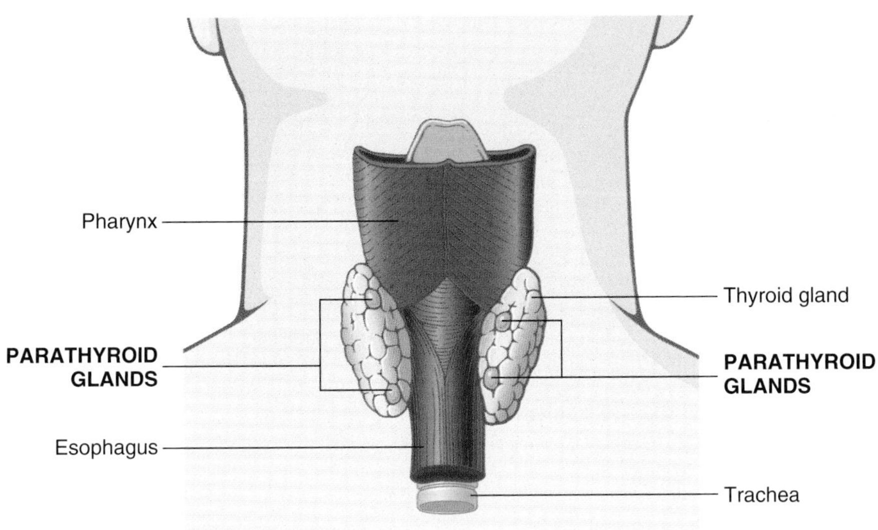

FIGURE 4-11 Parathyroid glands. These are four endocrine glands on the posterior (back side) of the thyroid gland.

poly-	many, much	polyuria ______
		polyneuropathy ______
		polydipsia ______ *Symptoms of diabetes mellitus are polyuria and polydipsia.*
post-	after, behind	postpartum ______
		postmortem ______
pre-	before	precancerous ______ *An example of a precancerous lesion is a* ***polyp*** *(benign growth), commonly found in the colon. Polyps are often removed via colonoscopy, because they may eventually become malignant.*
		prenatal ______

Polyuria and diuretics

Polyuria is the excretion of an abnormally large quantity of urine. Diuretics (DI- from DIA-, meaning "complete") are drugs that promote polyuria. They are used in the treatment of hypertension to lower blood pressure by removing excess fluid from the body.

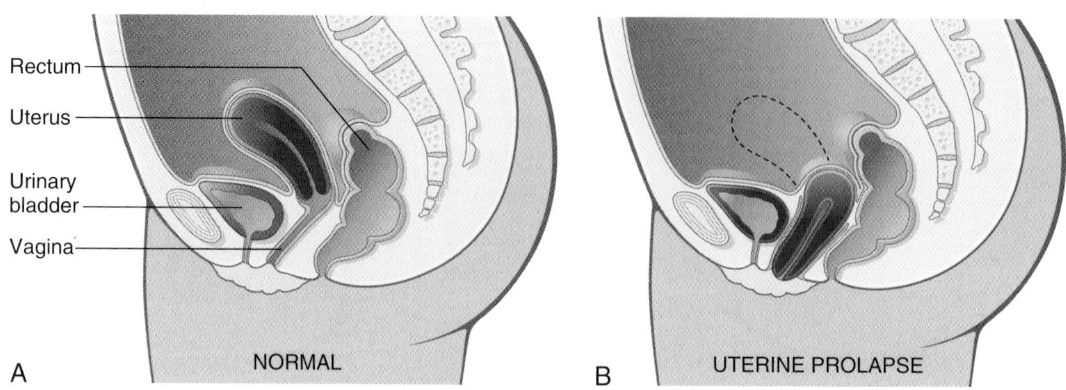

FIGURE 4-12 A. Normal uterus position. B. Uterine prolapse.

pro- before, forward prolapse ________________________

-LAPSE *means to slide. Figure 4-12 shows both the normal position of the uterus (tilted forward) and its position when prolapsed.*

pros- before, forward prosthesis ________________________

An artificial limb is a prosthesis—literally, something "placed before" (as a replacement). Figure 4-13 shows Amy Palmiero-Winters running with a sports prosthetic leg. Figure 4-14 shows a total hip replacement and a total knee joint replacement. See ***In Person: Total Knee Replacement*** *on page 151.*

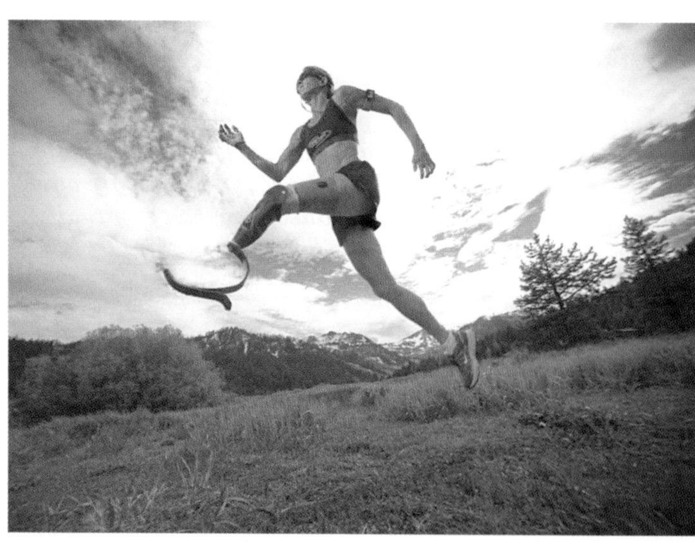

FIGURE 4-13 Amy Palmiero-Winters is the first female with a prosthetic leg to finish the Badwater 135, a 135-mile race from Badwater in Death Valley to Mount Whitney, California.

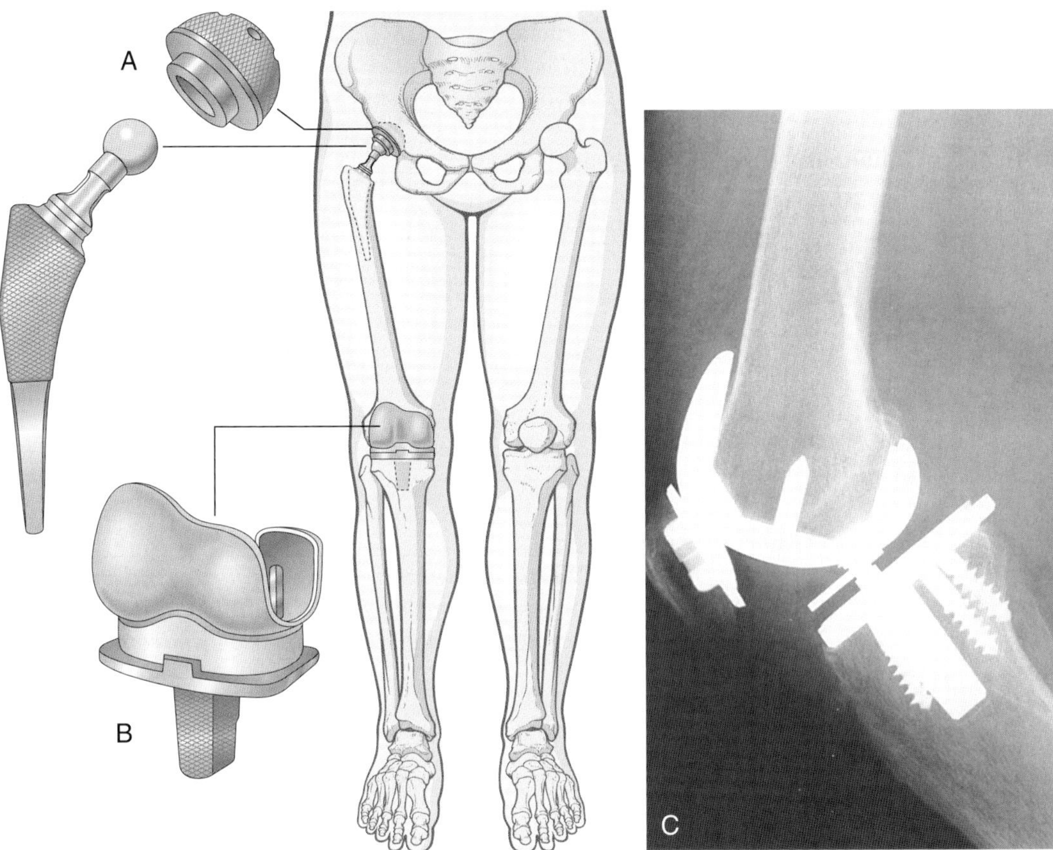

FIGURE 4-14 Total hip joint replacement and total knee joint replacement. A, In total hip joint replacement, a cementless prosthesis allows porous ingrowth of bone. **B,** In total knee joint replacement, the prosthesis includes a tibial metal retainer and a femoral component. The femoral component is chosen individually for each patient according to the amount of healthy bone present. **C,** X-ray image of knee replacement.

quadri- four

quadriplegia ______________________________

Paralysis of all four limbs.

re- back, behind

relapse ______________________________

Symptoms of disease return when a patient has a relapse. ***Exacerbation*** *is an increase in the severity of a disease or any of its symptoms.*

remission ______________________________

Symptoms of disease lessen when the disease goes into remission.

resection ______________________________

retro-	back, behind	retroperitoneal ________________ *The kidneys are retroperitoneal organs. (See Figure 2-4 on page 54.)*
sub-	under, less than	subcostal ________________
		subcutaneous ________________
		subtotal ________________ *A subtotal gastrectomy is a partial resection of the stomach.*
		subscapular ________________ *The scapula is the shoulder bone. Figure 4-15 shows its location.*
syn-	with, together	syndrome ________________ -DROME *means running or occurring. A syndrome is a group of symptoms and signs of illness that occur* ***together****. Table 4-4 gives examples of syndromes.*
tachy-	fast	tachycardia ________________
		tachypnea ________________

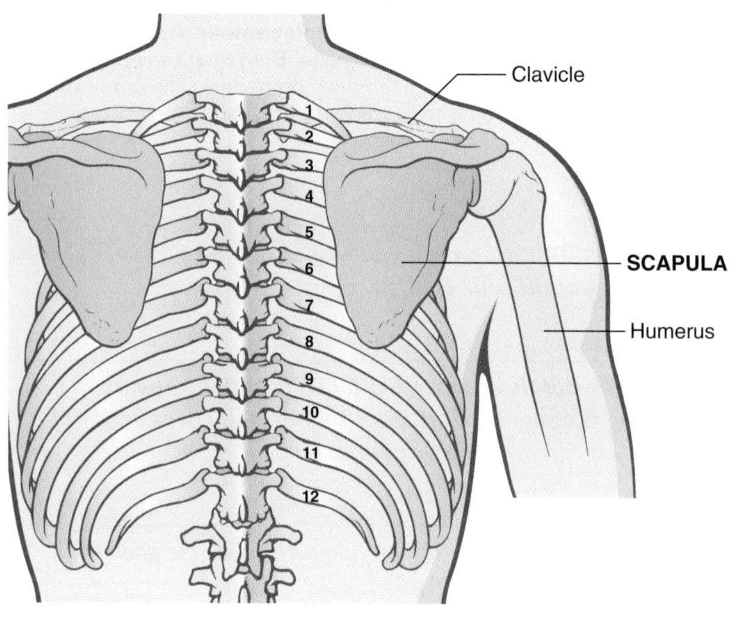

FIGURE 4-15 **Scapula (shoulder bone)**, posterior view. The clavicle is the collarbone, and the humerus is the upper arm bone.

TABLE 4-4 SYNDROMES

SYNDROME	SIGNS AND SYMPTOMS
acquired immunodeficiency syndrome (AIDS)	Severe infections, malignancy (Kaposi sarcoma and lymphoma), fever, malaise (discomfort), and gastrointestinal disturbances. It is caused by a virus that damages lymphocytes (white blood cells).
carpal tunnel syndrome	Pain, tingling, burning, and numbness of the hand and wrist. A nerve leading to the hand is compressed by connective tissue fibers in the wrist.
Down syndrome	Intellectual disabilities, flat face with a short nose, slanted eyes, broad hands and feet, stubby fingers, and protruding lower lip. The syndrome occurs when an extra chromosome is present in each cell of the body.
mitral valve prolapse syndrome	Abnormal sounds (murmurs) heard through a stethoscope placed on the chest. These murmurs indicate that the mitral valve is not closing properly. Chest pain, dyspnea (difficult breathing), and fatigue are other symptoms.
severe acute respiratory syndrome (SARS)	An infectious disease marked by fever and cough, which may progress to pneumonia. This syndrome is caused by the coronavirus; also called SARS-CoV-2.
toxic shock syndrome	High fever, vomiting, diarrhea, rash, hypotension (low blood pressure), and shock. It typically is caused by a bacterial infection in the vagina of menstruating women using superabsorbent tampons.

trans- across, through

transabdominal ____________________

transurethral ____________________

*In a **transurethral resection of the prostate gland (TURP),** pieces of the prostate gland are removed through the urethra. This procedure relieves symptoms of **benign prostatic hyperplasia (BPH).** See Figure 1-17 page 21.*

tri- three

tricuspid valve ____________________

-CUSPID *means "pointed end," as of a spear. The tricuspid valve is on the right side of the heart, while the mitral (bicuspid) valve is on the left side of the heart. Figure 4-16 shows the location of both valves and indicates the pathway of blood through the heart.*

ultra- beyond

ultrasonography____________________

Figure 4-17 shows an ultrasonogram (sonogram) of a fetus.

uni- one

unilateral ____________________

What is a symptom?

A symptom is an indication of disease observed by the patient (such as abdominal pain, fatigue, or loss of appetite.) Both SYM- and SYN- mean "with" or "together" and -PTOM means "a happening." The medical term **asymptomatic** means without symptoms. Often COVID-19 patients can transmit the coronavirus even if they are asymptomatic.

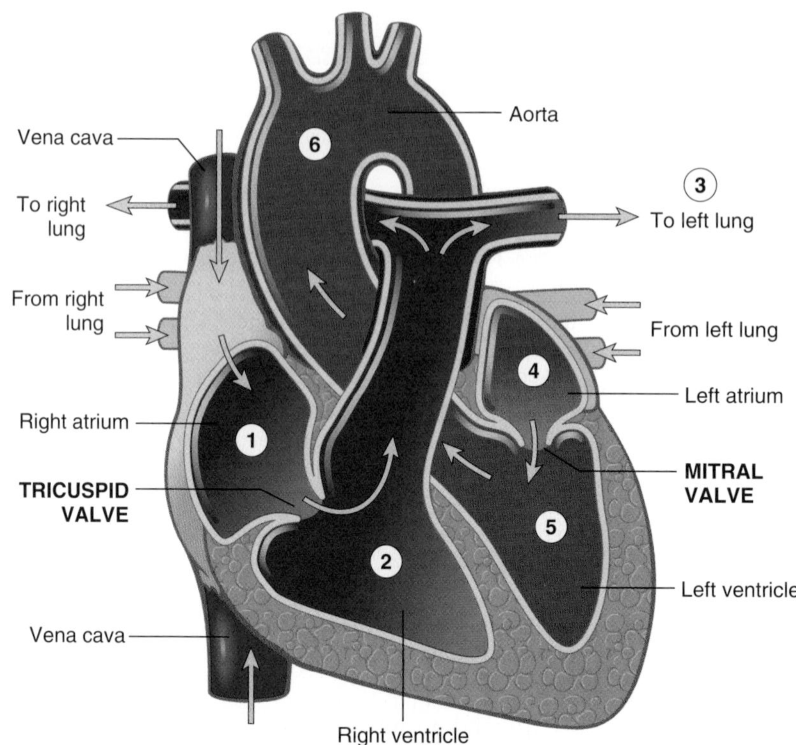

FIGURE 4-16 Tricuspid and mitral valves of the heart. Blood enters the ***right atrium*** of the heart (1) from the big veins (venae cavae) and passes through the ***tricuspid valve*** to the ***right ventricle*** (2). Blood then travels to the ***lungs*** (3), where it loses carbon dioxide (a gaseous waste) and picks up oxygen. Blood returns to the heart into the ***left atrium*** (4) and passes through the ***mitral valve*** to the ***left ventricle*** (5). It is then pumped from the left ventricle out of the heart into the largest artery, the ***aorta*** (6), which carries the blood to all parts of the body.

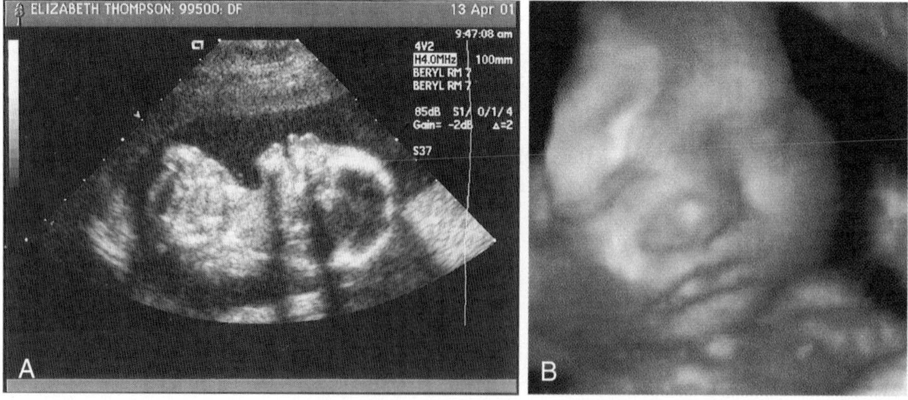

FIGURE 4-17 A, Ultrasonogram showing my grandson Samuel August "Gus" Thompson as a 19-week-old fetus. **B,** Three-dimensional sonogram.

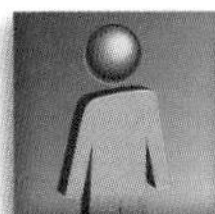

IN PERSON: TOTAL KNEE REPLACEMENT (TKR)

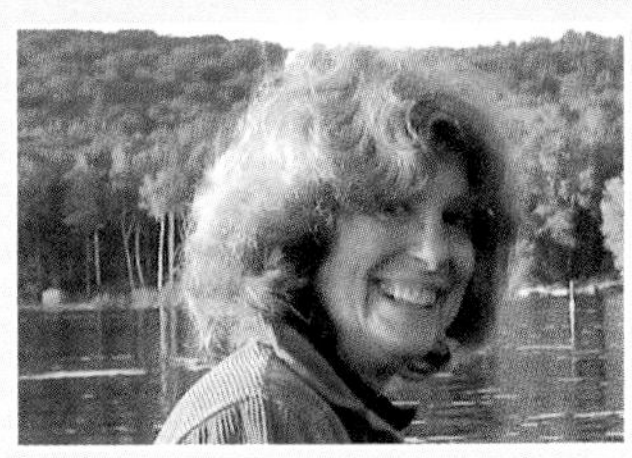

I had endured many years of diminishing mobility in my right leg, alleviated somewhat by occasional cortisone shots and two arthroscopic surgeries. While stitching the second arthroscopic wound, my orthopedist said, "Nothing more to be done with this one. ... Next stop: total knee replacement!" He was right! My TKR procedure was inevitable and indeed very radical.

It involved major trauma to all the supporting muscles, tendons, nerves, and blood vessels. Hence a long period of recuperation was involved. I took advantage of the extra day that was offered to me at MGH (bless Medicare!) for a total hospitalization of five days, during which I had to learn how to perform the most basic functions in new ways. I found, after many trials, that a walker is preferable to crutches. Both are hard on the hands, but the walker is more stable, and the attachable basket is a boon.

For those who are contemplating TKR, the question of where to do the rehab is crucial. If, as I did, you have the conditions to recover at home, that is preferable. The necessary conditions are, first, a partner or caregiver who is available 24/7 for the first few days and who doesn't decide to take a prolonged vacation after that. ... The second relates to the physical conditions at home. Preferably the living area should all be on one level; although climbing stairs becomes one of the protocols of physical therapy, it takes awhile to get to that point, and one is not very steady until that time. Easy access to bathrooms and to other living areas is crucial. The third necessary condition is the availability of the physical therapist. Living in the summer and fall months in rural New Hampshire, I was fortunate to qualify for the services of the local VNA [Visiting Nurse Association], and a marvelous physical therapist visited me three times a week for about six weeks. In between visits, I worked hard to win her approval, and although it seemed at first like tackling Everest to lift my leg even one inch off the floor, let alone walk, within about six weeks I could drive, even if I was getting around outside with crutches; within two months I had regained good mobility, and six months later I was as good as new, and ever so grateful. ...

Although I consider this procedure to be nothing short of miraculous, like any major elective surgery, one should not undertake it unless the pain of daily life outweighs its joys. ... When the doctors ask you about the pain, on a scale of 1 to 10, take them seriously. Don't undergo this surgery until it hovers around 8 or 9 ... and then—well, enjoy the results!

Sidra DeKoven Ezrahi is a professor emeritus of Comparative Literature at the Hebrew University and is a Guggenheim Fellow. She divides her time between Jerusalem, Israel, and Wilmot, New Hampshire.

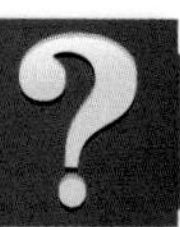

EXERCISES AND ANSWERS

Complete these exercises and check your answers. An important part of your success in learning medical terminology is checking your answers carefully with the Answers to Exercises beginning on page 160. Don't forget to wRite, Review, and Repeat!

A Give meanings for the following prefixes.

1. anti-____
2. ana-____
3. ad-____
4. bi-____
5. brady-____
6. ab-____
7. a-, an-____
8. ante-____
9. con-____
10. dia-____

B Complete the following sentences with the medical terms listed below.

analysis
anemia
antibiotic
antibody
antigen
apnea
atrophy
bilateral
bradycardia
diarrhea

1. A patient with hearing loss in both ears has a/an ____________________ condition.
2. When airways collapse or are blocked during sleep, a condition called sleep ____________________ may occur.
3. A protein produced by white blood cells in response to a foreign substance, such as a bacterium or virus, is a/an ____________________.

4

4. A foreign substance, such as a bacterium or virus, is a/an ______________________.
5. Decrease in hemoglobin in the blood to below the normal range produces a condition known as ______________________.
6. A condition of frequent loose, watery stools that seem to “flow through” the body is called ______________________.
7. The separation of substances into their component parts is known as ____________.
8. A medication produced from molds or synthesized in a laboratory to destroy microorganisms is a/an ______________________.
9. A condition in which the heart rate is less than 60 beats per minute is ___________.
10. Having an arm in a cast and not using it can cause ______________________.

C Give medical terms for the following meanings.

1. Without speech: ______________________
2. Lack of menstrual flow: ______________________
3. Before birth: ______________________
4. Glands located near the kidneys: ______________________ glands
5. An irregularity appearing with birth: ______________________ anomaly
6. Separation of waste materials from the blood when the kidneys fail: ______________

D Give meanings for the following prefixes.

1. ec-______________________
2. epi-______________________
3. hemi-______________________
4. hyper-______________________
5. hypo-______________________
6. dys-______________________
7. endo-______________________
8. ex-______________________
9. extra-______________________
10. in-______________________

E Complete the following sentences using the medical terms listed below.

dysmenorrhea
dysphagia
dysplasia
dyspnea
dysuria
endoscopy
epidermis
excision
extrahepatic
incision

1. Pain associated with menstrual flow is ______________________________.
2. Cutting into a part of the body is a/an ______________________________.
3. Any abnormal development in tissues or organs is ______________________________.
4. Cutting out of a part of the body is a/an ______________________________.
5. Painful burning sensation upon urination is ______________________________.
6. Painful breathing that may be caused by anxiety, strenuous exercise, or certain heart conditions is ______________________________.
7. The outer layer of skin is the ______________________________.
8. Pertaining to outside the liver is ______________________________.
9. Difficulty in swallowing is called ______________________________.
10. Visual examination (via an endoscope) of what is within an organ is ______________________________.

4

F Complete the following medical terms using the meanings provided.

1. High blood pressure is ____________________ **tension**.
2. A mass of blood above the membrane surrounding the brain is a/an ____________ **dural hemat** ____________.
3. A pregnancy that is out of its normal place is a/an __________ **topic pregnancy.**
4. A condition of excessive (too much) blood sugar is ____________________ **emia.**
5. A condition of deficient (too little) blood sugar is ____________________ **emia.**
6. Glands that secrete hormones within the body are ______________ **crine glands.**

7. Increase in development (size of cells) often caused by overuse of a muscle or organ is **hyper** ________________________.

8. Paralysis of half of the body related to a stroke is ________________________ **plegia.**

9. Excessive secretion from a gland in front of the trachea is **hyper** ________________.

10. Increased formation (numbers of cells) is **hyper** ________________________.

G Give meanings for the following prefixes.

1. intra-________________________
2. mal-________________________
3. para-________________________
4. peri-________________________
5. poly-________________________
6. inter-________________________
7. meta-________________________
8. neo-________________________
9. post-________________________
10. pre-________________________

H Give meanings for the following medical terms.

1. intervertebral________________________
2. metastasis________________________
3. metacarpals________________________
4. intravenous________________________
5. postmortem________________________
6. periosteum________________________
7. precancerous________________________
8. neonatal________________________
9. paraplegia________________________
10. malignant________________________

I **Complete each of the sentences that follow by selecting from the list of terms below. The bold words in each sentence should help you choose the correct term.**

adrenal glands	neoplasm	polyneuropathy
dyspnea	parathyroid glands	polyuria
extracranial	perianal	postpartum
hypoxia	polydipsia	
intrauterine		

1. An injury to the **outside** of the skull is a/an ______________________________ lesion.
2. Four small glands in the neck region **near** (posterior to) another endocrine gland are the ____________________________.
3. Common symptoms of diabetes are **much** urination, or ________________________, and **much** thirst, or ___________________________.
4. People who experience asthma often have **difficult** breathing, which is called ___________________________.
5. Bleeding can occur from cracks or sores **surrounding** the opening to the rectum. These are ____________________________ fissures.
6. Two glands each located **near** (above) a kidney are ______________________________.
7. A **new** growth, which can be malignant or benign, is a/an _______________________.
8. Disease of **many** nerves is known as a/an _____________________________________.
9. Any problem that affects the fetus **within** the womb is a/an ____________________ condition.
10. Women may experience moodiness and sad feelings **after** birth, a condition known as ____________________________ depression.
11. In some COVID-19 patients, breathing difficulties occur causing low oxygen levels called ______________.

J Give meanings for the following prefixes.

1. pro-________________
2. quadri-________________
3. sub-________________
4. tachy-________________
5. trans-________________
6. uni-________________
7. re-________________
8. pros-________________
9. retro-________________
10. syn-________________
11. ultra-________________
12. tri-________________

K Select from the list of terms below to complete each of the following sentences.

prolapse	remission	tachypnea
prosthesis	resection	tricuspid
quadriplegia	subtotal	ultrasonography
relapse	syndrome	unilateral

1. Removal or cutting out of an organ is a/an ________________.
2. Test that shows the structure of organs using sound waves beyond the normal range of hearing is ________________.
3. An artificial part of the body is a/an ________________.
4. Recurrence of symptoms of an illness is a/an ________________.
5. Recovery and disappearance of symptoms is a/an ________________.
6. Rapid breathing is ________________.
7. If the spinal cord is severed in the cervical region, paralysis of all four limbs, known as ________________, will result.
8. The ________________ valve has three parts and is on the right side of the heart, between the upper and lower chambers.
9. If a patient has a/an ________________ gastrectomy, less than the complete stomach is removed.
10. Pain, tingling, burning, and numbness of the hand are symptoms of carpal tunnel ________________.

L Define the following terms that describe parts of the body.

1. subscapular ____________________
2. transabdominal ____________________
3. retroperitoneal ____________________
4. subcutaneous ____________________
5. intervertebral ____________________

M Select from the terms listed below to complete the sentences that follow.

anemia	prolapse	tachycardia
aphasia	relapse	transurethral
paralysis	remission	

1. After her ninth child, muscles in Ms. Smith's uterine wall weakened, causing her uterus to fall and ____________________ through her vagina.
2. After Mr. Jones' heart attack, his cardiologist noticed a rapid heart rhythm, or ____________________.
3. A cerebrovascular accident (CVA) on the left side of the brain can cause a loss of speech, or ____________________.
4. Menorrhagia and lack of iron in Sharon's diet led to a condition of low hemoglobin and iron deficiency ____________________.
5. The operation to remove part of Bill's enlarged prostate gland involved placing a catheter through his urethra and removing pieces of the gland. The surgery, called a TURP, or ____________________ resection of the prostate gland, improved his ability to urinate. The prostate gland is at the base of the urinary bladder in males (see Figure 4-18).

4

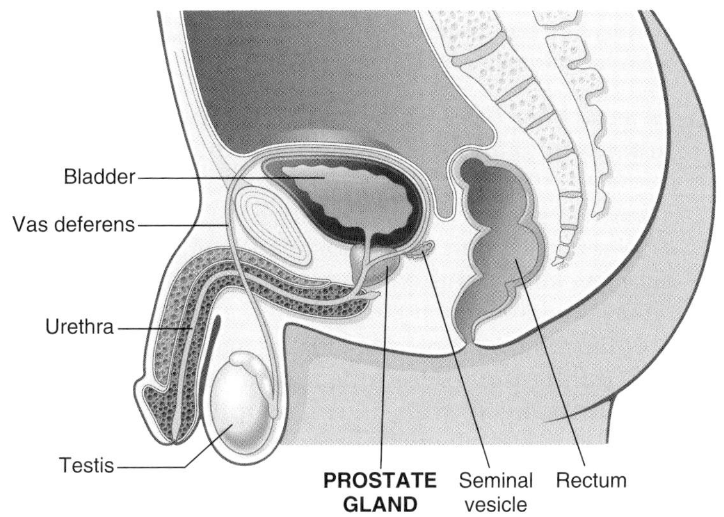

FIGURE 4-18 Prostate gland.

N Circle the correct meaning in bold in each of the following statements.

1. Dys- and mal- both mean (**outside, good, bad**).
2. Hypo- and sub- both mean (**under, above, outside**).
3. Epi- and hyper- both mean (**inside, beneath, above**).
4. Con- and syn- both mean (**apart, near, with**).
5. Ultra- and meta- both mean (**new, beyond, without**).
6. Ante-, pre-, and pro- all mean (**before, surrounding, between**).
7. Ec- and extra- both mean (**within, many, outside**).
8. Endo-, intra-, and in- all mean (**painful, within, through**).
9. Post-, re-, and retro- all mean (**behind, slow, together**).
10. Uni- means (**one, two, three**).
11. Tri- means (**one, two, three**).
12. Bi- means (**one, two, three**).

4

O **Circle the boldface term that best completes the meaning of the sentences in the following medical vignettes.**

1. As part of her **(intravenous, postpartum, prenatal)** care, Beatrix underwent **(ultrasonography, endoscopy, urinalysis)** to determine the age, size, and development of her fetus.
2. Ellen's pregnancy test was positive, but she had excruciating pelvic pain. After a careful pelvic exam and ultrasound scan, the doctors diagnosed a/an **(epidural, ectopic, subscapular)** pregnancy. She then underwent emergency surgery to remove the implanted tissue from the fallopian tube.
3. After noticing a suspicious-looking mole on her upper arm, Carole was diagnosed with **(malignant, benign, subtotal)** melanoma. This type of skin cancer is a/an **(intrauterine, extrahepatic, neoplastic)** process and has a high likelihood of **(paralysis, dysplasia, metastasis)** to other areas of the body.
4. Carole's daughter, Annabelle, found a mole on her back and quickly had it checked by her physician. Fortunately, after a biopsy, the pathologic examination revealed a **(transabdominal, precancerous, perianal)** nevus (mole) that was considered **(chronic, unilateral, benign)**. In the future, Annabelle will need close follow-up for other suspicious lesions.
5. Milton's blood pressure was 160/110 mm Hg. Normal blood pressure is 120/80 mm Hg. To reduce Milton's risk of stroke, his physician prescribed medication to treat his **(bradycardia, hypertension, dyspnea)**.

ANSWERS TO EXERCISES

A

1. against
2. up, apart
3. toward, near
4. two, both
5. slow
6. away from
7. no, not, without
8. before, forward
9. with, together
10. through, complete

B

1. bilateral
2. apnea
3. antibody
4. antigen
5. anemia
6. diarrhea
7. analysis
8. antibiotic
9. bradycardia
10. atrophy

C

1. aphasia
2. amenorrhea
3. antepartum or prenatal
4. adrenal
5. congenital
6. dialysis

D

1. out, outside
2. above, upon
3. half
4. excessive, too much, above
5. deficient, too little, below
6. bad, painful, difficult, abnormal
7. within, in, inner
8. out
9. outside of
10. in, into

E

1. dysmenorrhea
2. incision
3. dysplasia
4. excision
5. dysuria
6. dyspnea
7. epidermis
8. extrahepatic
9. dysphagia
10. endoscopy

F

1. **hyper**tension
2. **epi**dural hemat**oma**
3. **ec**topic
4. **hyperglyc**emia
5. **hypoglyc**emia
6. **endo**crine
7. hyper**trophy**
8. **hemi**plegia
9. hyper**thyroidism**
10. hyper**plasia**

G

1. within
2. bad
3. beside, near, along the side of
4. surrounding
5. many, much
6. between
7. change, beyond
8. new
9. after, behind
10. before

H

1. pertaining to between the vertebrae (backbones)
2. change of place or beyond control (spread of a cancerous tumor to a secondary location)
3. beyond the wrist bones (carpals); hand bones
4. pertaining to within a vein
5. after death
6. membrane surrounding a bone
7. pertaining to a condition that comes before malignancy—for example, dysplastic nevi (moles) that precede malignant melanoma
8. pertaining to new birth (a neonate is a newborn)
9. condition of paralysis of the lower half of the body
10. cancerous; not benign

I

1. extracranial
2. parathyroid glands
3. polyuria; polydipsia
4. dyspnea
5. perianal
6. adrenal glands
7. neoplasm
8. polyneuropathy
9. intrauterine
10. postpartum
11. hypoxia

J

1. before, forward
2. four
3. under, less than
4. fast
5. across, through
6. one
7. back, behind
8. before, forward
9. back, behind
10. with, together
11. beyond
12. three

K

1. resection
2. ultrasonography
3. prosthesis; literally, something "put forward"
4. relapse
5. remission
6. tachypnea
7. quadriplegia
8. tricuspid
9. subtotal
10. syndrome

L

1. pertaining to under the scapula (shoulder bone)
2. pertaining to across or through the abdomen
3. pertaining to behind the peritoneum
4. pertaining to under the skin
5. pertaining to between the vertebrae (backbones)

M

1. prolapse
2. tachycardia
3. aphasia
4. anemia
5. transurethral

N

1. bad
2. under
3. above
4. with
5. beyond
6. before
7. outside
8. within
9. behind
10. one
11. three
12. two

O

1. prenatal, ultrasonography
2. ectopic
3. malignant, neoplastic, metastasis
4. precancerous, benign
5. hypertension

4

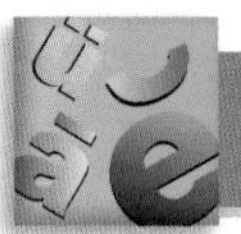

PRONUNCIATION OF TERMS

The terms that you have learned in this chapter are presented here with their pronunciations. The capitalized letters in **BOLDFACE** *represent the accented syllable. Pronounce each word out loud; then write its meaning in the space provided. All terms are defined in the* ***Mini-Dictionary,*** *beginning on page 363, and on the audio section of the Evolve website.*

4

Term	Pronunciation	Meaning
abnormal	ab-**NOR**-mal	__________
adrenal glands	ah-**DRE**-nal glanz	__________
analysis	ah-**NAL**-ih-sis	__________
anemia	ah-**NE**-me-ah	__________
antepartum	an-te-**PAR**-tum	__________
antibiotic	an-tih-bi-**OT**-ik	__________
antibody	**AN**-tih-bod-e	__________
antigen	**AN**-tih-jen	__________
aphasia	a-**FAY**-ze-ah	__________
apnea	**AP**-ne-ah	__________
atrophy	**AT**-ro-fe	__________
benign	be-**NIN**	__________
bilateral	bi-**LAT**-er-al	__________
bradycardia	bra-de-**KAR**-de-ah	__________
congenital anomaly	kon-**JEN**-ih-tal ah-**NOM**-ah-le	__________
dialysis	di-**AL**-ih-sis	__________
diarrhea	di-ah-**RE**-ah	__________
dysphagia	dis-**FAY**-jah	__________
dysplasia	dis-**PLAY**-zhah	__________
dyspnea	**DISP**-ne-ah *or* disp-**NE**-ah	__________
dysuria	dis-**U**-re-ah	__________
ectopic pregnancy	ek-**TOP**-ik **PREG**-nan-se	__________
endocrine glands	**EN**-do-krin glanz	__________

endoscopy	en-**DOS**-ko-pe	________
epidural hematoma	ep-ih-**DUR**-al he-mah-**TO**-mah	________
excision	ek-**SIZH**-un	________
extrahepatic	eks-tra-heh-**PAT**-ik	________
hemigastrectomy	heh-me-gast-**REK**-to-me	________
hemiplegia	heh-me-**PLE**-jah	________
hyperglycemia	hi-per-gli-**SE**-me-ah	________
hyperplasia	hi-per-**PLA**-zhah	________
hypertension	hi-per-**TEN**-shun	________
hyperthyroidism	hi-per-**THI**-royd-izm	________
hypertrophy	hi-**PER**-tro-fe	________
hypoxia	hi-**POX**-e-ah	________
hypoglycemia	hi-po-gli-**SE**-me-ah	________
incision	in-**SIZH**-un	________
intervertebral	in-ter-**VER**-teh-bral	________
intrauterine	in-trah-**U**-ter-in	________
intravenous	in-trah-**VE**-nus	________
malignant	mah-**LIG**-nant	________
metacarpal	met-ah-**KAR**-pal	________
metastasis	meh-**TAS**-tah-sis	________
neonatal	ne-o-**NA**-tal	________
neoplastic	ne-o-**PLAS**-tik	________
paralysis	pah-**RAL**-ih-sis	________
paraplegia	par-ah-**PLE**-jah	________
parathyroid glands	par-ah-**THI**-royd glanz	________
perianal	per-e-**A**-nal	________
periosteum	per-e-**OS**-te-um	________
polydipsia	pol-e-**DIP**-se-uh	________

polyneuropathy	pol-e-noo-**ROP**-ah-the ______
polyuria	pol-e-**UR**-e-ah ______
postmortem	post-**MOR**-tem ______
postpartum	post-**PAR**-tum ______
precancerous	pre-**KAN**-ser-us ______
prolapse	pro-**LAPS** ______
prosthesis	pros-**THE**-sis ______
quadriplegia	quah-drih-**PLE**-jah ______
relapse	re-**LAPS** ______
remission	re-**MISH**-un ______
resection	re-**SEK**-shun ______
retroperitoneal	reh-tro-per-ih-to-**NE**-al ______
subcostal	sub-**KOS**-tal ______
subcutaneous	sub-ku-**TA**-ne-us ______
subdural hematoma	sub-**DUR**-al he-mah-**TO**-mah ______
subscapular	sub-**SKAP**-u-lar ______
subtotal	**SUB**-to-tal ______
syndrome	**SIN**-drom ______
tachycardia	tak-eh-**KAR**-de-ah ______
tachypnea	tak-ip-**NE**-ah ______
transabdominal	trans-ab-**DOM**-ih-nal ______
transurethral	trans-u-**RE**-thral ______
tricuspid valve	tri-**KUS**-pid valv ______
ultrasonography	ul-trah-son-**OG**-rah-fe ______
unilateral	u-nih-**LAT**-er-al ______
urinalysis	u-rih-**NAL**-ih-sis ______

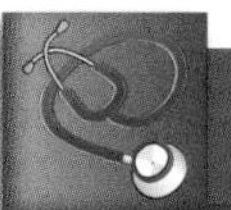

PRACTICAL APPLICATIONS

MATCHING

Match the abnormal condition in Column I with the organ, lesion, or body part in Column II that may be involved in or cause the condition. Answers are found on page 167.

Column I		Column II
1. aphasia	_______	A. urinary bladder
2. dysphagia	_______	B. colon
3. diarrhea	_______	C. uterine cervix
4. quadriplegia	_______	D. left-sided brain lesion
5. hyperglycemia	_______	E. pancreas
6. dysuria	_______	F. lungs
7. paraplegia	_______	G. heart
8. bradycardia	_______	H. cervical spinal cord lesion
9. dyspnea	_______	I. esophagus
10. dysplasia	_______	J. lumbar spinal cord lesion

4

DISEASE DESCRIPTION: HYPERTHYROIDISM

From the list below, select terms to complete the sentences in the paragraphs that follow.

antibiotics	exophthalmos	hypoplastic
antibodies	goiter	hyposecretion
bradycardia	hyperplastic	neoplastic
dyspnea	hypersecretion	tachycardia

1. Hyperthyroidism, also known as thyrotoxicosis or Graves disease, is marked by an excess of thyroid hormones. There is much evidence for a hereditary factor in the development of this condition, and some researchers consider it to be an autoimmune disorder caused by ________________ that bind to the surface of thyroid gland cells and stimulate ________________ of hormones (T3 and T4—triiodothyronine and thyroxine). On histologic examination, the enlarged gland is composed of ________________ follicles lined with hyperactive cells.

2. Signs and symptoms of hyperthyroidism include restlessness, insomnia, weight loss, sweating, and rapid heartbeat, or ________________. Abnormal protrusion of the eyes, known as ________________, is another clinical sign. The patient typically also has an enlarged thyroid gland, called a/an ________________.

WHAT'S YOUR DIAGNOSIS?

Case Study

A 22-year-old sexually active female presents to the ED [emergency department] with history of temperature of 104° F for 2 days, vomiting, diarrhea, and a red spotty rash over her chest and abdomen. She reports that she remembered not removing a tampon from her last menstrual cycle until a week after she had stopped menstruating. Other complaints include dysmenorrhea and dysuria.

Physical examination does not reveal an acute abdomen [sudden, severe abdominal pain] or any RLQ [right lower quadrant] tenderness. Blood test is negative for HCG [human chorionic gonadotropin or pregnancy test]; CBC [complete blood count] reveals elevated white blood cell count; blood cultures are positive for staphylococci.

The patient's fever and dehydration do not subside with initial emergency care, and she is subsequently admitted to the hospital. She is seen by a physician from ID [infectious disease], who confirms that the retained tampon has resulted in the above conditions. Her condition improves with IV fluids and antibiotics.

Using the information presented in this case study, what's your diagnosis? Answer is found on page 167.

A. Dehydration
B. Fever
C. Toxic shock syndrome (TSS) with *Staphylococcus aureus*
D. Rash
E. Nausea/vomiting

ANSWERS TO PRACTICAL APPLICATIONS

MATCHING

1. D	3. B	5. E	7. J	9. F
2. I	4. H	6. A	8. G	10. C

DISEASE DESCRIPTION: HYPERTHYROIDISM

1. antibodies, hypersecretion, hyperplastic
2. tachycardia, exophthalmos, goiter

WHAT'S YOUR DIAGNOSIS?

Answer: C. Toxic shock syndrome (TSS) with *Staphylococcus aureus*

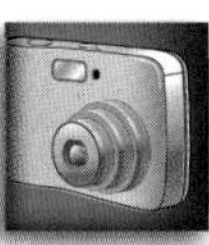

PICTURE SHOW

Answer the questions that follow each image. Correct answers are given on page 170.

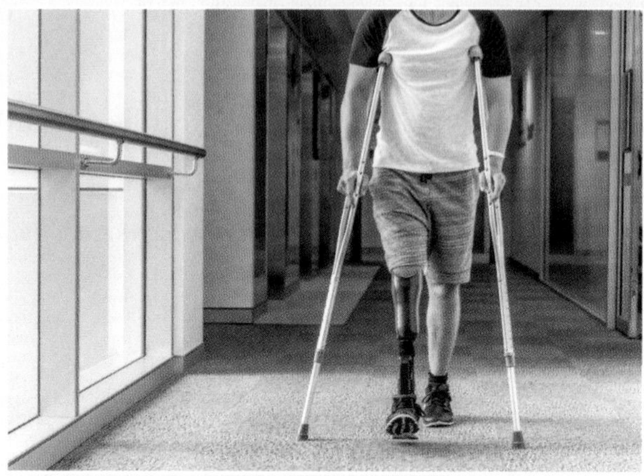

1. This man is walking with the assistance of a:
   a. polyneuropathy
   b. anastomosis
   c. prothesis
   d. metastasis

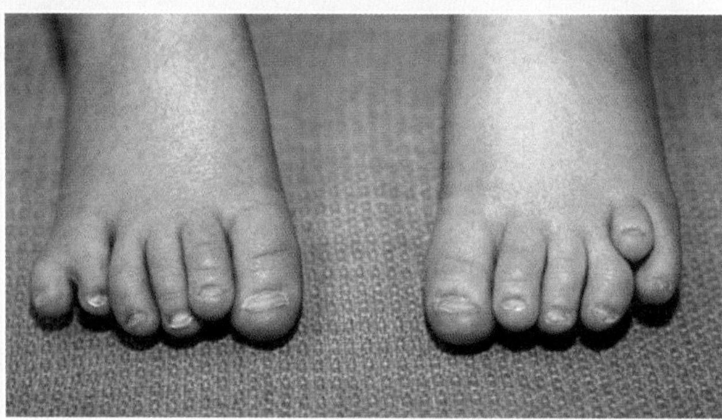

1. This image shows the feet of a child with a condition called: (HINT: The combining form for toes is DACTYL/O.)
   a. syndactyly
   b. condactyly
   c. transdactyly
   d. polydactyly

2. This condition occurs as a/an:
   a. neoplastic anomaly
   b. congenital anomaly
   c. hypertensive anomaly
   d. ectopic pregnancy

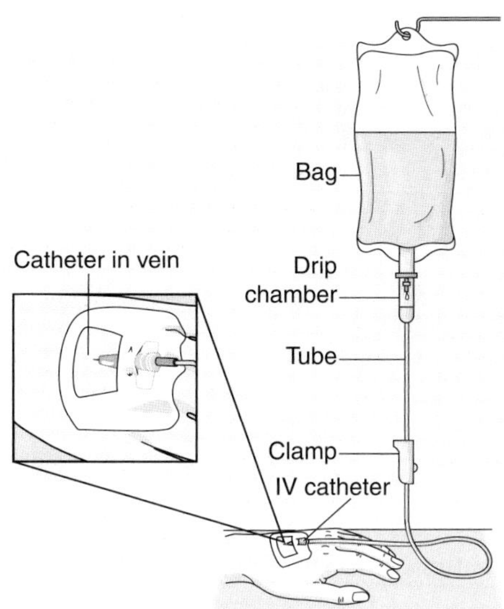

1. This equipment permits nutrients to enter the bloodstream and is used for:
   a. hemodialysis
   b. intrauterine feeding
   c. intravenous feeding
   d. peritoneal dialysis
2. Which term describes a condition or procedure that would be likely to make this equipment necessary?
   a. metacarpalgia
   b. hemigastrectomy
   c. polyneuropathy
   d. epidural hematoma
   e. ultrasonography

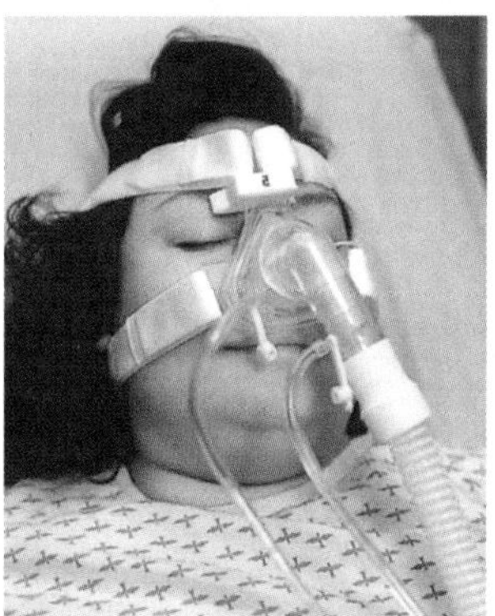

1. The image shows a woman using a device that helps her maintain adequate blood oxygen levels while sleeping. This method is called:
   a. airway prosthesis
   b. nasogastric intubation
   c. bronchoscopy
   d. continuous positive airway pressure (CPAP)
2. The condition that may require use of such a device during sleep is:
   a. bradycardia
   b. aphasia
   c. apnea
   d. dysphagia

E

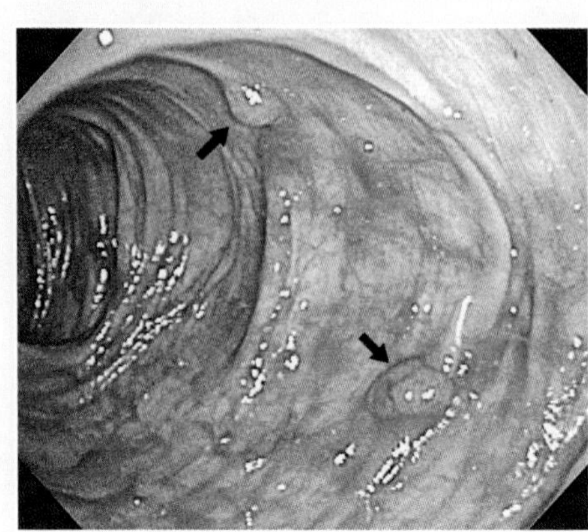

1. The arrows in this image show abnormal, precancerous, neoplastic lesions in the colon. They are:
   a. polyps
   b. fibroids
   c. prolapsed mitral valves
   d. metastases

2. This image was obtained using:
   a. intrauterine ultrasonography
   b. electrocardiography
   c. transabdominal ultrasonography
   d. endoscopy

ANSWERS TO PICTURE SHOW

A	1. c	
B	1. d	2. b
C	1. c	2. b
D	1. d	2. c
E	1. a	2. d

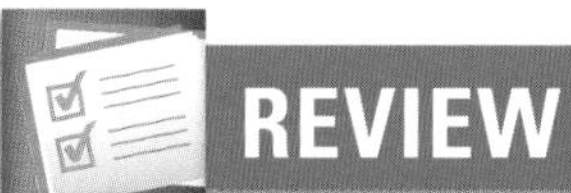

REVIEW

Write the meaning of each of the following word parts, and remember to check your answers with the Answers to Review on page 174.

PREFIXES

Prefix	Meaning
1. a-, an-	______
2. ab-	______
3. ad-	______
4. ana-	______
5. ante-	______
6. anti-	______
7. bi-	______
8. brady-	______
9. con-	______
10. dia-	______
11. dys-	______
12. ec-	______
13. endo-	______
14. epi-	______
15. ex-, extra-	______
16. hemi-	______
17. hyper-	______
18. hypo-	______
19. in-	______
20. inter-	______
21. intra-	______
22. mal-	______
23. meta-	______
24. neo-	______
25. para-	______
26. peri-	______
27. post-	______
28. pre-	______
29. pro-, pros-	______
30. quadri-	______
31. re-, retro-	______
32. sub-	______
33. syn-	______
34. tachy-	______
35. trans-	______
36. tri-	______
37. ultra-	______
38. uni-	______

COMBINING FORMS

Combining Form	Meaning	Combining Form	Meaning
1. abdomin/o	______	17. norm/o	______
2. an/o	______	18. oste/o	______
3. bi/o	______	19. ox/o	______
4. cardi/o	______	20. peritone/o	______
5. carp/o	______	21. plas/o	______
6. cis/o	______	22. ren/o	______
7. cost/o	______	23. scapul/o	______
8. crani/o	______	24. son/o	______
9. cutane/o	______	25. thyroid/o	______
10. dur/o	______	26. top/o	______
11. gen/o	______	27. troph/o	______
12. glyc/o	______	28. urethr/o	______
13. hemat/o	______	29. uter/o	______
14. later/o	______	30. ven/o	______
15. nat/i	______	31. vertebr/o	______
16. neur/o	______		

SUFFIXES

Suffix	Meaning	Suffix	Meaning
1. -al	______	21. -pathy	______
2. - ation	______	22. -phagia	______
3. -cision	______	23. -phasia	______
4. -crine	______	24. -plasia	______
5. -dipsia	______	25. -plasm	______
6. -emia	______	26. -plegia	______
7. -gen	______	27. -pnea	______
8. -graphy	______	28. -ptom	______
9. -ia	______	29. -rrhea	______
10. -ic	______	30. -scopy	______
11. -ine	______	31. -section	______
12. -ism	______	32. -stasis	______
13. -lapse	______	33. -tension	______
14. -lysis	______	34. -thesis	______
15. -meter	______	35. -tic	______
16. -mission	______	36. -trophy	______
17. -mortem	______	37. -um	______
18. -oma	______	38. -uria	______
19. -ous	______	39. -y	______
20. -partum	______		

ANSWERS TO REVIEW

PREFIXES

1. no, not, without
2. away from
3. toward
4. up, apart
5. before, forward
6. against
7. two
8. slow
9. with, together
10. through, complete
11. bad, painful, difficult, abnormal
12. out, outside
13. within, in, inner
14. above, upon
15. out, outside
16. half
17. excessive, above
18. below, under
19. in, into
20. between
21. within
22. bad
23. change, beyond
24. new
25. beside, near, along the side of
26. surrounding
27. after, behind
28. before
29. before, forward
30. four
31. back, behind
32. under, less than
33. with, together
34. fast
35. across, through
36. three
37. beyond
38. one

COMBINING FORMS

1. abdomen
2. anus
3. life
4. heart
5. wrist bones
6. to cut
7. ribs
8. skull
9. skin
10. dura mater
11. to produce
12. sugar
13. blood
14. side
15. birth
16. nerve
17. rule, order
18. bone
19. oxygen
20. peritoneum
21. formation, growth
22. kidney
23. shoulder blade (bone)
24. sound
25. thyroid gland
26. to put, place
27. development, nourishment
28. urethra
29. uterus
30. vein
31. vertebra (backbone)

SUFFIXES

1. pertaining to
2. process, condition
3. process of cutting
4. secretion
5. condition of thirst
6. blood condition
7. to produce
8. process of recording
9. condition
10. pertaining to
11. pertaining to
12. condition, process
13. to fall, slide
14. loosening, breakdown, separation, destruction
15. to measure
16. to send
17. death
18. tumor
19. pertaining to
20. birth
21. disease condition
22. to eat, swallow
23. to speak
24. formation
25. formation
26. paralysis
27. breathing
28. a happening
29. flow, discharge
30. process of visual examination
31. incision
32. to stand, place, stop, control
33. pressure
34. to put, place
35. pertaining to
36. nourishment; development
37. structure
38. urine condition
39. process, condition

4

TERMINOLOGY CHECKUP

In your own words, write the answers on the lines provided. Confirm your answers and check the box next to each item when you know you've "got" it!

☐ 1. What is the difference between **antigens, antibodies,** and **antibiotics?**

____

____

____

☐ 2. Explain the difference between a **primary malignant tumor** in the lung and a **breast cancer metastasis** in the lung.

____

____

____

☐ 3. What is the difference between a **remission** and a **relapse** of a disease?

____

____

____

☐ 4. Define the term **paralysis.** Give meanings for the following terms: **hemiplegia, quadriplegia,** and **paraplegia.**

____

____

____

☐ 5. What is a **syndrome** ? Name three syndromes.

____

____

____

ANSWERS TO TERMINOLOGY CHECKUP

1. **Antigens** are foreign substances (bacteria, viruses, fungi) that stimulate white blood cells to make **antibodies,** which destroy the antigens.
   Antibiotics, however, are medications produced ***outside*** the body to kill or inhibit the growth of antigens such as bacteria and other microorganisms.
2. A **primary malignant tumor** in the lung originates and grows in the lung. It is composed of lung cancer cells. A **breast cancer metastasis** in the lung originated in the breast and now has traveled to the lung. It is composed of breast cancer cells. A pathology report of the biopsy will reveal this distinction.
3. A **remission** is the ***lessening or absence of disease symptoms*** during an illness. Patients who have no signs or symptoms of illness are described as being "in remission."
   A **relapse** is the ***return of disease symptoms*** (-LAPSE meaning to fall or slide) after a period of time.
4. **Paralysis** is the ***loss of muscle function.*** It can be caused by a cerebrovascular accident (stroke) or nerve damage in any part of the body. The suffix **-plegia** means ***paralysis.*** For example, ***hemiplegia*** (hemi means half) is paralysis of one side of the body, as occurs with a stroke. ***Quadriplegia*** is paralysis of all four (QUADRI- means four) limbs of the body when spinal nerves in the neck are damaged. ***Paraplegia*** is paralysis of the lower part of the body when there is damage to lower regions of the spinal cord.
5. A **syndrome** is a group of signs and symptoms that occur together indicating a particular condition, the cause of which is not always known. Examples are: **mitral valve prolapse syndrome, carpal tunnel syndrome, acquired immunodeficiency syndrome (AIDS), and severe acute respiratory syndrome (SARS).**

CHAPTER 5

Medical Specialists and Case Reports

Chapter Sections

Introduction 178
Medical Specialists 178
Combining Forms and Vocabulary 181
Case Reports 186
In Person: Living With Crohn's 197
Exercises and Answers 198
Pronunciation of Terms 206
Practical Applications 209
Review 213
Terminology CheckUp 215

CHAPTER OBJECTIVES

- To describe the training process of physicians
- To identify medical specialists and describe their specialties
- To identify combining forms used in terms that describe specialists
- To decipher medical terminology as written in case reports

INTRODUCTION

This chapter reviews many of the terms you have learned in previous chapters and adds others related to medical specialists. In the following section, the training of physicians is described, and specialists are listed with their specialties. Next, on page 181, useful combining forms are presented with terminology to increase your medical vocabulary. Finally, short case reports beginning on page 186 illustrate the use of the medical language in context. As you read these reports, congratulate yourself on your understanding of medical terminology!

MEDICAL SPECIALISTS

Doctors complete 4 years of medical school and then pass national medical board examinations to receive an MD degree (MD stands for Latin *Medicinae Doctor,* "teacher [doctor] of medicine"). They may then begin postgraduate training, which lasts at least 3 years and in some cases longer. This postgraduate training is known as *residency training.* Examples of residency programs are:

Anesthesiology	Administration of agents capable of bringing about a loss of sensation
Dermatology	Diagnosis and treatment of skin disorders
Emergency medicine	Care of patients that requires sudden and immediate action
Family practice	Primary care of all members of the family on a continuing basis
Internal medicine	Diagnosis and treatment of usually complex, nonsurgical disorders in adults
Ophthalmology	Diagnosis and treatment of eye disorders
Pathology	Diagnosis of the cause and nature of disease
Pediatrics	Diagnosis and treatment of children's disorders
Psychiatry	Diagnosis and treatment of disorders of the mind
Radiology	Diagnosis using x-ray studies, including ultrasound and magnetic resonance imaging (MRI)
Surgery	Treatment by manual (SURG- means hand) or operative methods

Examinations are administered after the completion of each residency program to certify the doctor's competency in that specialty area.

A physician may then choose to specialize further by doing *fellowship training.* Fellowship programs (lasting 2 to 5 years) train doctors in *clinical* (patient care) and research (laboratory) skills. For example, an *internist* (specialist in internal medicine) may choose fellowship training in internal medicine specialties such as neurology, nephrology, endocrinology, or oncology. A surgeon interested in further specialization may do fellowship training in thoracic surgery, neurosurgery, or plastic surgery. On completion of training and examinations, the doctor is then recognized as a specialist in that area of medical practice.

Medical specialists with explanations of their specialties are listed below:

Medical Specialist	Area of Practice
allergist	Treatment of hypersensitivity reactions
anesthesiologist	Administration of agents to prevent pain and unpleasant awareness during surgical and other procedures
cardiologist	Treatment of heart disease
cardiovascular surgeon	Surgery on the heart and blood vessels
colorectal surgeon	Surgery on the colon and rectum
dermatologist	Treatment of skin disorders
emergency practitioner	Immediate evaluation and treatment of acute injury and illness in a hospital setting
endocrinologist	Treatment of endocrine gland disorders
family practitioner	Primary care treatment for families on a continuing basis
gastroenterologist	Treatment of stomach and intestinal disorders
geriatrician	Treatment of diseases of old age
gynecologist	Surgery and treatment for diseases of the female reproductive system
hematologist	Treatment of blood disorders
hospitalist	General medical care of hospitalized patients
infectious disease specialist	Treatment of diseases caused by micro organisms (bacteria, viruses, fungi, others)
internist	Adult comprehensive care in office of hospital setting
nephrologist	Treatment of kidney diseases
neurologist	Treatment of nerve disorders
neurosurgeon	Surgery on the brain, spinal cord, and nerves
obstetrician	Treatment of pregnant women; delivery of babies
oncologist	Diagnosis and treatment of malignant and benign tumors
ophthalmologist	Surgical and medical treatment of eye disorders
orthopedist	Surgical treatment of bone, muscle, and joint conditions
otolaryngologist	Surgical treatment of ear, nose, and throat disorders
pathologist	Diagnosis of disease by analysis of cells
pediatrician	Treatment of diseases of children
physiatrist	Treatment to restore function after injury or illness; physical medicine and rehabilitation specialist
psychiatrist	Treatment of mental disorders
pulmonologist	Treatment of lung diseases
radiologist	Examination of x-ray images for diagnosis; interpretation of ultrasound, MRI, and nuclear medicine studies
radiation oncologist	Treatment of disease with high-energy radiation
rheumatologist	Treatment of systemic diseases affecting joints and muscles
thoracic surgeon	Surgery on chest organs
urologist	Surgery on the urinary tract and for treatment of male reproductive disorders

Here are two groups of matching exercises for practice with this new terminology. *Answers are found on page 206.*

A **Match the medical specialists with the procedures and tests that they perform. Write the name of the specialist on the line provided.**

allergist	cardiovascular surgeon	gynecologist
anesthesiologist	endocrinologist	hematologist
cardiologist	gastroenterologist	ophthalmologist

Procedure/Test	Medical Specialist
1. Esophagoscopy and colonoscopy	______________________
2. Blood cell counts; bone marrow biopsy	______________________
3. Ultrasound examination of the heart; angioplasty	______________________
4. Skin testing to determine sensitivity to antigens	______________________
5. Serum (blood) level of hormones	______________________
6. Vision tests; retinoscopy	______________________
7. Coronary artery bypass grafting (CABG)	______________________
8. Catheter and IV line insertion for sedation during surgery	______________________
9. Pap smear (microscopic examination of cells from the cervix and organs); hysterectomy	______________________

5

B **Match the medical specialists with the procedures and tests that they perform. Write the name of the specialist on the line provided.**

neurologist	pathologist	radiologist
nephrologist	psychiatrist	radiation oncologist
orthopedist	pulmonologist	urologist

Procedure/Test	Medical Specialist
1. Nephrectomy; cystectomy; prostatectomy	______________________
2. Personality and mental function tests	______________________

3. Use of high-energy beams (photon and proton) to kill tumor cells ______________________

4. Fixation of bone fracture; arthroscopic surgery ______________________

5. Breathing function (spirometry) tests ______________________

6. Microscopic examination of biopsy samples; autopsies ______________________

7. CT scan; MRI; ultrasound examination ______________________

8. Kidney function tests; dialysis ______________________

9. Spinal and cranial nerve reflex tests ______________________

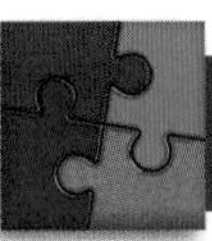

COMBINING FORMS AND VOCABULARY

5

The combining forms below should be familiar because they are found in the listed terms describing medical specialists. A medical term is included to illustrate the use of the combining form. Write the meaning of the medical term in the space provided. You can always check your answers with the ***Mini-Dictionary*** beginning on page 369.

Combining Form	Meaning	Medical Term	Meaning
cardi/o	heart	cardiomegaly	______________________
col/o	colon (large intestine)	colitis	______________________
dermat/o	skin	dermatitis	______________________
endocrin/o	endocrine glands	endocrinology	______________________
enter/o	intestines	enteritis	______________________

Ulcerative Colitis and Crohn Disease (Crohn's)

Both of these conditions are types of **inflammatory bowel disease (IBD)**, with similar signs and symptoms, such as abdominal pain, diarrhea, and bleeding from the rectum. While **ulcerative colitis** is confined to the colon, **Crohn's** commonly affects the last part of the small intestine and may involve other areas of the gastrointestinal tract. Lesions can be identified, but causes of both types of IBD are unknown. See ***In Person: Living with Crohn's*** on page 197.

esthesi/o	sensation	anesthesiology ______________
gastr/o	stomach	gastroscopy ______________
ger/o	old age	geriatrics ______________
gynec/o	woman, female	gynecology ______________
hemat/o	blood	hematoma ______________
iatr/o	treatment	iatrogenic ______________ IATR/O *means treatment by a physician or with medicines. An iatrogenic condition is produced (*-GENIC*) adversely by a treatment.*
laryng/o	voice box	laryngeal ______________
lymph/o	lymph	lymphadenopathy ______________ *Lymph "glands" are actually* ***lymph nodes****, located all over the body but especially in* ***axillary*** *(armpit),* ***inguinal*** *(groin),* ***cervical*** *(neck), and* ***mediastinal*** *(area between the lungs) regions. Lymphadenopathy often refers to the presence of malignant cells in lymph nodes.*
nephr/o	kidney	nephrostomy ______________ *A catheter (tube) is inserted into the kidney for drainage of fluid. This may be necessary if the ureter is injured or urine cannot pass from the kidney to the urinary bladder because of a blockage in the kidney. See Figure 5-1.*

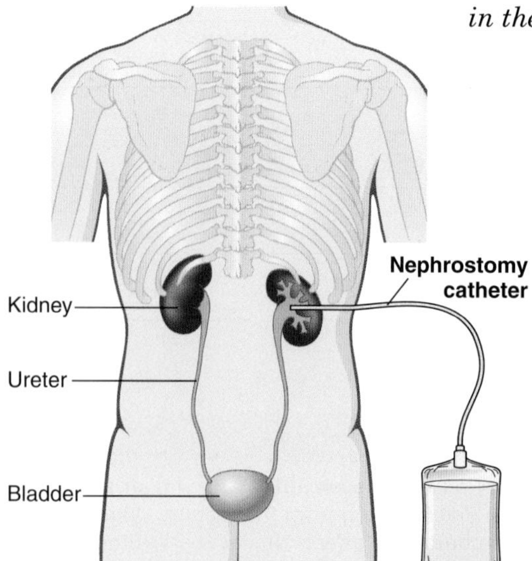

FIGURE 5-1 Nephrostomy. A **nephrostomy catheter** is placed to drain urine directly from the kidney.

neur/o	nerve	neuralgia ______________
nos/o	disease	nosocomial ______________ *A nosocomial infection is acquired during hospitalization (*COMI/O *means to care for).*
obstetr/o	midwife	obstetric ______________
odont/o	tooth	orthodontist ______________ ORTH/O *means straight.*
onc/o	tumor	oncogenic ______________ *Oncogenic viruses give rise to tumors.*
ophthalm/o	eye	ophthalmologist ______________
opt/o	eye	optometrist ______________ *An optometrist examines (*METR/O *means to measure) eyes and prescribes corrective lenses. Optometrists can detect abnormal eye conditions and prescribe medications to treat certain eye disorders.*
optic/o	eye	optician ______________ *Opticians grind lenses and fit glasses. Opticians are not permitted to diagnose or treat eye diseases.*
orth/o	straight	orthopedist ______________ PED/O *comes from* paidos, *the Greek word for "child." In the past, orthopedists were concerned with straightening bone deformities in children. Today, they treat bone, muscle, and joint disorders in adults as well.*
ot/o	ear	otitis ______________
path/o	disease	pathology ______________

Dental Specialists

The following are other specialists in dental medicine:

Dental Specialist	**Area of Expertise**
periodontist	Gums (PERI- means surrounding)
endodontist	Root canal therapy (the root canal is the inner part of a tooth containing blood vessels and nerves)
pedodontist	Children (PED/O means child)
prosthodontist	Replacement of missing teeth with artificial appliances (PROSTH/O = artificial replacement)

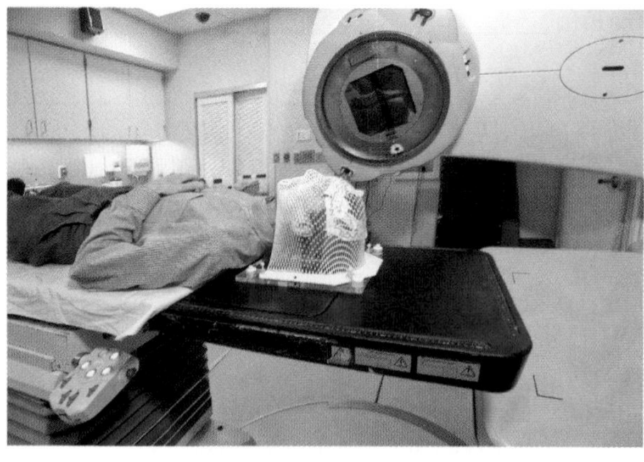

FIGURE 5-2 Radiation therapy. The patient is positioned to receive radiation to treat a tumor of the brain.

ped/o	child	pediatrics ____________
psych/o	mind	psychosis ____________
pulmon/o	lung	pulmonary ____________
radi/o	x-rays	radiotherapy ____________ *Radiotherapy is also called radiation therapy. It is used to treat (shrink) cancerous tumor. See Figure 5-2. Don't confuse radiotherapy with radiology, which is a diagnostic specialty using techniques such as x-rays, CT, MRI, and ultrasound.*
rect/o	rectum	rectocele ____________ -CELE *means a hernia or protrusion. The walls of the rectum weaken and bulge forward toward the vagina. See Figure 5-3.*

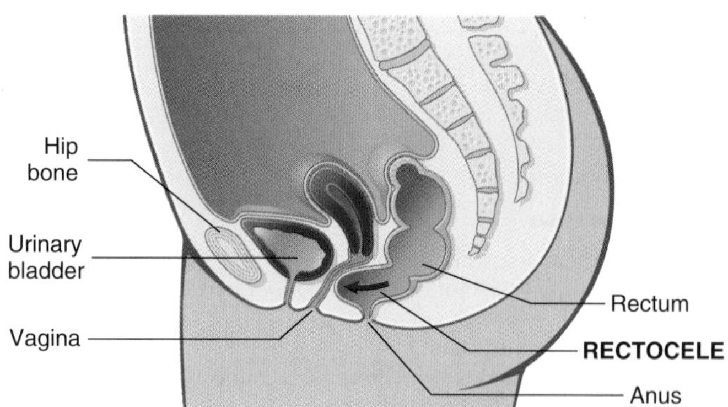

FIGURE 5-3 Rectocele.

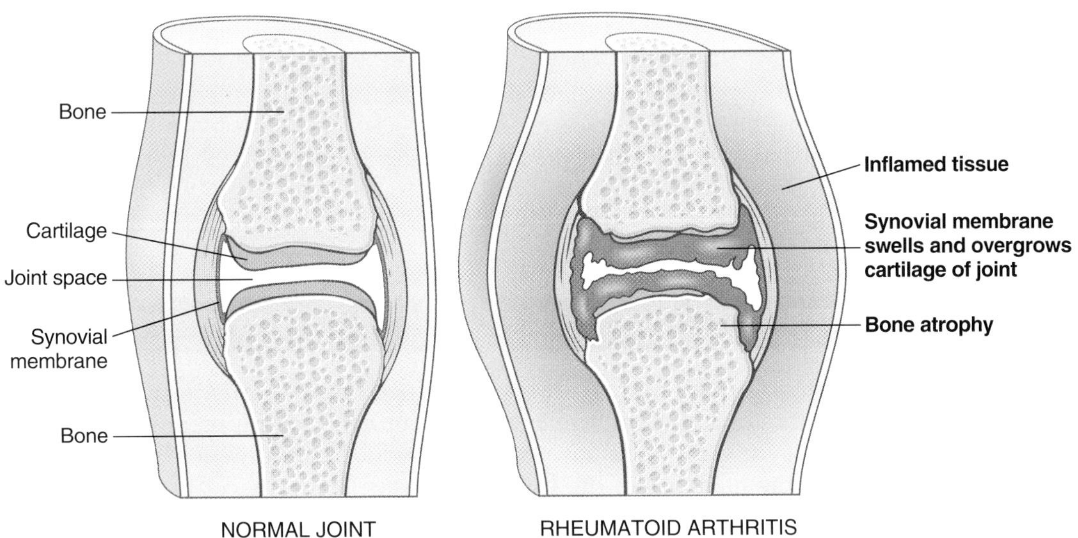

FIGURE 5-4 Differences between a normal joint and one affected by rheumatoid arthritis.

rheumat/o flow, fluid

rheumatology ______________________

Joints can fill with fluid when diseased—hence, RHEUMAT/O *indicates a problem with a swollen joint. Rheumatoid arthritis* ◪ *is a chronic inflammatory disease of joints and connective tissues that leads to deformation of joints. See Figures 5-4 and 5-5.*

Rheumatoid Arthritis and Osteoarthritis

Rheumatoid arthritis first appears when patients (often women) are young, and it has an autoimmune component (antibodies are found that destroy joint tissue). **Osteoarthritis** most often appears in older patients (both men and women) and is marked by degenerative changes that cause destruction of the joint space (see Chapter 1, page 13). Knee and hip replacements may be helpful treatments for patients with osteoarthritis.

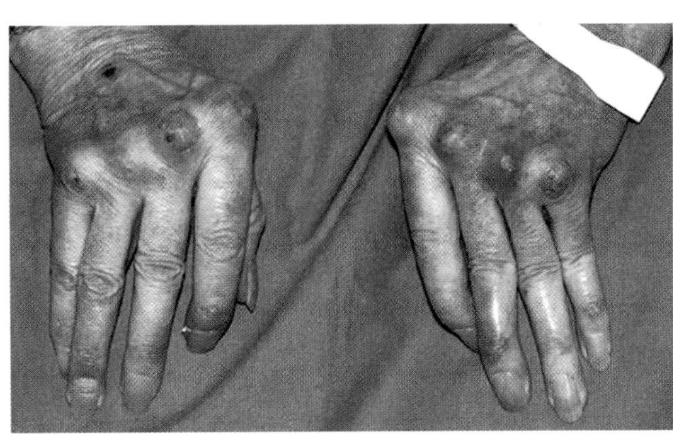

FIGURE 5-5 Advanced rheumatoid arthritis of the hands. Notice the soft tissue swelling and deformed joints—fingers, knuckles, and wrist. Atrophy of muscles and tendons (connecting muscles to bones) allows one joint surface to slip past the other (subluxation).

rhin/o	nose	rhinorrhea ______________________
thorac/o	chest	thoracotomy ______________________
ur/o	urinary tract	urology ______________________
vascul/o	blood vessels	vasculitis ______________________

CASE REPORTS

Here are short case reports related to medical ***specialties***. Many of the terms will be familiar to you; others are explained in the ***Mini-Dictionary*** (beginning on page 363). For more information about each system, refer to Appendix 1 beginning on page 217. In each case report, write the meaning of the **boldface** terms in the spaces provided.

CASE 1 *Cardiology*

5

Mr. Rose was admitted to the cardiac care unit (CCU) with **angina** and a history of **hypertension.**

A **coronary angiogram** (Figure 5-6, *A*) showed **spasm** of the right coronary artery (arrow), causing **acute myocardial ischemia**. An electrocardiogram (ECG) showed **ventricular arrhythmias** as well.

Nitroglycerin was administered, and within minutes, the angiogram showed reversal of the spasm (Figure 5-6, *B*). The ECG recorded reversal of the life-threatening arrhythmias as well. To prevent further ischemia and **myocardial infarction,** Mr. Rose's treatment will include **antiarrhythmic, diuretic,** and **anticoagulant** drugs. In the future, he may need an additional procedure to place a **stent** in his coronary artery to keep it open.

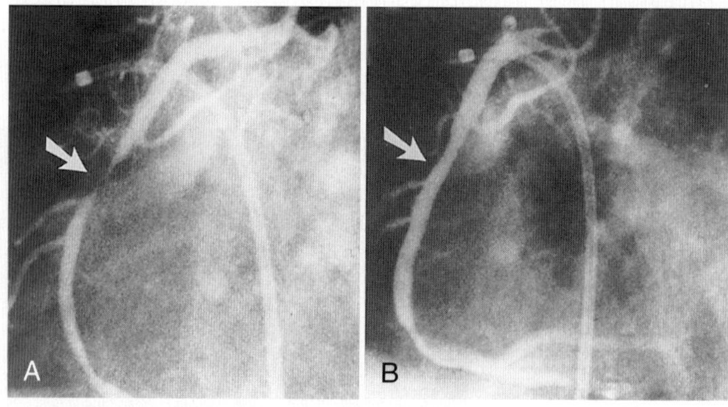

FIGURE 5-6 A, Coronary angiogram showing spasm of the right coronary artery (arrow). **B,** Angiogram showing reversal of the spasm (arrow).

CASE 1 *Cardiology (Continued)*

acute myocardial ischemia ______________________________

angina ______________________________

antiarrhythmic ______________________________

anticoagulant ______________________________

coronary angiogram ______________________________

diuretic ______________________________

hypertension ______________________________

myocardial infarction ______________________________

nitroglycerin ______________________________

spasm ______________________________

stent ______________________________

ventricular arrhythmias ______________________________

CASE 2 *Gynecology*

Ms. Sessions has had **dysmenorrhea** and **menorrhagia** for several months. She is also **anemic.** Because of the presence of a **large fibroid,** as seen on a **pelvic ultrasound** (**sonogram**) (see Figure 5-7, *A*), a **hysterectomy** was recommended. After it was removed, the uterus was opened to reveal multiple fibroids (**leiomyomas**) bulging into the uterine cavity and displaying a firm, white appearance. See Figure 5-7, *B*.

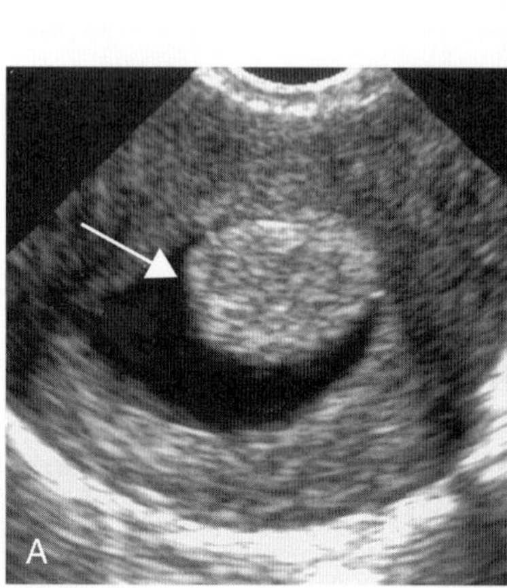

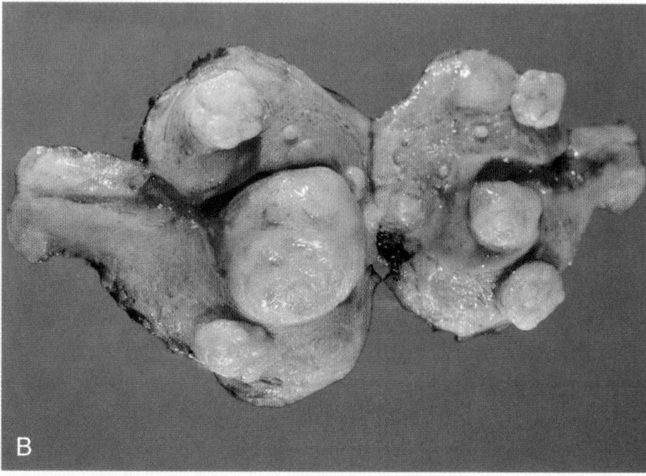

FIGURE 5-7 A, Pelvic sonogram. B, Fibroids (leiomyomas). These are benign tumors of the uterus.

5

anemic ____________________

dysmenorrhea ____________________

fibroid ____________________

hysterectomy ____________________

leiomyomas ____________________

menorrhagia ____________________

pelvic ultrasound ____________________

sonogram ____________________

CASE 3 *Oncology*

John Smith, a 26-year-old law student, was admitted to the hospital after experiencing several months of **fatigue,** low-grade fevers, chest pain, and night sweats. A chest **MRI** scan (see Figure 5-8) revealed large **mediastinal** masses, as shown by arrows. **Needle biopsy** confirmed a **diagnosis** of **Hodgkin lymphoma.** There was no evidence of **lymphadenopathy** or **hepatic** involvement. Treatment included **chemotherapy** followed by **radiotherapy** to the chest. Mr. Smith's **prognosis** is good.

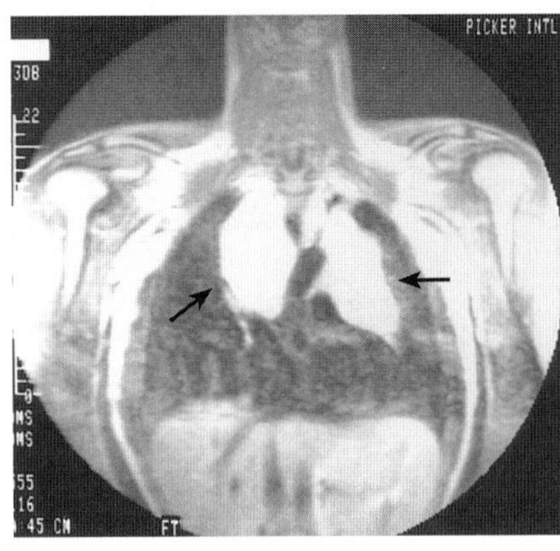

FIGURE 5-8 Magnetic resonance imaging of the upper body.

chemotherapy ____

diagnosis ____

fatigue ____

hepatic ____

Hodgkin lymphoma ____

lymphadenopathy ____

mediastinal ____

MRI ____

needle biopsy ____

prognosis ____

radiotherapy ____

CASE 4 *Urology*

Scott Jones has a history of lower back pain, associated with **hematuria** and **dysuria.** An abdominal x-ray film (Figure 5-9, *A*) shows a **renal calculus** (black arrow). His doctor tells him that renal calculi should be suspected any time a calcification is seen within the renal outline or along the expected course of the **ureter** (dotted lines).

Treatment with shock wave **lithotripsy** (Figure 5-9, *B*) is expected to crush the stone and relieve his **signs and symptoms.**

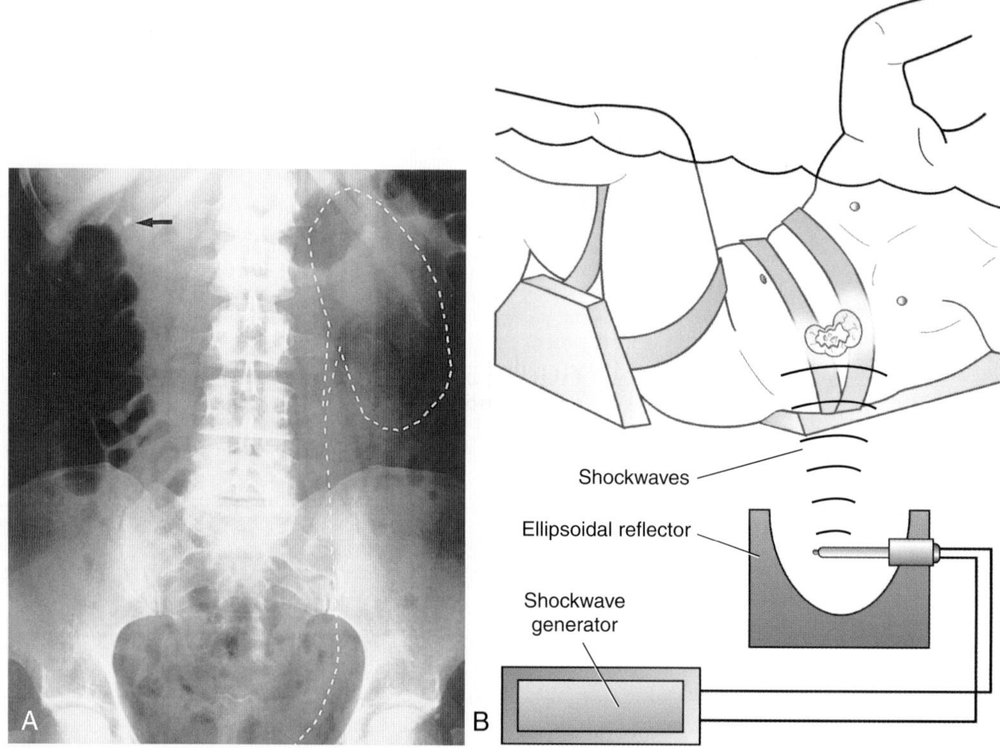

FIGURE 5-9 **A,** An abdominal x-ray image showing a **renal calculus** (arrow). **B, Lithotripsy.**

dysuria ____________________

hematuria ____________________

lithotripsy ____________________

renal calculus ____________________

signs and symptoms ____________________

ureter ____________________

CASE 5 *Gastroenterology*

Mr. Pepper suffers from **dyspepsia,** acid reflux, and sharp **abdominal** pain. A recent episode of **hematemesis** has left him very weak and **anemic. Gastroscopy** and an **upper GI series** with **barium** revealed the presence of a large **peptic ulcer.** Figure 5-10 is a photograph of a peptic ulcer located in the stomach. Mr. Pepper will be admitted to the hospital and treated with medication to reduce gastric acid output and with antibiotics to control a bacterium (*Helicobacter*, or *H. pylori*) known to cause ulcers. If his condition does not improve, he may be scheduled for a partial **gastrectomy.**

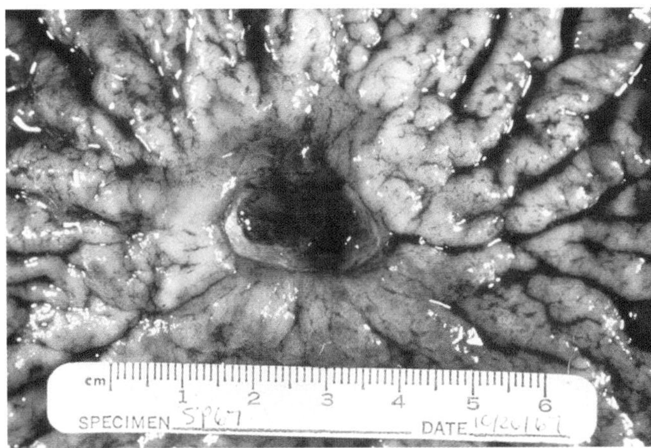

FIGURE 5-10 **Peptic (gastric) ulcer.**

abdominal ______________________________

anemic ______________________________

barium ______________________________

dyspepsia ______________________________

gastrectomy ______________________________

gastroscopy ______________________________

hematemesis ______________________________

peptic ulcer ______________________________

upper GI series ______________________________

5

CASE 6 *Radiology*

Evaluation of David Green's **posteroanterior** chest x-ray film (Figure 5-11, *A*) shows an ill-defined mass near the right **hilum** (see arrows). The **lateral** view (Figure 5-11, *B*) also shows the mass, and its shaggy outline is very suggestive of **carcinoma.** Further evaluation by **CT scan** (Figure 5-11, C) clearly shows the mass in relation to the **mediastinal** structures such as the **pulmonary artery** (PA) and **aorta** (Ao).

Impression: Lung cancer.

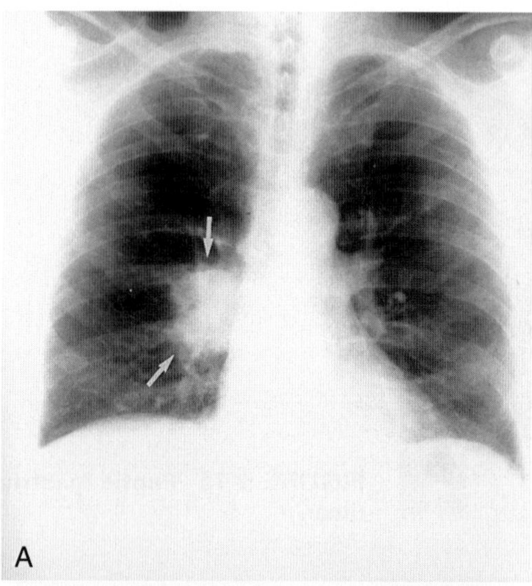

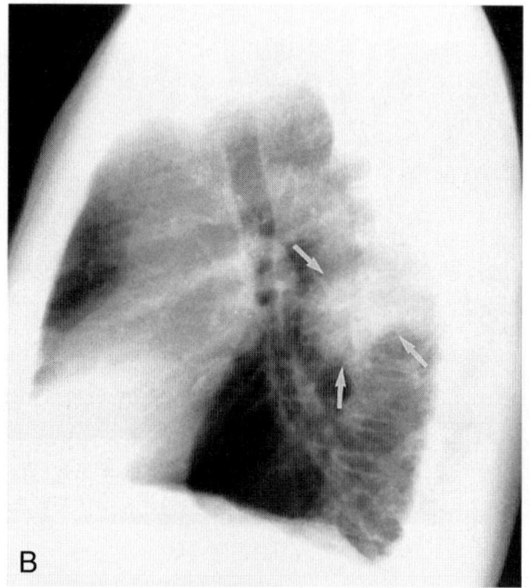

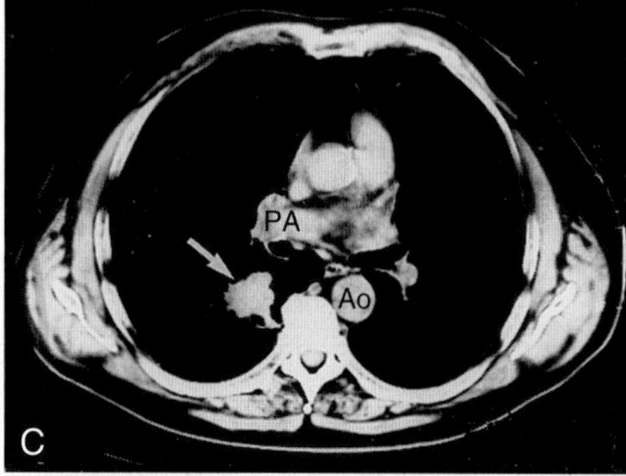

FIGURE 5-11 **A, Posteroanterior chest x-ray** view shows an ill-defined mass (arrows). **B, Lateral chest x-ray** view clearly shows the mass to be posterior to the hilum. **C, Computed tomography** image clearly shows the mass (arrow) in relation to the mediastinal structures.

5

CASE 6 *Radiology (Continued)*

aorta ________________________________

carcinoma ________________________________

CT scan ________________________________

hilum ________________________________

lateral ________________________________

mediastinal ________________________________

posteroanterior ________________________________

pulmonary artery ________________________________

CASE 7 *Endocrinology*

A 36-year-old woman known to have **type 1 diabetes mellitus** was brought to the emergency department after being found collapsed at home. She had experienced 3 days of extreme weakness, **polyuria,** and **polydipsia.** It was discovered that a few days before her admission, she had discontinued use of her external **insulin pump** (see Figure 5-12).

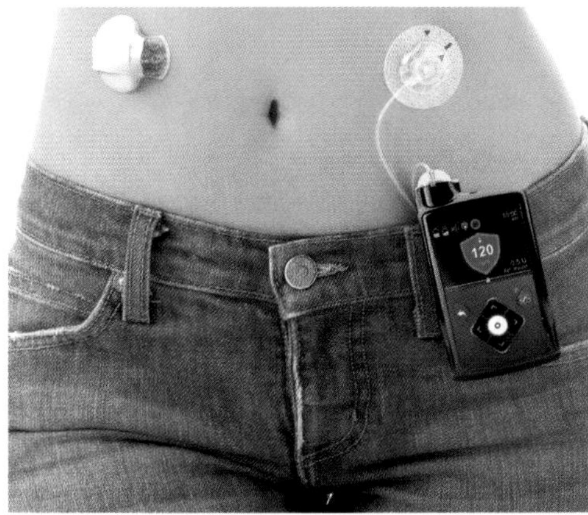

FIGURE 5-12 External insulin pump. The device on the patient's right side is an insulin sensor that continuously monitors insulin levels and communicates with the insulin pump.

insulin pump ________________________________

polydipsia ________________________________

polyuria ________________________________

type 1 diabetes mellitus ________________________________

CASE 8 *Orthopedics*

A 20-year-old male patient was admitted to the hospital after a motorcycle accident. He was found to have a **fracture** of the right **fibula** (see Fig 5-13, *A*) and right **femur**, along with **pelvic** and **intra-abdominal** injuries. He was taken to surgery, and internal **fixation** of the right femur was performed. A cast was applied to the femur for immobilization, and the fibula healed on its own with **callus** formation (Figure 5-13, *B*).

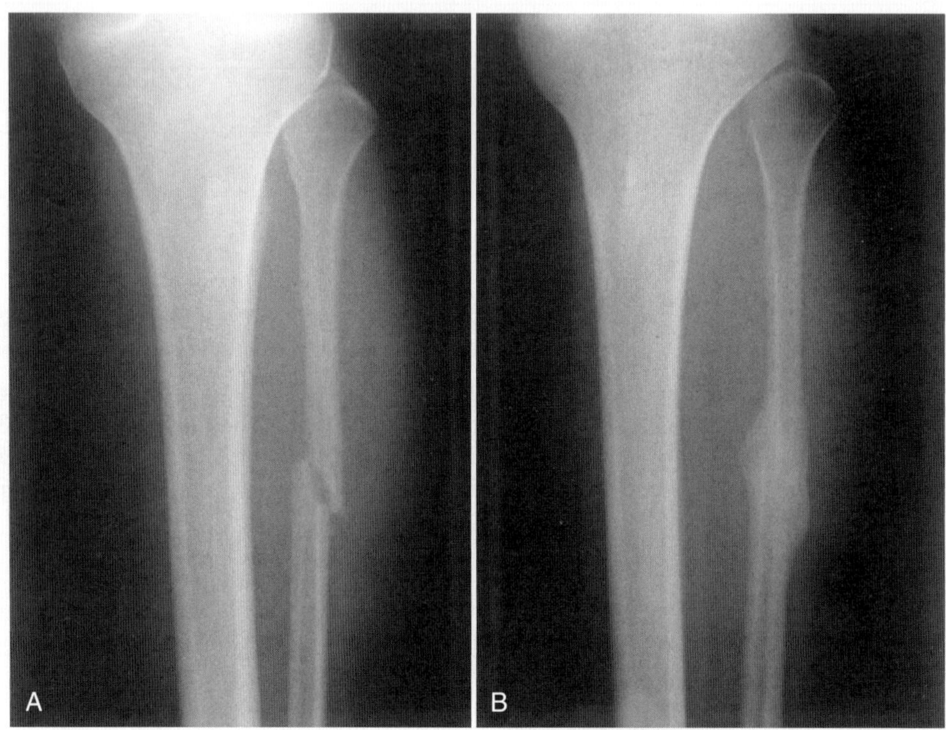

FIGURE 5-13 **A,** Fracture of the fibula. **B,** Callus formation, **6 weeks later.**

callus ______________________________

femur ______________________________

fibula ______________________________

fixation ______________________________

fracture ______________________________

intra-abdominal ______________________________

pelvic ______________________________

CASE 9 *Nephrology*

A 52-year-old woman with **chronic renal failure** secondary to long-standing **hypertension** has been maintained on **hemodialysis** for the past 18 months. An **arteriovenous fistula** (Figure 5-14) was created surgically to provide long-term vascular access for hemodialysis. For the past 3 weeks, during the dialysis sessions, she has become moderately **hypotensive,** with symptoms of dizziness. Consequently, we have decided to withhold her **antihypertensive** medications before dialysis.

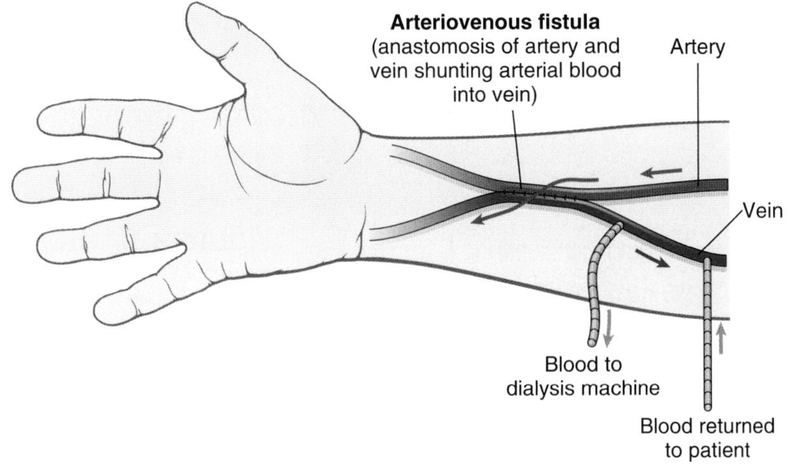

FIGURE 5-14 Arteriovenous fistula created for hemodialysis.

antihypertensive ______________________________

arteriovenous fistula ______________________________

chronic ______________________________

hemodialysis ______________________________

hypertension ______________________________

hypotensive ______________________________

renal failure ______________________________

CASE 10 *Neurology*

Ms. Kindrick is admitted with severe, throbbing **unilateral frontal cephalgia** that has lasted for 2 days. Light makes her cringe, and she has **nausea.** Before the onset of these symptoms, she saw zigzag lines for about 20 minutes and a **scotoma** (see Figure 5-15). Diagnosis is **acute migraine** with **aura.** A **vasoconstrictor** is prescribed, and Ms. Kindrick's condition is improving. [Migraine headaches are thought to be caused by sudden **dilation** of blood vessels.]

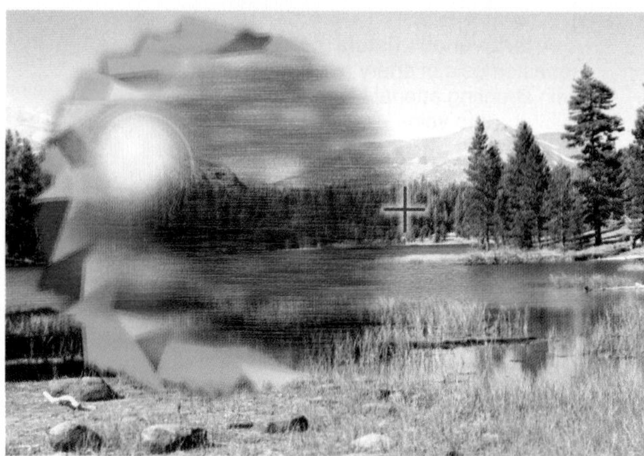

FIGURE 5-15 Scotoma. This abnormal area of the visual field is both "positive" (consisting of bright flickering imagery) and "negative" (displaying a relatively dark area that obscures the visual field). It is called a scintillating scotoma.

acute ______________________________

aura ______________________________

cephalgia ______________________________

dilation ______________________________

frontal ______________________________

migraine ______________________________

nausea ______________________________

scotoma ______________________________

unilateral ______________________________

vasoconstrictor ______________________________

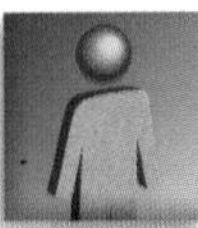

IN PERSON: LIVING WITH CROHN'S

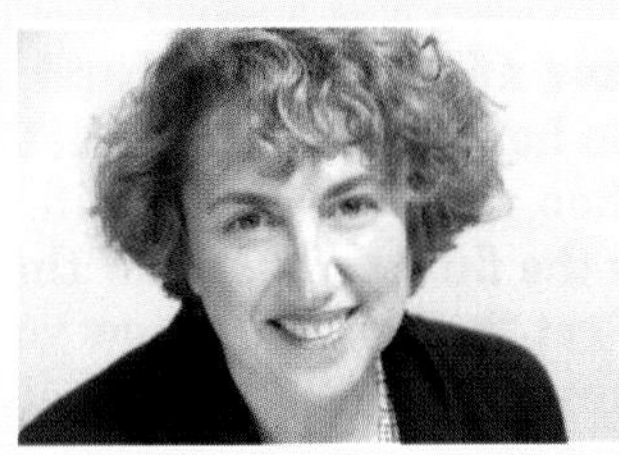

When a friend told me she was felled by the flu yesterday, I was jealous. To someone with a chronic illness, like me, having something acute always seems luxurious. Lie in bed, read glossy magazines, take over-the-counter meds, sleep it off, and in a matter of days you're okay. I have Crohn disease, a chronic inflammation of the small intestine, which is characterized by flare-ups and remission. During flare-ups, I've experienced fever, diarrhea, vomiting, pain, and intestinal obstruction. Even in remission I am never "okay."

Right now I have been in remission two years after a third surgery to remove yet another portion of my small bowel. This time internal bleeding, a rather rare symptom of Crohn's, necessitated the surgery. I was enduring weekly iron infusions, which turned into bimonthly blood transfusions, as my hemoglobin plummeted to 6 (12 is normal). It was no way to live. After the surgery, the bleeding stopped, but I had bouts of urgent, watery diarrhea for a year. That was no way to live either, and unfortunately, as wonderful as my doctor is, I've found that few physicians want to address after-effects of small bowel surgery. After visiting several doctors and by trial-and-error, I finally got these symptoms under control with codeine, Lomotil, and Metamucil, but I will never be able to absorb vitamin B_{12}, so I must inject it monthly for the rest of my life. In addition to taking medicine to cope with having less and less small bowel, I take medicine in the hopes of preventing the next flare-up. Every few weeks, I inject myself with a biologic medicine, Humira, but I must eventually be weaned off this drug because it has possible long-term side effects, the scariest of which is lymphoma. At 52 and with two school-age children, however, I have learned to think of valuing my present quality of life the most, over possible unknown dangers lurking in the future.

I do often think about the past. What would my life be like if our family doctor hadn't told my parents that my constant episodes of diarrhea—which occurred since I was a child—were caused by "nerves"? By the time I was 21, my weight had dropped below 100 pounds, and I was twisted in pain after every meal. My dad arranged for me to visit his own doctor, who gave me a small bowel series that showed I had Crohn's and that a portion of my small intestine was "as narrow as a pencil." By then it was too late for even prednisone (then the drug of choice despite side effects ranging from puffy face to psychosis) to open up the inflamed passage, and I had my first surgery just months after I was diagnosed. Thinking of those times—as well as all the other flare-up times—makes me flinch. While you can never relive pain, you can remember what it felt like. In my case, it was as if a large metal bike lock chain was being forced through my tender gut.

Before that first surgery, I was just out of college and longing to make my mark on the world, but I spent most of my evenings curled up in my small bedroom, listening to the soothing strains of "Make Believe Ballroom Hour" on the radio. Or, because vomiting and diarrhea usually accompanied the pain, I lay with my back pressed against the cold tiles of the bathroom floor. Later on, as a mom with two

Continued

young children, I would lie on the couch watching life swirl around me, feeling guilty that I could not take part.

There was a silver lining to those flare-ups, and that is the tender affection of those around me: husband, family, and friends. When you have Crohn's, no one knows you have it until things get unbearable. It's not the kind of illness you discuss, but when you have pain and fever, you can kind of approximate those times of being felled by the flu. Yet you know that it will take more than a dose of Nyquil or a night's sleep to get "better." You know you'll face another course of medications—often untried ones—or that you will likely end up in the hospital undergoing yet another surgery.

Nancy J. Brandwein is a writer, editor, and food columnist.

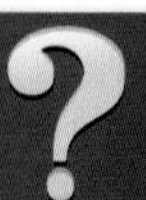

EXERCISES AND ANSWERS

Complete these exercises and check your answers. An important part of your success in learning medical terminology is checking your answers carefully with the Answers to Exercises beginning on page 205.

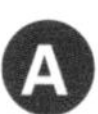

A Match each of the listed residency programs to its description that follows.

anesthesiology
dermatology
emergency medicine
family practice
internal medicine
ophthalmology
pathology
pediatrics
psychiatry
radiology
surgery

1. Treatment by operation or manual (hand) methods ________________
2. Diagnosis and treatment of often complex medical disorders in adult patients ________________
3. Diagnosis and treatment of disorders of the mind ________________
4. Primary care of all family members on a continuing basis ________________
5. Diagnosis and treatment of skin disorders ________________
6. Diagnosis and treatment of eye disorders ________________
7. Diagnosis of disease using x-rays ________________
8. Diagnosis and treatment of children's disorders ________________
9. Care of patients with illness that requires immediate action ________________
10. Administration of agents that produce loss of sensation/awareness ________________
11. Diagnosis of disease by examining cells and tissues ________________

B **Name the physician who treats the following problems (first letters are given).**

1. kidney diseases: **n**________________________
2. tumors: **o**________________________
3. broken bones: **o**________________________
4. female diseases: **g**________________________
5. eye disorders: **o**________________________
6. heart disorders: **c**________________________
7. nerve disorders: **n**________________________
8. lung disorders: **p**________________________
9. mental disorders: **p**________________________
10. stomach and intestinal disorders: **g**________________________

5

C **Match the medical specialists in Column I to their area of practice in Column II.**

Column I		Column II
1. urologist	________	A. operates on the large intestine
2. thoracic surgeon	________	B. treats blood disorders
3. radiation oncologist	________	C. treats thyroid and pituitary gland disorders
4. colorectal surgeon	________	D. rehabilitates after spinal injuries
5. endocrinologist	________	E. treats disorders of childhood
6. obstetrician	________	F. operates on the urinary tract
7. radiologist	________	G. treats disorders of the skin
8. pediatrician	________	H. delivers babies
9. hematologist	________	I. operates on the chest
10. dermatologist	________	J. examines x-ray images to diagnose disease
11. physiatrist	________	K. treats tumors using high-energy radiation

D Complete each of the sentences that follow using a term from the list below.

clinical	oncologist	research
geriatrician	ophthalmologist	surgeon
hospitalist	optician	orthopedist
infectious disease specialist	optometrist	
	pathologist	

1. A doctor who diagnoses and treats diseases that are caused by micro organisms is a/an ______________________.
2. A doctor who performs bone surgery is a/an ______________________.
3. A doctor who takes care of patients practices ______________________ medicine.
4. A medical professional who grinds lenses and fills prescriptions for eye glasses is a/an ______________________.
5. A doctor who reads biopsy samples and performs autopsies is a/an ______________________.
6. A doctor who treats cancerous tumors is a/an ______________________.
7. A medical professional (nonphysician) who examines eyes, prescribes eyeglasses, and treats eye disorders is a/an ______________________.
8. A doctor who operates on patients is a/an ______________________.
9. A doctor who does experiments with test tubes and laboratory equipment is interested in ______________________ medicine.
10. A doctor who specializes in surgery and medical treatment of disorders of the eye is a/an ______________________.
11. A doctor who specializes in the treatment of older people is a/an ______________________.
12. A physician who cares for hospitalized patients is a/an ______________________.

E **Which medical specialist would you consult for the following medical conditions? The first letter of the specialist is given.**

1. Arthritis: **r**____________________________________
2. Otitis media: **o**____________________________________
3. Anemia: **h**____________________________________
4. Urinary bladder cancer: **u**____________________________________
5. Chronic bronchitis: **p**____________________________________
6. Cerebrovascular accident: **n**____________________________________
7. Breast cancer: **o**____________________________________
8. Coronary artery blockages (bypass surgery): **c**____________________________________
9. Dislocated shoulder bone: **o**____________________________________
10. Thyroid gland enlargement: **e**____________________________________
11. Kidney disease: **n**____________________________________
12. Acne (skin disorder): **d**____________________________________
13. Hay fever (hypersensitivity reaction): **a**____________________________________
14. Viral and bacterial diseases: **i**____________________________________
15. Rehabilitation after herniated disc: **p**____________________________________

F **Give the meaning for each of the following medical terms.**

1. neuralgia ______________________________
2. pathology ______________________________
3. cardiomegaly ______________________________
4. nephrostomy ______________________________
5. thoracotomy ______________________________
6. laryngeal ______________________________
7. otitis ______________________________
8. colitis ______________________________
9. pulmonary ______________________________
10. iatrogenic ______________________________
11. gastroscopy ______________________________
12. radiotherapy ______________________________
13. anesthesiology ______________________________
14. enteritis ______________________________
15. nosocomial ______________________________

G Use the following combining forms and suffixes to make the medical terms called for.

Combining Forms		Suffixes	
aden/o	onc/o	-algia	-pathy
col/o	ophthalm/o	-ectomy	-scopy
laryng/o	ot/o	-genic	-stomy
lymph/o	path/o	-itis	-therapy
nephr/o	psych/o	-logy	-tomy
neur/o	thorac/o	-osis	

1. Inflammation of the ear: ____________________
2. Removal of a nerve: ____________________
3. Incision of the chest: ____________________
4. Study of tumors: ____________________
5. Pertaining to producing disease: ____________________
6. Inflammation of the voice box: ____________________
7. Opening of the large intestine to the outside of the body: ____________________
8. Visual examination of the eye: ____________________
9. Abnormal condition of the mind: ____________________
10. Inflammation of the kidney: ____________________
11. Removal of the large intestine: ____________________
12. Pain in the ear: ____________________
13. Treatment of the mind: ____________________
14. Pertaining to producing tumors: ____________________
15. Disease of lymph glands (nodes): ____________________

5

H Circle the bold term that best completes the meaning of the sentences in the following medical vignettes.

1. Dr. Butler is a physician who operates on hearts. He trained as a **(neurologic, cardiovascular, pulmonary)** surgeon. Often, his procedures require that Dr. Smith, a/an **(gynecologic, ophthalmic, thoracic)** surgeon, assist him when the surgical problem involves the chest and lungs.

2. Pauline noticed a rash over most of her body. First she saw Dr. Cole, her **(family practitioner, oncologist, radiologist)**, who performs her yearly physicals. Dr. Cole, who is not a/an **(endocrinologist, orthopedist, dermatologist)** by training, referred her to a skin specialist to make the proper diagnosis and treat the rash.

3. Dr. Liu is a/an **(internist, obstetrician, pediatrician)** as well as a/an **(nephrologist, urologist, gynecologist)** and can take care of her female patients before, during, and after their pregnancies.

4. After her sixth pregnancy, Sally developed an abnormal condition at the lower end of her colon. She went to a/an **(gastroenterologist, hematologist, optometrist)**, who made the diagnosis of protrusion of the rectum into the vagina. She then consulted colorectal and gynecologic surgeons to make an appropriate treatment plan for her condition, known as a **(vasculitis, rectocele, colostomy).**

5. In the cancer clinic, patients often see a medical **(oncologist, orthopedist, rheumatologist)**, who prescribes and monitors chemotherapy, and a/an **(pulmonologist, radiation oncologist, radiologist)**, a physician who prescribes and supervises the use of **(drugs, surgery, radiation)** to treat tumors with high-energy beams.

6. During a lengthy hospitalization, Janet developed a cough and fever (unrelated to any treatment or procedure she received). Her surgeon ordered a chest x-ray, which showed a/an **(oncogenic, nosocomial, iatrogenic)** pneumonia. A/an **(anesthesiologist, neurologist, infectious disease specialist)** was called in to diagnose and treat the hospital-acquired disease condition.

7. Sam had noticed bright red rectal bleeding for several days when he finally saw his family practitioner. This physician referred him to a/an **(endocrinologist, urologist, gastroenterologist).** A **(laparoscopy, colonoscopy, bronchoscopy)** was scheduled, which revealed a large pedunculated (on a stalk) polyp (benign growth) in the descending colon. See Figure 5-16. The polyp was resected and sent to the **(pathology, hematology, infectious disease)** department for evaluation. Fortunately, it was a noncancerous or **(malignant, metastatic, benign)** lesion. Sam will need follow-up **(laparotomy, endoscopy, laparoscopy)** in a year.

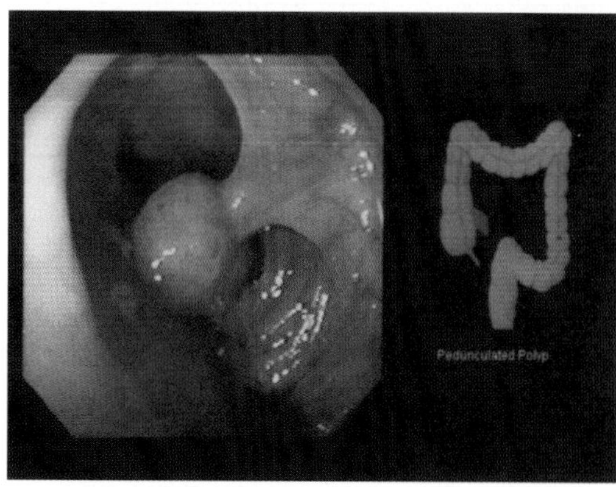

FIGURE 5-16 Pedunculated polyp in the descending colon. It arises from the mucosal surface of the colon and is projecting into the lumen of the colon.

ANSWERS TO EXERCISES

A

1. surgery
2. internal medicine
3. psychiatry
4. family practice
5. dermatology
6. ophthalmology
7. radiology
8. pediatrics
9. emergency medicine
10. anesthesiology
11. pathology

B

1. nephrologist
2. oncologist
3. orthopedist
4. gynecologist
5. ophthalmologist
6. cardiologist (internist) or cardiovascular surgeon (surgeon)
7. neurologist
8. pulmonary specialist
9. psychiatrist
10. gastroenterologist

C

1. F
2. I
3. K
4. A
5. C
6. H
7. J
8. E
9. B
10. G
11. D

D

1. infectious disease specialist
2. orthopedist
3. clinical
4. optician
5. pathologist
6. oncologist
7. optometrist
8. surgeon
9. research
10. ophthalmologist
11. geriatrician
12. hospitalist

E

1. rheumatologist
2. otolaryngologist
3. hematologist
4. urologist
5. pulmonary specialist
6. neurologist
7. oncologist
8. cardiovascular surgeon
9. orthopedist
10. endocrinologist
11. nephrologist
12. dermatologist
13. allergist
14. infectious disease specialist
15. physiatrist

F

1. nerve pain
2. study of disease
3. enlargement of the heart
4. opening from the kidney to the outside of the body
5. incision of the chest
6. pertaining to the voice box
7. inflammation of the ear
8. inflammation of the colon
9. pertaining to the lungs
10. pertaining to an abnormal condition that is produced by treatment
11. process of visual examination of the stomach (using an endoscope)
12. treatment of disease using high-energy radiation
13. study of loss of sensation or feeling
14. inflammation of the intestines (usually small intestine)
15. pertaining to a disease acquired in the hospital

G

1. otitis
2. neurectomy
3. thoracotomy
4. oncology
5. pathogenic
6. laryngitis
7. colostomy
8. ophthalmoscopy
9. psychosis
10. nephritis
11. colectomy
12. otalgia
13. psychotherapy
14. oncogenic
15. lymphadenopathy

H

1. cardiovascular, thoracic
2. family practitioner, dermatologist
3. obstetrician, gynecologist
4. gastroenterologist, rectocele
5. oncologist, radiation oncologist, radiation
6. nosocomial, infectious disease specialist
7. gastroenterologist, colonoscopy, pathology, benign, endoscopy

MEDICAL SPECIALISTS MATCHING EXERCISES (ON PAGES 180-181)

A

1. gastroenterologist
2. hematologist
3. cardiologist
4. allergist
5. endocrinologist
6. ophthalmologist
7. cardiovascular surgeon
8. anesthesiologist
9. gynecologist

B

1. urologist
2. psychiatrist
3. radiation oncologist
4. orthopedist
5. pulmonologist
6. pathologist
7. radiologist
8. nephrologist
9. neurologist

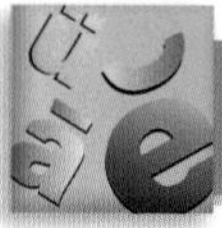

PRONUNCIATION OF TERMS

The terms that you have learned in this chapter are presented here with their pronunciations. The capitalized letters in **BOLDFACE** *represent the accented syllable. Pronounce each word out loud; then write the meaning in the space provided. Meanings of all terms can be checked with the* ***Mini-Dictionary*** *beginning on page 363 and on the audio section of the Evolve website.*

Term	Pronunciation	Meaning
anesthesiology	an-es-the-ze-**OL**-o-je	____________
cardiologist	kar-de-**OL**-o-jist	____________
cardiovascular surgeon	kar-de-o-**VAS**-ku-lar **SUR**-jun	____________
clinical	**KLIN**-ih-kal	____________
colitis	ko-**LI**-tis	____________
colorectal surgeon	ko-lo-**REK**-tal **SUR**-jun	____________
dermatologist	der-mah-**TOL**-o-jist	____________
dermatology	der-mah-**TOL**-o-je	____________
emergency medicine	e-**MER**-jen-se **MED**-ih-sin	____________
endocrinologist	en-do-krih-**NOL**-o-jist	____________
enteritis	en-teh-**RI**-tis	____________
family practitioner	**FAM**-ih-le prak-**TIH**-shun-er	____________
gastroenterologist	gas-tro-en-ter-**OL**-o-jist	____________
gastroscopy	gas-**TROS**-ko-pe	____________

geriatric	jer-e-**AH**-trik ____________
geriatrician	jer-e-ah-**TRISH**-un ____________
gynecologist	gi-neh-**KOL**-o-jist ____________
gynecology	gi-neh-**KOL**-o-je ____________
hematologist	he-mah-**TOL**-o-jist ____________
hematoma	he-mah-**TO**-mah ____________
hospitalist	**HOS**-pih-tah-list ____________
iatrogenic	i-ah-tro-**JEN**-ik ____________
infectious disease	in-**FEK**-shus dih-**ZEZ** ____________
internal medicine	in-**TER**-nal **MED**-ih-sin ____________
laryngitis	lah-rin-**JI**-tis ____________
lymphadenopathy	limf-ah-deh-**NOP**-ah-the ____________
nephrologist	neh-**FROL**-o-jist ____________
nephrostomy	neh-**FROS**-to-me ____________
neuralgia	nu-**RAL**-jah ____________
neurologist	nu-**ROL**-o-jist ____________
neurosurgeon	nu-ro-**SUR**-jun ____________
nosocomial	nos-o-**KO**-me-al ____________
obstetrician	ob-steh-**TRISH**-an ____________
obstetrics	ob-**STET**-riks ____________
oncogenic	ong-ko-**JEN**-ik ____________
oncologist	ong-**KOL**-o-jist ____________
ophthalmologist	of-thal-**MOL**-o-jist ____________
ophthalmology	of-thal-**MOL**-o-je ____________
optician	op-**TISH**-an ____________

Term	Pronunciation	
optometrist	op-**TOM**-eh-trist	____________
orthopedist	or-tho-**PE**-dist	____________
otitis	o-**TI**-tis	____________
otolaryngologist	o-to-lah-rin-**GOL**-o-jist	____________
pathologist	pah-**THOL**-o-jist	____________
pathology	pah-**THOL**-o-je	____________
pediatric	pe-de-**AT**-rik	____________
pediatrician	pe-de-ah-**TRISH**-un	____________
physiatrist	fih-**ZI**-ah-trist	____________
psychiatrist	si-**KI**-ah-trist	____________
psychosis	si-**KO**-sis	____________
pulmonary specialist	**PUL**-mo-nair-e **SPESH**-ah-list	____________
radiation oncologist	ra-de-**A**-shun ong-**KOL**-o-jist	____________
radiologist	ra-de-**OL**-o-jist	____________
radiotherapy	ra-de-o-**THER**-ah-pe	____________
rectocele	**REK**-to-sel	____________
research	**RE**-surch	____________
rheumatologist	roo-mah-**TOL**-o-jist	____________
rheumatology	roo-mah-**TOL**-o-je	____________
rhinorrhea	ri-no-**RE**-ah	____________
surgery	**SUR**-jer-e	____________
thoracic surgeon	tho-**RAS**-ik **SUR**-jun	____________
thoracotomy	tho-rah-**KOT**-o-me	____________
urologist	u-**ROL**-o-jist	____________
vasculitis	vas-ku-**LI**-tis	____________

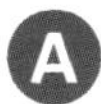

PRACTICAL APPLICATIONS

ALLIED HEALTH SPECIALISTS

This section provides three groups of exercises on allied health specialists and their job descriptions. Answers are on page 212. ***Appendix 6, Health Professions Resource****, beginning on page 353, lists health professions with education requirements, national association information, and certificate and licensing requirements.*

A Match each allied health specialist to the appropriate job description. Write your answer on the blank line.

- audiologist
- blood bank technologist
- chiropractor
- clinical laboratory technician
- dental assistant
- dental hygienist
- diagnostic medical sonographer
- dietitian/nutritionist
- nurse anesthetist
- nurse practitioner

1. Treats health problems associated with the muscular, nervous, and skeletal systems, especially the spine ____________
2. Examines, diagnoses, and treats patients under the direct supervision of a physician ____________
3. Works with people who have hearing problems by using testing devices to measure hearing loss ____________
4. Provides preventive dental care and teaches the practice of good oral hygiene ____________
5. Collects, types, and prepares blood and its components for transfusions ____________
6. Aids in the delivery of anesthesia during surgery ____________
7. Assists a dentist with dental procedures ____________
8. Performs diagnostic ultrasound procedures ____________
9. Plans nutrition programs and supervises the preparation and serving of meals ____________
10. Performs tests to examine and analyze body fluids, tissues, and cells ____________

5

B Select from the list of specialists to match the job description.

- ECG technician
- emergency medical technician/paramedic
- health information management professional
- home health aide
- licensed practical nurse
- medical assistant
- medical laboratory technician
- nuclear medicine technologist
- nursing aide
- occupational therapist

1. Cares for elderly, disabled, and ill persons in their own homes, helping them live there instead of in an institution ____________________

2. Performs routine tests and laboratory procedures ____________________

3. Designs, manages, and administers the use of heath care data and information ____________________

4. Operates an electrocardiograph to record ECGs and for Holter monitoring and stress tests ____________________

5. Performs radioactive tests and procedures under the supervision of a nuclear medicine physician, who interprets the results ____________________

6. Gives immediate care to acutely ill or injured persons and transports them to medical facilities ____________________

7. Helps physicians examine and treat patients and performs tasks to keep offices running smoothly ____________________

8. Cares for the sick, injured, convalescing, and handicapped under the direct supervision of physicians and registered nurses; provides basic bedside care ____________________

9. Helps individuals with mentally, physically, developmentally, or emotionally disabling conditions to develop, recover, or maintain daily living and working skills____________________

10. Helps care for physically or mentally ill, injured, or disabled patients confined to nursing, hospital, or residential care facilities; also known as nursing assistants or hospital attendants ____________________

C **Match the specialist to the appropriate job description.**

- ophthalmic medical technician
- phlebotomist
- physical therapist
- physician assistant
- radiation therapist
- radiographer/radiologic technologist
- registered nurse
- respiratory therapist
- speech-language pathologist
- surgical technologist

1. Evaluates, treats, and cares for patients with breathing disorders

   ____

2. Draws and tests blood under the supervision of a medical technologist or laboratory manager _______________

3. Cares for sick and injured people by assessing and recording symptoms, assisting physicians during treatments and examinations, and administering medications

   ____

4. Prepares cancer patients for treatment and administers prescribed doses of ionizing radiation to specific areas of the body _______________

5. Helps ophthalmologists provide medical eye care _______________

6. Examines, diagnoses, and treats patients under the direct supervision of a physician _______________

7. Assists in operations under the supervision of surgeons or registered nurses

   ____

8. Improves mobility, relieves pain, and prevents or limits permanent physical disabilities in patients with injuries or disease _______________

9. Produces x-ray images of parts of the body for use in diagnosing medical problems

   ____

10. Assesses and treats persons with speech, language, voice, and fluency disorders

    ____

ANSWERS TO PRACTICAL APPLICATIONS

A

1. chiropractor
2. nurse practitioner
3. audiologist
4. dental hygienist
5. blood bank technologist
6. nurse anesthetist
7. dental assistant
8. diagnostic medical sonographer
9. dietitian/nutritionist
10. clinical laboratory technician

B

1. home health aide
2. medical laboratory technician
3. health information management professional
4. ECG technician
5. nuclear medicine technologist
6. emergency medical technician/paramedic
7. medical assistant
8. licensed practical nurse
9. occupational therapist
10. nursing aide

C

1. respiratory therapist
2. phlebotomist
3. registered nurse
4. radiation therapist
5. ophthalmic medical technician
6. physician assistant
7. surgical technologist
8. physical therapist
9. radiographer/radiologic technologist
10. speech-language pathologist

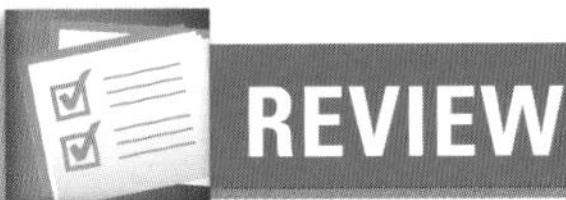

REVIEW

Test your understanding of the combining forms and suffixes used in this chapter by completing this review. Remember to check your responses with the Answers to Review on page 214.

COMBINING FORMS

Combining Form	Meaning
1. aden/o	______
2. cardi/o	______
3. col/o	______
4. dermat/o	______
5. endocrin/o	______
6. enter/o	______
7. esthesi/o	______
8. gastr/o	______
9. ger/o	______
10. gynec/o	______
11. hemat/o	______
12. iatr/o	______
13. laryng/o	______
14. lymph/o	______
15. nephr/o	______
16. neur/o	______
17. nos/o	______
18. obstetr/o	______

Combining Form	Meaning
19. onc/o	______
20. ophthalm/o	______
21. opt/o, optic/o	______
22. orth/o	______
23. ot/o	______
24. path/o	______
25. ped/o	______
26. physi/o	______
27. psych/o	______
28. pulmon/o	______
29. radi/o	______
30. rect/o	______
31. rheumat/o	______
32. rhin/o	______
33. thorac/o	______
34. ur/o	______
35. vascul/o	______

5

SUFFIXES

Suffix	Meaning	Suffix	Meaning
1. -algia	__________	10. -oma	__________
2. -ary	__________	11. -osis	__________
3. -cele	__________	12. -pathy	__________
4. -eal	__________	13. -rrhea	__________
5. -genic	__________	14. -scopy	__________
6. -ist	__________	15. -stomy	__________
7. -itis	__________	16. -therapy	__________
8. -logy	__________	17. -tomy	__________
9. -megaly	__________		

ANSWERS TO REVIEW

COMBINING FORMS

1. gland
2. heart
3. colon
4. skin
5. endocrine glands
6. intestines
7. sensation
8. stomach
9. old age
10. woman
11. blood
12. treatment
13. voice box
14. lymph
15. kidney
16. nerve
17. disease
18. midwife
19. tumor
20. eye
21. eye
22. straight
23. ear
24. disease
25. child
26. function
27. mind
28. lung
29. x-rays
30. rectum
31. flow, fluid
32. nose
33. chest
34. urinary tract
35. blood vessels

SUFFIXES

1. pain
2. pertaining to
3. hernia, protrusion
4. pertaining to
5. pertaining to producing
6. specialist
7. inflammation
8. study of
9. enlargement
10. mass, tumor
11. abnormal condition
12. disease, emotion
13. flow
14. process of visual examination
15. opening
16. treatment
17. incision

TERMINOLOGY CHECKUP

Give the difference between the following pairs of medical specialists. Write the answers on the lines provided. Confirm your answers and check the box next to each item when you know you've "got" it!

☐ 1. **orthopedist** ____________________

rheumatologist ____________________

☐ 2. **nephrologist** ____________________

urologist ____________________

☐ 3. **cardiologist** ____________________

cardiovascular surgeon ____________________

☐ 4. **pulmonologist** ____________________

otolaryngologist ____________________

thoracic surgeon ____________________

☐ 5. **neurologist** ____________________

neurosurgeon ____________________

☐ 6. **pathologist** ____________________

oncologist ____________________

hematologist ____________________

☐ 7. **radiologist** ____________________

radiation oncologist ____________________

☐ 8. **gynecologist** ____________________

obstetrician ____________________

☐ 9. **physiatrist** ____________________

psychiatrist ____________________

ANSWERS TO TERMINOLOGY CHECKUP

1. An **orthopedist** is a surgeon who diagnoses and treats bone, muscle, and joint conditions, whereas a **rheumatologist** is an internal medicine specialist who primarily diagnoses and treats disorders of joints.

2. A **nephrologist** is an internal medicine specialist who diagnoses and treats disorders of the kidneys, whereas a **urologist** is a surgeon who operates on the kidneys, urinary tract, and male reproductive organs.

3. A **cardiologist** is an internal medicine specialist who diagnoses and treats disorders of the heart, whereas a **cardiovascular surgeon** operates on the heart and blood vessels.

4. A **pulmonologist** is an internal medicine specialist who diagnoses and treats diseases of the lungs, whereas an **otolaryngologist** is a surgeon who operates on the ear, nose, throat, head, and neck. A **thoracic surgeon**, however, operates on organs in the chest, such as the heart, lungs, and esophagus.

5. A **neurologist** is an internal medicine specialist who diagnoses and treats disorders of the brain, spinal cord, and nerves, whereas a **neurosurgeon** operates on the brain, nerves, and spinal cord.

6. A **pathologist** is an internal medicine specialist who examines dead bodies (performs autopsies) and specimens of living cells (biopsies) to determine the correct diagnosis. An **oncologist**, also a specialist in internal medicine, diagnoses and treats malignant tumors. A **hematologist** is a specialist in internal medicine who diagnoses and treats disorders of the blood.

7. A **radiologist** is primarily a diagnostic physician who examines images from x-ray, CT, ultrasound, and MRI studies, whereas a **radiation oncologist** treats malignancies with high-energy radiation (photons and protons).

8. A **gynecologist** is a surgical specialist who treats diseases of the female reproductive system. An **obstetrician** specializes in the treatment of pregnant women and delivery of infants.

9. A **physiatrist** restores function after injury or illness and is also known as a physical medicine and rehabilitation specialist. A **psychiatrist** treats mental disorders.

APPENDIX 1

Body Systems

This appendix contains full-color diagrams of body systems. For each system, the material presented is divided into seven sections. **Anatomy** shows major organs and structures with labels and combining forms (in parentheses) for each body part. The parts of the body are defined and explained in the ***Mini-Dictionary*** (beginning on page 363). **Terminology** reviews combining forms and their meanings and gives examples of medical terminology using each combining form. **Pathology** explains terms related to common pathological conditions. **Laboratory Tests and Diagnostic Procedures** presents common tests and procedures, which can be cross-referenced for additional information in ***Appendix 3, Diagnostic Tests and Procedures***. **Treatment Procedures** explains therapies that treat abnormal conditions in each system. **Abbreviations** lists selected abbreviations for easy reference. **Matching Exercises** review the terminology to reinforce your understanding; answers to all exercises are provided, beginning on page 293.

Use this appendix both as a study guide for classroom work and as a reference for your work in the medical field.

Cardiovascular System 218

Digestive System 226

Endocrine System 234

Female Reproductive System 240

Lymphatic System 246

Male Reproductive System 250

Musculoskeletal System 255

Nervous System 265

Respiratory System 271

Skin and Sense Organs 279

Urinary System 287

CARDIOVASCULAR SYSTEM

ANATOMY

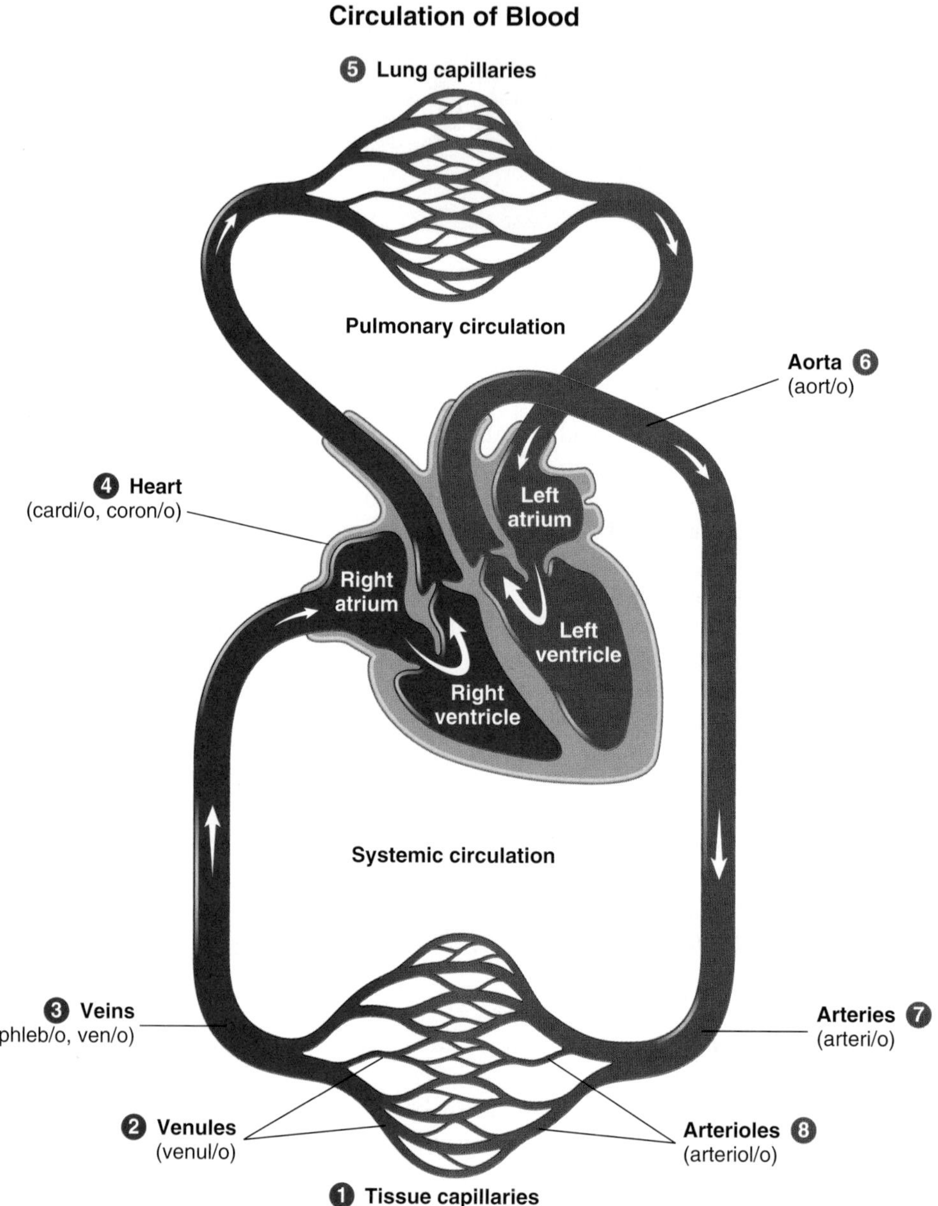

Red vessels contain blood that is rich in oxygen. Blue vessels contain blood that is oxygen-poor. Arrows show the path of blood flow from the **tissue capillaries** ❶ through **venules** ❷ and **veins** ❸ toward the **heart** ❹, to the **lung capillaries** ❺, back to the heart, out of the **aorta** ❻ to the **arteries** ❼ and **arterioles** ❽, and then back to the tissue capillaries.

TERMINOLOGY

Meanings for terminology are found in the ***Mini-Dictionary***, beginning on page 363.

Combining Form	Meaning	Terminology	Meaning
angi/o	vessel	angioplasty	_______________
aort/o	aorta	aortic stenosis	_______________
arteri/o	artery	arteriosclerosis	_______________
arteriol/o	arteriole	arteriolitis	_______________
cardi/o	heart	cardiomyopathy	_______________
		pericardium	_______________
coron/o	heart	coronary arteries	_______________
phleb/o	vein	phlebotomy	_______________
ven/o	vein	intravenous	_______________
venul/o	venule	venulitis	_______________

PATHOLOGY

Definitions for additional terms in **boldface** are found in the ***Mini-Dictionary***.

Aneurysm: Local widening of an artery caused by weakness in the arterial wall or breakdown of the wall from **atherosclerosis.**

Angina: Chest pain caused by decreased blood flow to heart muscle. Also called angina pectoris (PECT/O means chest). *See page 186 for a case report related to a patient with angina.*

Arrhythmia: Abnormal heartbeat (rhythm); **fibrillation** and **flutter** are examples.

Atherosclerosis: Hardening of arteries with a collection of cholesterol-like plaque.

Congestive heart failure: Inability of the heart to pump its required amount of blood. Blood accumulates in the lungs, causing **pulmonary edema.**

Hypertension: High blood pressure. Essential hypertension is high blood pressure with no apparent cause. In secondary hypertension, another illness (kidney disease or an adrenal gland disorder) is the cause of the high blood pressure.

Myocardial infarction: Heart attack. An **infarct** is an area of dead (**necrotic**) tissue.

Shock: Group of signs and symptoms (paleness of skin, weak and rapid pulse, shallow breathing) indicating poor oxygen supply to tissues and insufficient return of blood to the heart.

LABORATORY TESTS AND DIAGNOSTIC PROCEDURES

Consult ***Appendix 3***, beginning on page 307, for pronunciation of terms and additional information.

Angiography: Recording (via x-ray images) blood vessels after the injection of contrast into the bloodstream.
Cardiac catheterization: Introducing a catheter (flexible, tubular instrument) into coronary blood vessels to measure pressure and flow patterns of blood.
Cardiac enzyme tests: Measurements of enzymes released into the bloodstream after a heart attack (myocardial infarction).
Doppler ultrasound: Measuring blood flow in vessels via sound waves.
Echocardiography: Images of the heart are produced using sound waves.
Electrocardiography: Recording electricity flowing through the heart.
Holter monitoring: Detection of abnormal heart rhythms (**arrhythmias**) that involves having a patient wear a compact version of an electrocardiograph for 24 hours.
Lipid tests: Measurements of cholesterol and triglyceride levels in the blood.
Lipoprotein tests: Measurements of **high-density lipoprotein (HDL)** and **low-density lipoprotein (LDL)** in the blood.
Magnetic resonance imaging (MRI): Producing an image, by beaming magnetic waves at the heart, that gives detailed information about congenital heart disease, cardiac masses, and disease within large blood vessels.
MUGA scan: Imaging the motion of heart wall muscles and assessing the function of the heart via a multiple-gated acquisition scan, which uses radioactive chemicals.
Positron emission tomography (PET) scan: Radioactive chemicals, which release radioactive particles, are injected into the bloodstream and travel to the heart. Cross-sectional images show the flow of blood and the functional activity of the heart muscle.
Stress test: An electrocardiogram plus blood pressure and heart rate measurements shows the heart's response to physical exertion (treadmill test).
Technetium Tc 99m sestamibi scan: A radioactive pharmaceutical (sestamibi "tagged" with technetium-99m) is injected intravenously to show perfusion (flow) of blood in heart muscle. It is taken up in the area of a myocardial infarction, producing "hot spots." In an ETT-MIBI exercise tolerance test, an intravenous radioactive substance is given before the patient reaches maximal heart rate on a treadmill.
Thallium-201 scan: A radioactive test that shows where injected thallium-201 (a radioactive substance) localizes in heart muscle.

TREATMENT PROCEDURES

Cardiac catheter ablation: Flexible tube is threaded through blood vessels into the heart to destroy (ablate) abnormal tissue that causes arrhythmias.
Cardioversion: Brief discharges of electricity passing across the chest to stop a cardiac **arrhythmia.** Also called **defibrillation.**
Coronary artery bypass grafting (CABG): Vessels taken from the patient's legs or chest are connected to coronary arteries to make detours around blockages.

Endarterectomy: Surgical removal of the innermost lining of an artery to remove fatty deposits and clots.
Heart transplantation: A donor heart is transferred to a recipient.
Percutaneous coronary intervention (PCI): A balloon-tipped catheter (a flexible, tubular instrument) is threaded into a coronary artery to compress fatty deposits and open the artery. **Stents** (expandable slotted tubes) create wider openings that make the recurrence of blockages less likely. Also called **balloon angioplasty.**
Thrombolytic therapy: Drugs such as tPA (tissue plasminogen activator) and streptokinase are injected into a patient's bloodstream to dissolve clots that may cause a heart attack.

ABBREVIATIONS

See ***Appendix 4***, beginning on page 329, for a more complete list of medical abbreviations.

AAA	Abdominal aortic aneurysm
ACS	Acute coronary syndrome (disease changes in coronary arteries leading to plaque/clot formation and heart attack or other heart problems)
AED	Automated external defibrillator (electronic device that can diagnose and treat serious arrhythmias)
AMI	Acute myocardial infarction (heart attack)
BP	Blood pressure
CABG	Coronary artery bypass grafting (surgical placement of vessels, either vein or artery, to detour blocked coronary arteries)
CAD	Coronary artery disease
CCU	Coronary care unit
CHF	Congestive heart failure (heart is unable to pump its required amount of blood)
CPR	Cardiopulmonary resuscitation
ECG	Electrocardiography
ECHO *or* **Echo**	Echocardiography
HDL	High-density lipoprotein
HTN	Hypertension (high blood pressure)
ICD	Implantable cardioverter-defibrillator
LDL	Low-density lipoprotein (combination of fat and protein; high cholesterol content and associated with formation of plaque in arteries)
MI	Myocardial infarction (heart attack)
PCI	Percutaneous coronary intervention (placement of a catheter and stent in a coronary artery to open the artery; balloon angioplasty)

MATCHING EXERCISES

The following exercises will help you review terminology related to the cardiovascular system. Answers begin on page 293.

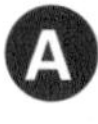 **Match the term in Column I with its meaning in Column II. These terms are illustrated in the diagram on page 218 and are defined in the *Mini-Dictionary,* beginning on page 363.**

Column I		Column II
1. aorta	______	A. Blood vessels that carry blood to the heart from the body tissues
2. lung capillaries	______	B. Largest artery in the body
3. arteries	______	C. Tiny blood vessels that lie near cells and through whose walls gases, food, and wastes can pass
4. arterioles	______	
5. venules	______	D. Small veins
6. veins	______	E. Small arteries
7. pulmonary circulation	______	F. Blood vessels that carry blood away from the heart
8. systemic circulation	______	G. Passage of blood from the heart to the body tissues and back
9. tissue capillaries	______	H. Hollow muscular organ that pumps blood all over the body
10. heart	______	I. Tiny blood vessels surrounding lung tissue through which gases pass into and out of the blood
		J. Passage of blood from the heart to the lungs and back to the heart

B Match the combining form in Column I with its meaning in Column II.

Column I		Column II
1. phleb/o	_____	A. Artery
2. arteriol/o	_____	B. Vessel
3. angi/o	_____	C. Heart
4. venul/o	_____	D. Vein
5. arteri/o	_____	E. Small artery
6. coron/o	_____	F. Small vein

C Match the medical term in Column I with its meaning in Column II.

Column I		Column II
1. intravenous	_____	A. Inflammation of small veins
2. arteriosclerosis	_____	B. Narrowing of the largest artery
3. phlebotomy	_____	C. Disease of heart muscle
4. cardiomyopathy	_____	D. Pertaining to within a vein
5. angioplasty	_____	E. Inflammation of small arteries
6. arteriolitis	_____	F. Hardening of arteries
7. venulitis	_____	G. Incision of a vein
8. aortic stenosis	_____	H. Surgical repair of blood vessels
9. pericardium	_____	I. Pertaining to the heart
10. coronary	_____	J. Membrane surrounding the heart

D Match the pathologic condition in Column I with its meaning in Column II.

Column I		Column II
1. hypertension	_____	A. Abnormal heartbeat
2. atherosclerosis	_____	B. Local widening of an artery
3. angina	_____	C. Heart attack
4. shock	_____	D. Chest pain
5. myocardial infarction	_____	E. High blood pressure
6. arrhythmia	_____	F. Inability of the heart to pump its required amount of blood
7. congestive heart failure	_____	G. Group of signs and symptoms: pale skin, weak rapid pulse, and shallow respirations
8. aneurysm	_____	H. Hardening of arteries with cholesterol-like plaque

E Match the test or procedure in Column I with its description in Column II.

Column I		Column II
1. lipid tests	_____	A. Sound waves produce images of the heart
2. MUGA scan	_____	B. X-ray images of blood vessels after contrast is injected into the bloodstream
3. lipoprotein tests	_____	C. Measurement of HDL and LDL in blood
4. Holter monitoring	_____	D. Recording electricity through the heart
5. angiography	_____	E. Measurement of substances in the blood that indicate a heart attack
6. cardiac enzyme test	_____	F. Sound waves measure blood flow in vessels
7. electrocardiography	_____	G. Abnormal heart rhythms are detected with a compact ECG over a 24-hour period
8. echocardiography	_____	H. Radioactive test to detect blood perfusion in heart muscle
9. sestamibi scan	_____	I. Measurement of triglyceride and cholesterol levels in the blood
10. Doppler ultrasound	_____	J. Radioactive chemicals and a scanner produce images of the motion of the heart wall

F **Match the treatment procedure in Column I with its description in Column II.**

Column I		Column II
1. cardioversion	_____	A. Surgery to detour around blockages in coronary arteries
2. thrombolytic therapy	_____	B. Drugs such as tPA dissolve clots that may cause a heart attack
3. heart transplantation	_____	C. Balloon-tipped catheter with stent opens coronary arteries
4. endarterectomy	_____	D. Flexible tube is threaded into the heart; abnormal tissue is destroyed
5. CABG	_____	E. Brief discharges of electricity stop a cardiac arrhythmia
6. PCI	_____	F. Removal of innermost lining of an artery to eliminate fatty deposits
7. cardiac catheter ablation	_____	G. Donor heart is transferred to a recipient

DIGESTIVE SYSTEM

ANATOMY

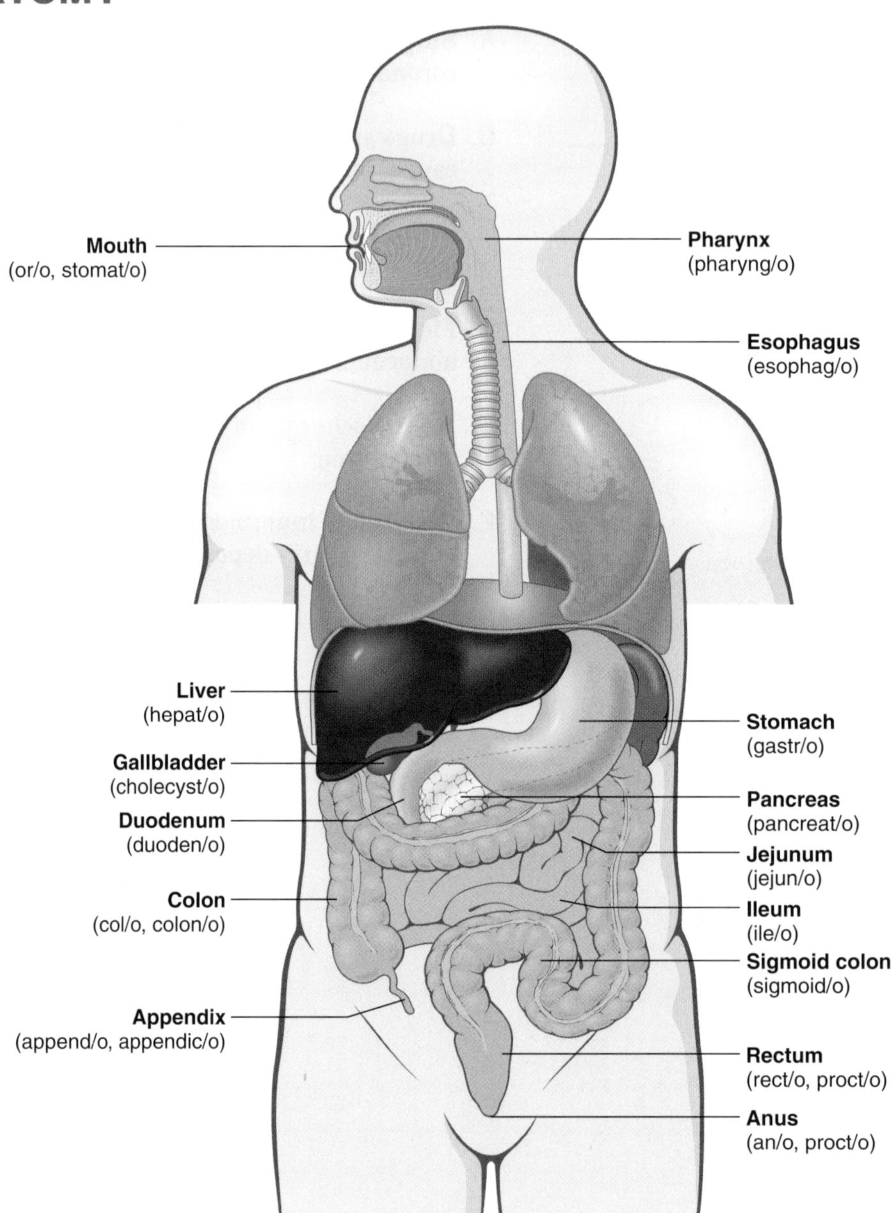

Food enters the body via the mouth and travels through the **pharynx**, **esophagus**, and **stomach** to the small intestine (**duodenum**). The **liver**, **gallbladder**, and **pancreas** make and store chemicals that aid in the digestion of foods. Digested (broken-down) food is absorbed into the bloodstream through the walls of the small intestine (**jejunum** and **ileum**). Any substance that cannot be absorbed continues into the **colon** (large intestine) and leaves the body through the **rectum** and **anus**. *(Modified from Chabner D-E:* The Language of Medicine, *ed 12, St. Louis, 2021, Elsevier.)*

TERMINOLOGY

Meanings for terminology are found in the ***Mini-Dictionary***.

Combining Form	Meaning	Terminology	Meaning
an/o	anus	anal	______
append/o	appendix	appendectomy	______
appendic/o	appendix	appendicitis	______
cholecyst/o	gallbladder	cholecystectomy	______
col/o	colon	colostomy	______
colon/o	colon	colonoscopy	______
duoden/o	duodenum	duodenal	______
esophag/o	esophagus	esophageal	______
gastr/o	stomach	gastralgia	______
hepat/o	liver	hepatomegaly	______
ile/o	ileum	ileostomy	______
jejun/o	jejunum	gastrojejunostomy	______
or/o	mouth	oral	______
pancreat/o	pancreas	pancreatitis	______
pharyng/o	pharynx	pharyngeal	______
proct/o	anus and rectum	proctoscopy	______
rect/o	rectum	rectocele	______
sigmoid/o	sigmoid colon	sigmoidoscopy	______
stomat/o	mouth	stomatitis	______

PATHOLOGY

Definitions for additional terms in **boldface** are found in the ***Mini-Dictionary***.

Cholelithiasis: Abnormal condition of gallstones.
Cirrhosis: Chronic disease of the liver with degeneration of liver cells.
Colonic polyposis: Condition in which **polyps** protrude from the mucous membrane lining the colon.
Diverticulosis: Abnormal condition of small pouches or sacs (**diverticula**) in the wall of the intestine (often the colon). **Diverticulitis** is inflammation and infection within diverticula.
Gastroesophageal reflux disease (GERD): A condition in which contents of the stomach flow back into the esophagus.
Hepatitis: Inflammation of the liver.
Inflammatory bowel disease (IBD): Inflammation of the terminal (last) portion of the ileum (**Crohn disease**) or inflammation of the colon (**ulcerative colitis**).
Irritable bowel syndrome (IBS): Signs and symptoms are cramping, abdominal bloating, constipation, and diarrhea. Although IBS causes distressing symptoms, it does not permanently harm the intestine. Its cause is unknown.
Hepatocellular carcinoma (HCC): Cancer (primary) of the liver.
Jaundice: Yellow-orange coloration of the skin and other tissues, from high levels of **bilirubin** in the bloodstream (**hyperbilirubinemia**).
Peptic ulcer: Open sore (lesion) that develops in the lining of the stomach (gastric ulcer) or the first part of the small intestine (duodenal ulcer). *See page 191 for a case report related to peptic ulcers.*

LABORATORY TESTS AND DIAGNOSTIC PROCEDURES

Consult ***Appendix 3*** for pronunciation of terms and additional information.

Abdominal computed tomography (CT) scan: A series of cross-sectional x-ray images that show abdominal organs.
Abdominal magnetic resonance imaging (MRI): Magnetic and radio waves create images of abdominal organs and tissues in all three planes of the body.
Abdominal ultrasonography: Process of beaming sound waves into the abdomen to produce images of organs, such as the gallbladder. **Endoscopic ultrasonography** is useful to detect enlarged lymph nodes and tumors in the upper abdomen.
Barium tests: X-ray examinations using a liquid barium mixture to locate disorders of the gastrointestinal tract. In a **barium enema (lower GI series),** barium is injected into the anus and rectum, and x-ray images are taken of the colon. In an **upper GI series (barium swallow),** barium is taken in through the mouth, and x-ray images reveal the esophagus, stomach, and small intestine.
Cholangiography: X-ray examination of the bile ducts (CHOLANGI/O-) after the injection of contrast material through the liver (**percutaneous transhepatic cholangiography**) or through a catheter (a flexible, tubular instrument) from the mouth, esophagus, and stomach into the bile ducts (**endoscopic retrograde cholangiopancreatography,** or **ERCP**).

Gastrointestinal endoscopy: Visual examination of the gastrointestinal tract with an endoscope. Examples are **esophagoscopy, gastroscopy, colonoscopy,** and **sigmoidoscopy.**
Hemoccult test: Feces are placed on paper containing the chemical guaiac, which reacts with hidden (occult) blood. This is an important screening test for colon cancer.
Laparoscopy: Visual examination of the abdominal cavity through an endoscope inserted in the abdomen.
Liver function tests (LFTs): Measurements of liver enzymes and other substances in the blood. Enzyme levels increase when the liver is damaged (as in hepatitis). Examples of liver enzymes are **ALT, AST,** and **alkaline phosphatase (alk phos).** High **bilirubin** (blood pigment) levels indicate **jaundice** caused by liver disease or other problems affecting the liver.
Stool culture: Feces (stools) are placed in a growth medium (culture) to test for microorganisms (such as bacteria).

TREATMENT PROCEDURES

Anastomosis: Surgical creation of an opening between two gastrointestinal organs. Examples are gastrojejunostomy, cholecystojejunostomy, and choledochoduodenostomy (CHOLEDOCH/O means common bile duct).
Colostomy: Surgical creation of a new opening of the colon to the outside of the body.
Ileostomy: Surgical creation of a new opening of the ileum to the outside of the body.
Laparoscopic surgery: Removal of organs or tissues via a laparoscope (instrument inserted into the abdomen through a small incision). Examples are **laparoscopic cholecystectomy** and **laparoscopic appendectomy,** which are types of **minimally invasive surgery or keyhole surgery.**

ABBREVIATIONS

ALT, AST Alanine transaminase and aspartate transaminase (liver enzymes measured as part of LFTs)
BE Barium enema (barium, a contrast agent, is introduced through the rectum, and x-ray pictures of the colon are taken)
ERCP Endoscopic retrograde cholangiopancreatography
GB Gallbladder
GERD Gastroesophageal reflux disease
GI Gastrointestinal
HCC Hepatocellular carcinoma
IBD Inflammatory bowel disease (Crohn disease and ulcerative colitis)
IBS Irritable bowel syndrome
LFTs Liver function tests (ALT, AST, bilirubin)
NPO Nothing by mouth (Latin, *nil per os*)
TPN Total parenteral nutrition (intravenous solutions are given to maintain nutrition)

MATCHING EXERCISES

The following exercises will help you review terminology related to the digestive system. Answers begin on page 293.

A Match the term in Column I with its description in Column II.

Column I		Column II
1. mouth	_____	A. Organ that receives food from the esophagus and sends it to the intestine
2. pharynx	_____	B. Third part of the small intestine
3. esophagus	_____	C. Throat
4. stomach	_____	D. Second part of the small intestine
5. duodenum	_____	E. Large intestine
6. jejunum	_____	F. First part of the small intestine
7. ileum	_____	G. Opening that is the beginning of the digestive system
8. colon	_____	H. Tube that carries food to the stomach

B Match the term in Column I with its description in Column II.

Column I		Column II
1. sigmoid colon	_____	A. Opening of the colon to the outside of the body
2. rectum	_____	B. Sac that stores bile
3. anus	_____	C. S-shaped lower portion of the large intestine
4. appendix	_____	D. Organ that makes bile, stores sugar, and produces proteins to clot blood
5. liver	_____	E. Gland that makes both digestive juices and insulin (hormone)
6. gallbladder	_____	F. Small sac that hangs from the beginning of the large intestine
7. common bile duct	_____	G. Tube that carries bile from the liver and gallbladder to the intestine
8. pancreas	_____	H. Final section of the colon

C Match the combining form in Column I with its meaning in Column II.

Column I		Column II
1. gastr/o	_____	A. Mouth
2. col/o	_____	B. Endocrine and exocrine gland near the stomach
3. proct/o	_____	C. Third part of the small intestine
4. cholecyst/o	_____	D. Stomach
5. pharyng/o	_____	E. Liver
6. or/o	_____	F. First part of the small intestine
7. hepat/o	_____	G. Large intestine
8. duoden/o	_____	H. Anus and rectum
9. ile/o	_____	I. Gallbladder
10. pancreat/o	_____	J. Throat

D Match the term in Column I with its meaning in Column II.

Column I		Column II
1. hepatomegaly	_____	A. Pertaining to the tube leading from the throat to the stomach
2. cholecystectomy	_____	B. Pain of the stomach
3. proctoscopy	_____	C. Enlargement of the liver
4. ileostomy	_____	D. Inflammation of the mouth
5. stomatitis	_____	E. Pertaining to the first part of the small intestine
6. gastrojejunostomy	_____	F. Removal of the gallbladder
7. pancreatitis	_____	G. Visual examination of the anus and rectum
8. duodenal	_____	H. New opening of the third part of the small intestine to the outside of the body
9. esophageal	_____	I. New opening between the stomach and second part of the small intestine
10. gastralgia	_____	J. Inflammation of a gland adjacent to the stomach

E Match the pathologic condition in Column I with its meaning in Column II.

Column I		Column II
1. hepatitis	_____	A. Yellow-orange coloration of the skin and other tissues
2. cirrhosis	_____	B. Abnormal condition of small pouches or sacs in the wall of the intestine
3. cholelithiasis	_____	C. Ulcerative colitis and Crohn disease
4. colonic polyposis	_____	D. Inflammation of the liver
5. jaundice	_____	E. Abnormal condition of gallstones
6. inflammatory bowel disease	_____	F. Chronic disease of the liver with degeneration of liver cells
7. diverticulosis	_____	G. Small growths protrude from the mucous membrane lining the intestine
8. irritable bowel syndrome	_____	H. Contents of the stomach flow backwards into the esophagus
9. hepatocellular carcinoma	_____	I. Signs and symptoms of GI distress, but no lesions found in the GI tract
10. gastroesophageal reflux disease	_____	J. Primary cancer of the liver

F Match the test or procedure in Column I with its description in Column II.

Column I		Column II
1. LFTs	_____	A. X-ray examination of bile ducts
2. abdominal CT	_____	B. Minimally invasive surgery of the abdomen
3. cholangiography	_____	C. Visual examination of the gastrointestinal tract (colonoscopy)
4. stool culture	_____	D. Feces are placed in a growth medium and tested for microorganisms
5. GI endoscopy	_____	E. Cholecystojejunostomy
6. hemoccult test	_____	F. Magnetic waves create images of abdominal organs in three planes of the body
7. barium tests	_____	G. Measurements of liver enzymes (ALT, AST, alk phos) and other substances
8. abdominal MRI	_____	H. Feces are tested for blood; stool guaiac test
9. anastomosis	_____	I. Series of cross-sectional x-ray images that shows abdominal organs
10. laparoscopic surgery	_____	J. X-ray images of the GI tract obtained after introduction of a radiopaque liquid into the rectum or mouth

ENDOCRINE SYSTEM

ANATOMY

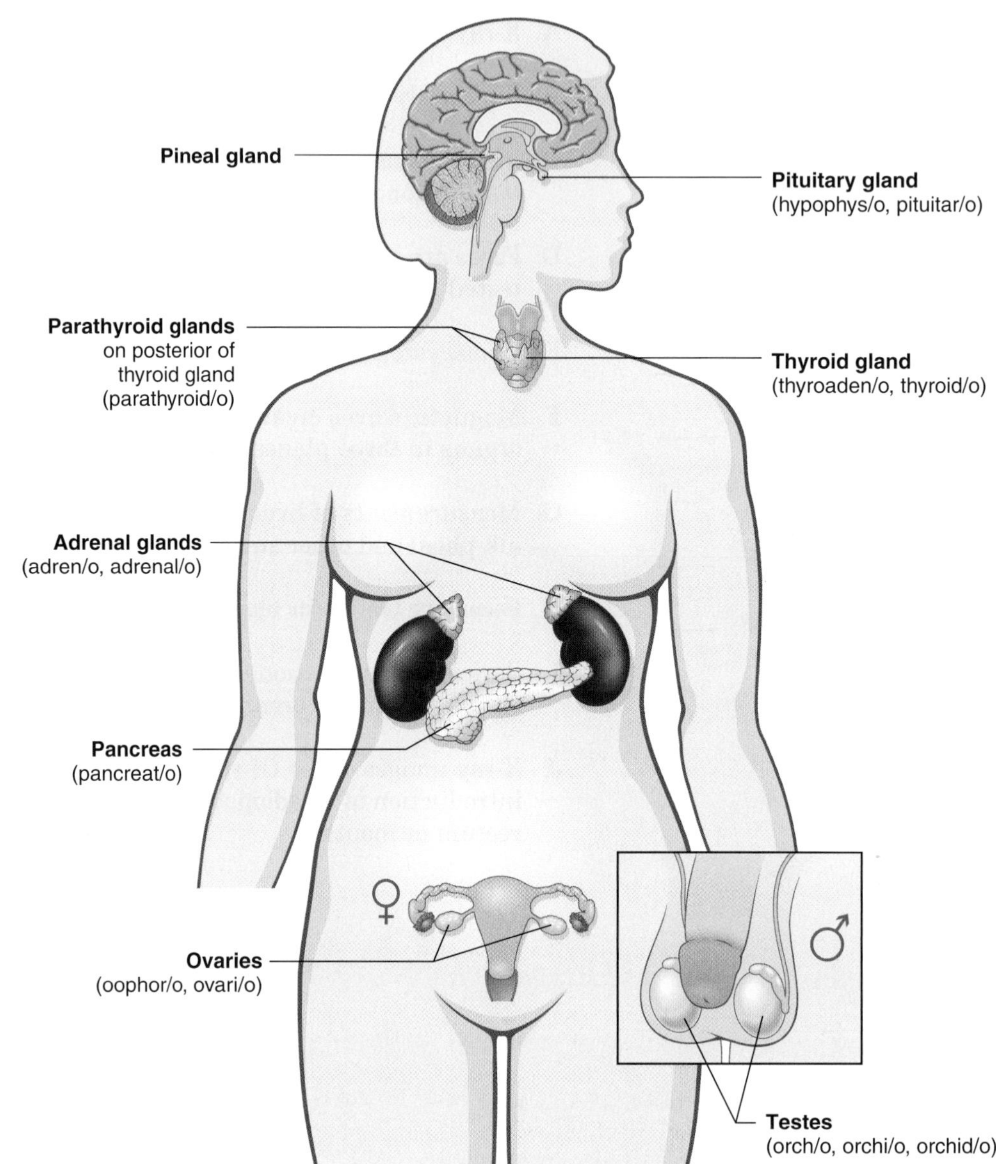

Endocrine glands secrete (form and give off) hormones into the bloodstream. The hormones travel throughout the body, affecting organs (including other endocrine glands) and controlling their actions. *(Modified from Chabner D-E:* The Language of Medicine, *ed 12, St. Louis, 2021, Elsevier.)*

TERMINOLOGY

Meanings for terminology are found in the ***Mini-Dictionary.***

Combining Form	Meaning	Terminology
adren/o	adrenal gland	adrenopathy ________________
adrenal/o	adrenal gland	adrenalectomy ________________
hypophys/o	pituitary gland	hypophyseal ________________
oophor/o	ovary	oophoritis ________________
ovari/o	ovary	ovarian cyst ________________
orch/o	testis	orchitis ________________
orchi/o	testis; testicle	orchiopexy ________________
orchid/o	testis; testicle	orchidectomy ________________
pancreat/o	pancreas	pancreatectomy ________________
parathyroid/o	parathyroid gland	hyperparathyroidism ________________
pituitar/o	pituitary gland	hypopituitarism ________________
thyroaden/o	thyroid gland	thyroadenitis ________________
thyroid/o	thyroid gland	thyroidectomy ________________

PATHOLOGY

Definitions for additional terms in **boldface** are found in the ***Mini-Dictionary***.

Acromegaly: Enlargement of extremities caused by hypersecretion from the anterior portion of the pituitary gland after puberty.

Cushing syndrome: Group of clinical features produced by excess secretion of **cortisol** from the adrenal cortex. These signs and symptoms include obesity, moon-like facies (fullness of the face), **hyperglycemia,** and **osteoporosis.**

Diabetes mellitus: Disorder of the pancreas that causes an increase in blood glucose levels (hyperglycemia). **Type 1 diabetes,** with onset usually in childhood, involves complete deficiency of **insulin** in the body. **Type 2 diabetes,** with onset usually in adulthood, involves some insulin deficiency and resistance of tissues to the action of insulin. *See page 193 for a case report of a patient with type 1 diabetes.*

Goiter: Enlargement of the thyroid gland.
Hyperthyroidism: Overactivity of the thyroid gland; also called **Graves disease** or **exophthalmic** (eyeballs bulge outward) **goiter.**

LABORATORY TESTS AND DIAGNOSTIC PROCEDURES

Consult ***Appendix 3*** for pronunciation of terms and additional information.

Computed tomography (CT scan): Cross-sectional x-ray images of the pituitary gland and other endocrine organs.
Exophthalmometry: Measurement of eyeball protrusion (**exophthalmos**) as an indicator of **Graves disease** (**hyperthyroidism**).
Fasting blood sugar (glucose) test: Measurement of glucose levels in a blood sample taken from a fasting patient and in specimens taken 30 minutes, 1 hour, 2 hours, and 3 hours after the ingestion of 75 g of glucose. Delayed return of blood glucose to normal levels indicates **diabetes mellitus.**
Magnetic resonance imaging (MRI): Magnetic waves produce images of the **hypothalamus,** pituitary gland, and other endocrine organs in all three planes of the body.
Radioactive iodine uptake: Measurement of how much of a radioactive element (iodine) is absorbed by the thyroid gland. The radioactive iodine is given by mouth and measured as evidence of thyroid function.
Serum and urine tests: Measurement of hormones, **electrolytes** (such as sodium and potassium), and glucose levels in blood (serum) and urine as indicators of endocrine function.
Thyroid function tests: Measurement of levels of T4 (thyroxine), T3 (triiodothyronine), and TSH (thyroid-stimulating hormone) in the bloodstream.
Thyroid scan: Procedure in which a radioactive compound, injected intravenously, localizes in the thyroid gland. A scanning device produces an image showing the presence of tumors or nodules in the gland.

BODY SYSTEMS

ABBREVIATIONS

ACTH Adrenocorticotropic hormone (from the pituitary gland)
DM Diabetes mellitus
GH Growth hormone (secreted by the pituitary gland)
GTT Glucose tolerance test (measures the ability to respond to a glucose load; test for diabetes mellitus)
HbA1c Hemoglobin A1c measures the average amount of glucose in red blood cells. Useful to follow control of glucose in diabetic patients.
K+ Potassium (an electrolyte)
Na+ Sodium (an electrolyte)
RAIU Radioactive iodine uptake (test for thyroid function)
T3 Triiodothyronine (hormone from the thyroid gland)
T4 Thyroxine (hormone from the thyroid gland)
TSH Thyroid-stimulating hormone (from the pituitary gland)

MATCHING EXERCISES

The following exercises will help you review terminology related to the endocrine system. Answers begin on page 293.

A Match the term in Column I with its location in Column II.

Column I		Column II
1. thyroid gland	_____	A. Two paired male glands located in the scrotal sac
2. ovaries	_____	B. Organ at the base of the brain in the sella turcica (round depression at the base of the skull)
3. testes	_____	C. Gland in the neck on either side of the trachea
4. parathyroid glands	_____	D. Two glands, one above each kidney
5. pituitary gland	_____	E. Gland adjacent to the stomach
6. pancreas	_____	F. Four glands behind the thyroid gland
7. adrenal glands	_____	G. Two paired organs in the female abdomen

B **Match the combining form in Column I with the secretion or function in Column II.**

Column I		Column II
1. hypophys/o	_____	A. Regulates calcium in the blood and bones
2. orchid/o	_____	B. Secretes epinephrine (adrenaline) and cortisol
3. oophor/o	_____	C. Secretes insulin, which allows sugar to enter cells
4. thyroaden/o	_____	D. Secretes testosterone
5. pancreat/o	_____	E. Secretes growth hormone and hormones that control the thyroid gland, ovaries, and testes
6. adren/o	_____	F. Secretes estrogen and progesterone
7. parathyroid/o	_____	G. Secretes thyroxine (T4), which increases metabolism of body cells

C **Match the medical term in Column I with its meaning in Column II.**

Column I		Column II
1. thyroadenitis	_____	A. Disease of the adrenal glands
2. oophoritis	_____	B. Pertaining to the pituitary gland
3. orchiopexy	_____	C. Inflammation of the thyroid gland
4. hyperparathyroidism	_____	D. Removal of the thyroid gland
5. thyroidectomy	_____	E. Surgical fixation of an undescended testicle
6. adrenopathy	_____	F. Increased secretion of parathyroid hormone
7. hypophyseal	_____	G. Inflammation of an ovary

D Match the pathologic condition in Column I with its description in Column II.

Column I		Column II
1. diabetes mellitus	_____	A. Enlargement of the thyroid gland
2. acromegaly	_____	B. Hypersecretion of cortisone from the adrenal glands
3. goiter	_____	C. Deficiency of insulin leading to high blood sugar levels
4. Cushing syndrome	_____	D. Enlargement of extremities caused by increased growth hormone from the pituitary gland
5. hyperthyroidism	_____	E. Overactivity of the thyroid gland

E Match the test or procedure in Column I with its description in Column II.

Column I		Column II
1. thyroid scan	_____	A. Measures blood glucose levels
2. exophthalmometry	_____	B. Radioactive compound, injected intravenously, localizes in the thyroid gland; images are produced
3. fasting blood sugar	_____	C. Measures hormones, electrolytes, and sugar in blood and urine
4. thyroid function testing	_____	D. Measures localization of an element necessary for making thyroid hormone
5. CT scan	_____	E. Measures eyeball protrusion
6. serum and urine testing	_____	F. Cross-sectional x-ray images of endocrine organs
7. radioactive iodine uptake	_____	G. Measures T3, T4, and TSH levels in the blood

FEMALE REPRODUCTIVE SYSTEM

ANATOMY

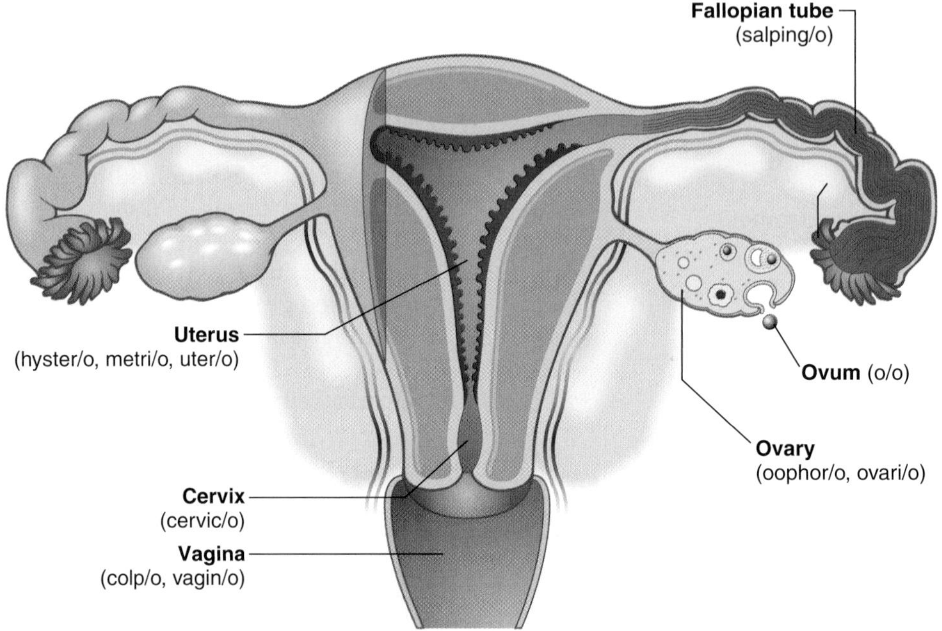

An egg cell **(ovum)** is produced in the **ovary** and travels through the **fallopian tube**. If a sperm cell is present and fertilization (the union of the egg and sperm cell) takes place, the resulting cell (embryo) may implant in the lining of the **uterus.** The embryo (later called the fetus) develops in the uterus for nine months and is delivered from the body through the **cervix** and **vagina**. *(Modified from Chabner D-E:* The Language of Medicine, *ed 12, St. Louis, 2021, Elsevier.)*

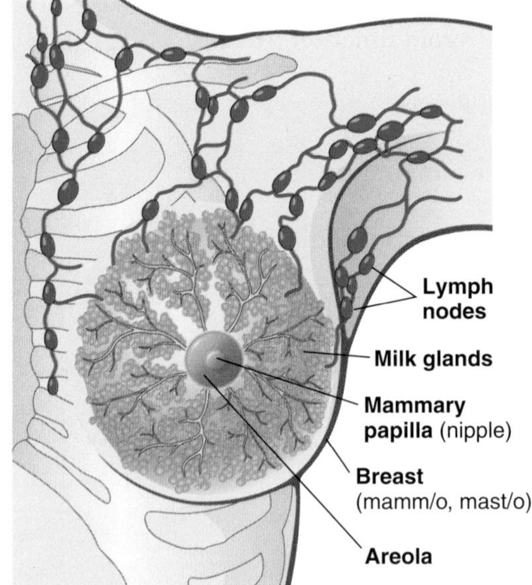

The **breast** contains glandular tissue that produces milk after delivery of an infant. The **areola** is the dark-pigmented area surrounding the **mammary papilla** (breast nipple). There are numerous **lymph nodes** around the breast and in the underarm (axilla). *(Modified from Chabner D-E:* The Language of Medicine, *ed 12, St. Louis, 2021, Elsevier.)*

TERMINOLOGY

Meanings for terminology are found in the ***Mini-Dictionary***.

Combining Form	Meaning	Terminology	Meaning
cervic/o	cervix	cervical	
colp/o	vagina	colposcopy	
vagin/o	vagina	vaginitis	
hyster/o	uterus	hysterectomy	
mamm/o	breast	mammogram	
mast/o	breast	mastectomy	
metri/o	uterus	endometrium	
uter/o	uterus	uterine	
o/o	egg	oocyte	
oophor/o	ovary	oophorectomy	
ovari/o	ovary	ovarian cancer	
salping/o	fallopian tube	salpingectomy	

PATHOLOGY

Definitions for additional terms in **boldface** are found in the ***Mini-Dictionary***.

Amenorrhea: Absence of menstrual flow.
Dysmenorrhea: Painful menstrual flow.
Ectopic pregnancy: Pregnancy (gestation) that is not in the uterus; usually occurs in a fallopian tube.
Endometriosis: Tissue from the inner lining of the uterus (**endometrium**) is found abnormally in other pelvic or abdominal locations (**fallopian tubes, ovaries,** or **peritoneum**).
Fibroids: Benign tumors in the uterus. Also called **leiomyomas;** LEI/O means smooth (referring to **visceral muscle** within an internal organ). *See page 188 for a case report related to fibroids.*
Menorrhagia: Excessive discharge of blood (-RRHAGIA) from the uterus during menstruation.
Pelvic inflammatory disease: Inflammation (often caused by bacterial infection) in the region of the pelvis. Because the condition primarily affects the fallopian tubes, it is also called **salpingitis.**

LABORATORY TESTS AND DIAGNOSTIC PROCEDURES

Consult ***Appendix 3*** for pronunciation of terms and additional information.

Amniocentesis: Puncture of the amnion (sac surrounding the developing fetus).
Aspiration: Withdrawal of fluid from a cavity or sac. In breast aspiration, a needle is used to remove fluid from cystic lesions in the breast. The fluid is analyzed for the presence of malignant cells.
Colposcopy: Visual examination of the vagina and cervix with a colposcope (a small magnifying instrument resembling a mounted pair of binoculars).
Conization: Removal of a wedged-shaped section (cone) of the cervix for **biopsy.**
Hysterosalpingography: X-ray imaging of the uterus and fallopian tubes after injection of a contrast agent into the uterus.
Mammography: X-ray imaging (recording) of the breast.
Pap smear: Insertion of an instrument (spatula) into the vagina to obtain a sample of cells from the cervix (neck of the uterus). Microscopic analysis of the smear can detect the presence of cervical cancer.
Pelvic ultrasonography: Recording (imaging) of sound waves as they impact organs in the region of the hip. In transvaginal ultrasound, a sound probe is placed in the vagina.
Pregnancy test: Measurement of human chorionic gonadotropin (HCG), a hormone in blood and urine that indicates pregnancy.

TREATMENT PROCEDURES

Cauterization: Heat is used to destroy abnormal tissue, for example, in the lining of the **cervix** (lower neck-like region of the uterus).
Cryosurgery: Use of cold temperatures (often liquid nitrogen) to freeze and destroy tissue (such as the lining of the cervix).
Dilation and curettage (D&C): Widening (dilation or dilatation) of the opening of the cervix and scraping (curettage) of the lining of the uterus to remove tissue and stop prolonged or heavy uterine bleeding.
Hysterectomy: Excision of the uterus either through the abdominal wall (abdominal hysterectomy) or through the vagina (vaginal hysterectomy)
Myomectomy: The surgical removal of **fibroid (myoma)** tissue from the uterus. **Uterine artery embolization** may be used instead to shrink the fibroids. Tiny pellets are injected into the uterine artery. The pellets act as emboli to block blood flow to fibrous tissue.
Tubal ligation: Fallopian tubes are tied off (ligated) and cut to prevent pregnancy.

ABBREVIATIONS

CS	Cesarean section (fetus is removed through an abdominal incision)
D&C	Dilation and curettage
DUB	Dysfunctional uterine bleeding (not associated with menstruation)
GYN	Gynecology
HRT	Hormone replacement therapy (estrogen and progesterone)
IVF	In vitro fertilization (egg and sperm are combined outside the body in a laboratory container; fertilized eggs are injected into the uterus for pregnancy)
OB	Obstetrics (labor and delivery of a fetus)
PID	Pelvic inflammatory disease (salpingitis, oophoritis, endometritis; leading causes are sexually transmitted infections)
STI	Sexually transmitted infection; also called STD (sexually transmitted disease)
TAH-BSO	Total abdominal hysterectomy with bilateral salpingo-oophorectomy (entire uterus and both fallopian tubes and ovaries are removed)

MATCHING EXERCISES

The following exercises will help you review terminology related to the female reproductive system. Answers begin on page 294.

A Match the term in Column I with its meaning in Column II.

Column I		Column II
1. ovary	_____	A. Muscular passageway from the uterus to the outside of the body
2. cervix	_____	B. Neck (lower portion) of the uterus
3. fallopian tube	_____	C. One of two paired organs in the female abdomen that produce egg cells and hormones
4. vagina	_____	D. One of two paired tubes that lead from the ovaries to the uterus
5. uterus	_____	E. One of two paired organs containing glands that produce milk after childbirth
6. breast	_____	F. Muscular organ that holds and provides nourishment for the developing fetus

B Match the combining form in Column I with its meaning in Column II.

Column I		Column II
1. oophor/o	_____	A. Uterus
2. colp/o	_____	B. Fallopian tube
3. salping/o	_____	C. Neck of the uterus
4. hyster/o	_____	D. Ovary
5. cervic/o	_____	E. Vagina
6. mast/o	_____	F. Breast

C Match the medical term in Column I with its meaning in Column II.

Column I		Column II
1. salpingectomy	_____	A. Visual examination of the vagina
2. mammography	_____	B. Pertaining to the lower, neck-like region of the uterus
3. vaginitis	_____	C. Inflammation of the breast
4. colposcopy	_____	D. Removal of a fallopian tube
5. hysterectomy	_____	E. Inner lining of the uterus
6. cervical	_____	F. X-ray imaging of the breast
7. endometrium	_____	G. Resection of the uterus
8. mastitis	_____	H. Inflammation of the vagina

D Match the pathologic condition in Column I with its meaning in Column II.

Column I		Column II
1. fibroids	_____	A. Absence of menstrual flow
2. dysmenorrhea	_____	B. Excessive discharge of blood from the uterus during menstruation
3. endometriosis	_____	C. Leiomyomas (benign muscle growths) in the uterus
4. ectopic pregnancy	_____	D. Uterine tissue found in sites (ovary, fallopian tubes) other than in the uterus
5. amenorrhea	_____	E. Painful menstrual flow
6. pelvic inflammatory disease	_____	F. Salpingitis
7. menorrhagia	_____	G. Embryo develops outside the uterus

E Match the test or procedure in Column I with its description in Column II.

Column I		Column II
1. pregnancy test	_____	A. Endoscopic visual examination of the vagina
2. pelvic ultrasonography	_____	B. Withdrawal of fluid from a cavity or sac
3. conization	_____	C. Removal of a section of the cervix for biopsy
4. colposcopy	_____	D. X-ray imaging of the breast
5. mammography	_____	E. X-ray examination of the uterus and fallopian tubes
6. Pap smear	_____	F. Sound wave image of organs in the hip region
7. hysterosalpingography	_____	G. Secretions from the vagina and cervix are examined microscopically
8. aspiration	_____	H. Measurement of HCG levels
9. amniocentesis	_____	I. Puncture to remove fluid from the sac surrounding the fetus

F Match the treatment procedure in Column I with its description in Column II.

Column I		Column II
1. myomectomy	_____	A. Use of cold temperatures to freeze and destroy tissue
2. cryosurgery	_____	B. Fallopian tubes are tied to prevent pregnancy
3. cauterization	_____	C. Removal of fibroids from the uterus
4. tubal ligation	_____	D. Widening the cervix and scraping the lining of the uterus
5. D&C	_____	E. Use of heat to destroy abnormal tissue

LYMPHATIC SYSTEM

ANATOMY

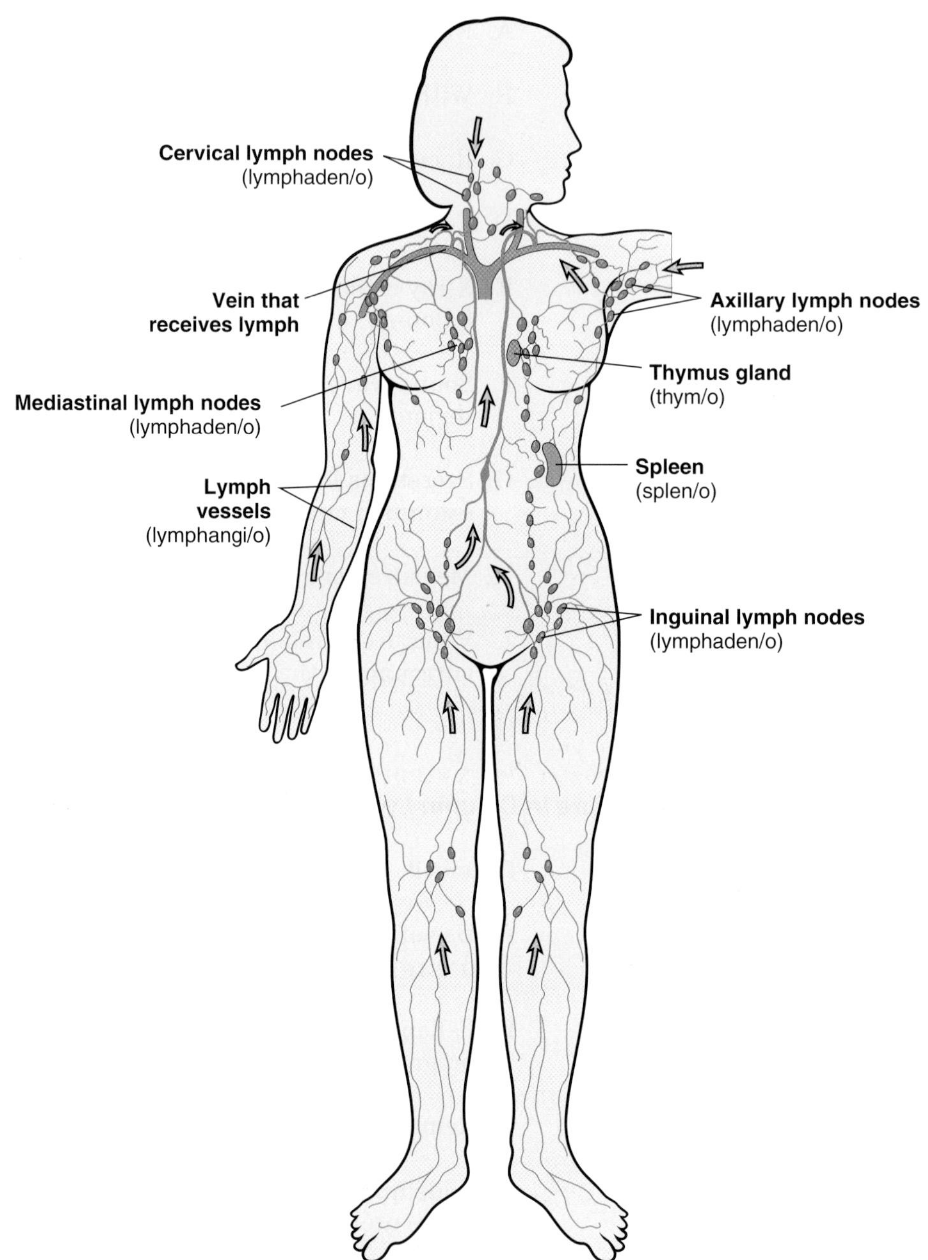

Lymph originates in the tissue spaces around cells and travels in **lymph vessels** and through **lymph nodes** to a large vein in the neck, where it enters the bloodstream. Arrows in the figure indicate the direction of lymph flow. Lymph contains white blood cells (lymphocytes), which help the body fight disease. The **spleen** produces lymphocytes and disposes of dying blood cells. The **thymus gland** stimulates the production of lymphocytes. *(Modified from Chabner D-E:* The Language of Medicine, *ed 12, St. Louis, 2021, Elsevier.)*

TERMINOLOGY

Meanings for terminology are found in the ***Mini-Dictionary.***

Combining Form	Meaning	Terminology	Meaning
lymph/o	lymph fluid	lymphedema	_______________
lymphaden/o	lymph node ("gland")	lymphadenectomy	_______________
		lymphadenopathy	_______________
lymphangi/o	lymph vessel	lymphangiectasis	_______________
splen/o	spleen	splenomegaly	_______________
thym/o	thymus gland	thymoma	_______________

PATHOLOGY

Definitions for additional terms in **boldface** are found in the ***Mini-Dictionary.***

Acquired immunodeficiency syndrome (AIDS): Suppression or deficiency of the immune response (destruction of **lymphocytes**) caused by exposure to **human immunodeficiency virus (HIV).**

Lymphoma: Malignant tumor of lymph nodes and lymphatic tissue. **Hodgkin lymphoma** is an example of a lymphoma. *See page 189 for a case report related to Hodgkin lymphoma.*

Mononucleosis: Acute infectious disease with enlargement of lymph nodes and increased numbers of **lymphocytes** and **monocytes** in the bloodstream.

Sarcoidosis: Inflammatory disease in which small nodules, or tubercles, form in lymph nodes and other organs. SARC/O means flesh, and -OID means resembling.

LABORATORY TESTS AND DIAGNOSTIC PROCEDURES

Consult ***Appendix 3*** for pronunciation of terms and additional information.

Computed tomography (CT) scan: X-ray views in the transverse plane for the diagnosis of abnormalities in lymphoid organs (lymph nodes, spleen, and thymus gland).

ELISA (enzyme-linked immunosorbent assay): Test to screen for antibodies to the **human immunodeficiency virus (HIV),** which causes **acquired immunodeficiency syndrome (AIDS).**

Western blot test: A blood test to detect the presence of antibodies to specific antigens, such as the **human immunodeficiency virus.** It is regarded as a more precise test than the ELISA.

TREATMENT PROCEDURES

Chemotherapy: Treatment with powerful drugs to kill cancer cells (**Hodgkin lymphoma, non-Hodgkin lymphoma,** and **multiple myeloma**) and viruses such as the **human immunodeficiency virus.**

Radiotherapy (radiation therapy): Treatment with high-dose radiation to destroy malignant lesions in the body.

ABBREVIATIONS

AIDS	Acquired immunodeficiency syndrome
ELISA	Enzyme-linked immunosorbent assay (test to detect anti-HIV antibodies)
HAART	Highly active antiretroviral therapy (for AIDS)
HIV	Human immunodeficiency virus
IgA, IgD, IgE, IgG, IgM	Immunoglobulins (antibodies)
MAC	*Mycobacterium avium* complex (a group of pathogens that cause lung disease in patients with depressed immune systems)
PCP	*Pneumocystis* pneumonia (opportunistic infection seen in patients with AIDS)

MATCHING EXERCISES

The following exercises will help you review terminology related to the lymphatic system. Answers begin on page 294.

A Match the term in Column I with its meaning in Column II.

Column I		Column II
1. lymph nodes	_____	A. Blood-forming organ in early life; later a storage organ for red blood cells and a source of lymphocytes
2. thymus	_____	B. Gland in the mediastinum; produces lymphocytes, which play an important role in immunity.
3. lymph	_____	C. Stationary collections of lymph tissue throughout the body
4. spleen	_____	D. Clear fluid, present in tissue spaces, that circulates in lymph vessels
5. lymph vessels	_____	E. Small tubes that carry lymph fluid throughout the body

B Match the combining form in Column I with its meaning in Column II.

Column I		Column II
1. thym/o	_____	A. Spleen
2. lymphangi/o	_____	B. Lymph fluid
3. lymphaden/o	_____	C. Thymus gland
4. splen/o	_____	D. Lymph vessels
5. lymph/o	_____	E. Lymph nodes (glands)

C Match the medical term in Column I with its meaning in Column II.

Column I		Column II
1. lymphadenopathy	_____	A. Malignant tumor of lymph nodes and lymphatic tissue
2. lymphangiectasis	_____	B. Acute infectious disease with enlargement of lymph nodes and increase in lymphocytes and monocytes
3. splenomegaly	_____	C. Accumulation of lymph fluid in tissue spaces, causing swelling
4. lymphoma	_____	D. Widening, dilation of lymph vessels
5. lymphadenectomy	_____	E. Enlargement of an abdominal organ that produces lymphocytes
6. mononucleosis	_____	F. Excision of lymph nodes
7. lymphedema	_____	G. Disease of lymph nodes

D Match the procedure or test in Column I with its description in Column II.

Column I		Column II
1. ELISA	_____	A. Treatment with high-dose radiation to destroy malignant tissue
2. Western blot	_____	B. X-ray images in a cross-sectional plane for diagnosis of lymph node abnormalities
3. chemotherapy	_____	C. Precise blood test to detect antibodies to specific antigens, as in HIV infection
4. CT scan	_____	D. Screening test for antibodies to the AIDS virus
5. radiotherapy	_____	E. Treatment with powerful drugs to kill cancer cells

MALE REPRODUCTIVE SYSTEM

ANATOMY

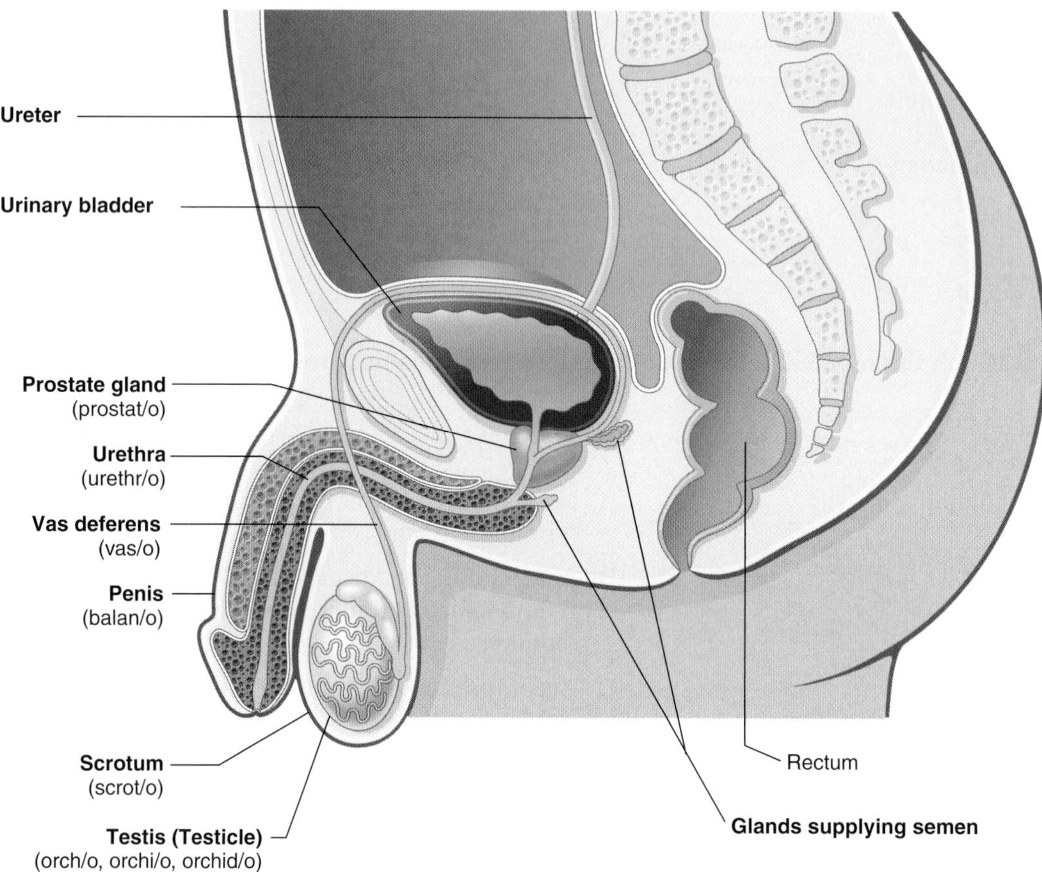

Sperm cells are produced in the testes (*singular:* **testis**) and travel up into the body, through the **vas deferens,** and around the urinary bladder. The vas deferens unites with the **urethra,** which opens to the outside of the body through the **penis.** The **prostate gland** and the other glands near the **urethra** produce a fluid (semen) that leaves the body with sperm cells. *(Modified from Chabner D-E:* The Language of Medicine, *ed 12, St. Louis, 2021, Elsevier.)*

TERMINOLOGY

Meanings for terminology are found in the ***Mini-Dictionary.***

Combining Form	Meaning	Terminology	Meaning
balan/o	penis	balanitis	______________
orch/o **orchi/o**	testis; pl. testes	orchitis	______________
		orchiectomy	______________
orchid/o	testis	orchidectomy	______________
prostat/o	prostate gland	prostatectomy	______________
scrot/o	scrotum	scrotal	______________
urethr/o	urethra	urethritis	______________
vas/o	vas deferens	vasectomy	______________

PATHOLOGY

Definitions for additional terms in **boldface** are found in the ***Mini-Dictionary.***

Benign prostatic hyperplasia: Noncancerous enlargement of the prostate gland.
Cryptorchism: Condition of undescended testis. The testis is not in the scrotal sac at birth. CRYPT/O means hidden.
Hydrocele: Sac of clear fluid (swelling) in the scrotum. HYDR/O means water, and -CELE indicates a hernia (a bulging or swelling).
Prostatic carcinoma: Cancer of the prostate gland (prostate cancer).
Sexually transmitted infections: These affect both males and females and are spread by sexual or other genital contact. Examples are **chlamydial infection, gonorrhea, herpes genitalis,** and **syphilis.**
Testicular carcinoma: Malignant tumor of the testis. An example is a **seminoma.**
Varicocele: Enlarged, swollen veins near a testicle. VARIC/O means swollen veins.

LABORATORY TESTS AND DIAGNOSTIC PROCEDURES

Consult ***Appendix 3*** for pronunciation of terms and additional information.

Digital rectal examination (DRE): Examination of the prostate gland with finger palpation through the rectum.
Prostate-specific antigen (PSA): Measurement of the amount of PSA in the blood. Higher than normal levels are associated with prostate enlargement and cancer.
Semen analysis: Measurement of the number, shape, and motility of sperm cells.

TREATMENT PROCEDURES

Orchiopexy: Surgical fixation (-PEXY) of an undescended testicle in a young male infant.

Transurethral resection of the prostate gland (TURP): The removal of portions of the prostate gland with an **endoscope** inserted into the urethra. **Photoselective vaporization of the prostate** (GreenLight PVP) is a newer technique that uses a laser to treat benign prostatic hyperplasia.

Vasectomy: Procedure in which the vas deferens on each side is cut, a piece is removed, and the free ends are folded and ligated (tied) with sutures. Vasectomy produces sterilization so that sperm are not released with semen.

ABBREVIATIONS

BPH	Benign prostatic hyperplasia
DRE	Digital rectal examination
GU	Genitourinary
PSA	Prostate-specific antigen
STI	Sexually transmitted infection; also called STD (sexually transmitted disease)
TURP	Transurethral resection of the prostate gland

MATCHING EXERCISES

The following exercises will help you review terminology related to the male reproductive system. Answers begin on page 294.

A Match the term in Column I with its meaning in Column II.

Column I

1. scrotum _____
2. penis _____
3. vas deferens _____
4. testis _____
5. prostate _____

Column II

A. One of two paired male organs in the scrotum that produces sperm cells and male hormones

B. External male organ, containing the urethra, through which both urine and semen (sperm cells and fluid) leave the body

C. Sac on the outside of the body that contains the testes

D. One of two tubes that carry sperm cells from the testes to the outside of the body

E. Male organ that surrounds the base of the urinary bladder and produces fluid that leaves the body together with sperm

B Match the combining form in Column I with its meaning in Column II.

Column I		Column II
1. prostat/o	_____	A. Tube leading from the urinary bladder to the outside of the body
2. vas/o	_____	B. Gland that produces fluid portion of semen
3. orch/o	_____	C. Penis
4. scrot/o	_____	D. Testis
5. balan/o	_____	E. Tube carrying sperm cells from the testis to the ejaculatory duct and urethra
6. urethr/o	_____	F. Sac containing the testes

C Match the medical term in Column I with its meaning in Column II.

Column I		Column II
1. urethritis	_____	A. Resection of the prostate gland
2. scrotal	_____	B. Inflammation of the penis
3. vasectomy	_____	C. Inflammation of a testis
4. orchitis	_____	D. Inflammation of the urethra
5. prostatectomy	_____	E. Pertaining to the sac containing the testes
6. orchidectomy	_____	F. Resection of a piece of each vas deferens
7. balanitis	_____	G. Excision of a testicle

D Match the pathologic condition in Column I with its meaning in Column II.

Column I		Column II
1. varicocele	_____	A. Undescended testicle
2. benign prostatic hyperplasia	_____	B. Malignant tumor of the prostate gland
3. hydrocele	_____	C. Hernia (collection of fluid) in the scrotal sac
4. testicular carcinoma	_____	D. Malignant tumor; one type is a seminoma
5. prostatic carcinoma	_____	E. Swollen, twisted veins near the testis
6. cryptorchism	_____	F. Nonmalignant enlargement of the prostate gland

E Match the test or procedure in Column I with its description in Column II.

Column I		Column II
1. orchiopexy	_____	A. Measurement of the number, shape, and motility of sperm cells
2. vasectomy	_____	B. Measures blood levels of prostate-specific antigen
3. TURP	_____	C. Examination of the prostate gland with finger palpation through the rectum
4. DRE	_____	D. Removal of portions of the prostate gland with an endoscope inserted into the urethra
5. semen analysis	_____	E. Surgical fixation of an undescended testicle
6. PSA test	_____	F. Two tubes that carry sperm from the testicles are cut and tied off

MUSCULOSKELETAL SYSTEM

ANATOMY

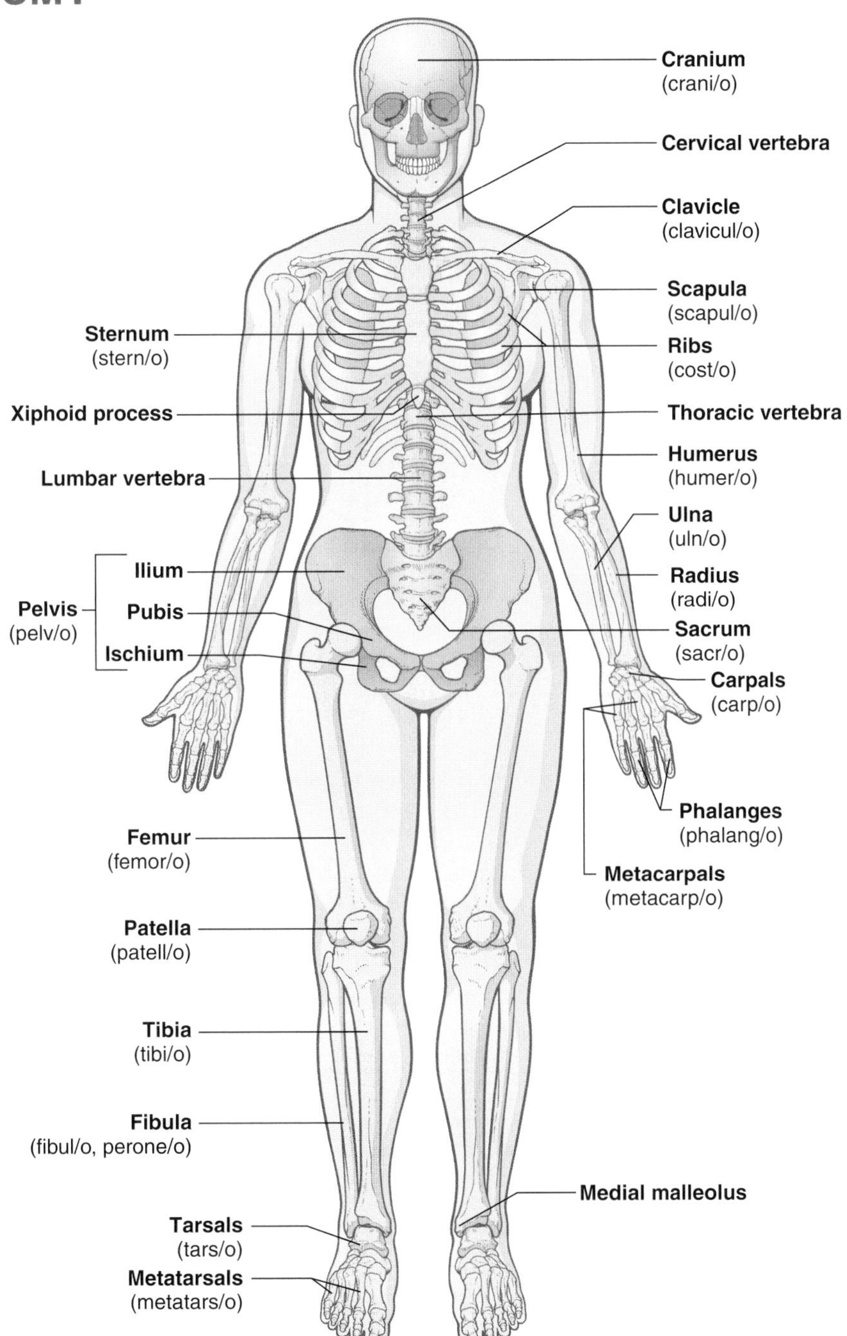

Bones are connected to **muscles** that contract to move the body. **Joints** are the spaces between bones. Near the joints are **ligaments** that connect bones to other bones and **tendons** that connect bones to muscles. *(Modified from Chabner D-E:* The Language of Medicine*, ed 12, St. Louis, 2021, Elsevier.)*

For your reference, included here are anterior and posterior views of superficial muscles in the body.

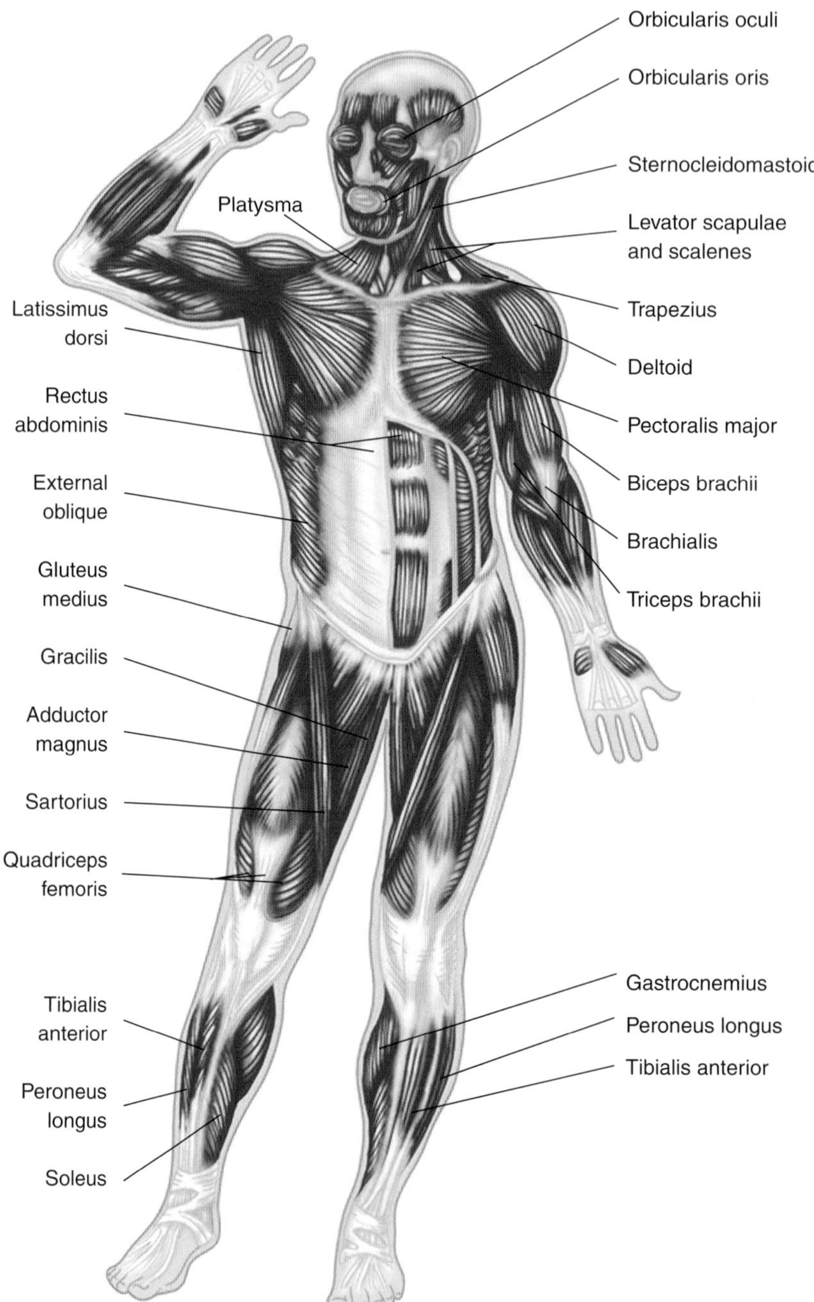

The **anterior superficial muscles.** *(Modified from* Miller-Keane Encyclopedia & Dictionary of Medicine, Nursing, & Allied Health*, ed 7, Philadelphia, 2003, Elsevier.)*

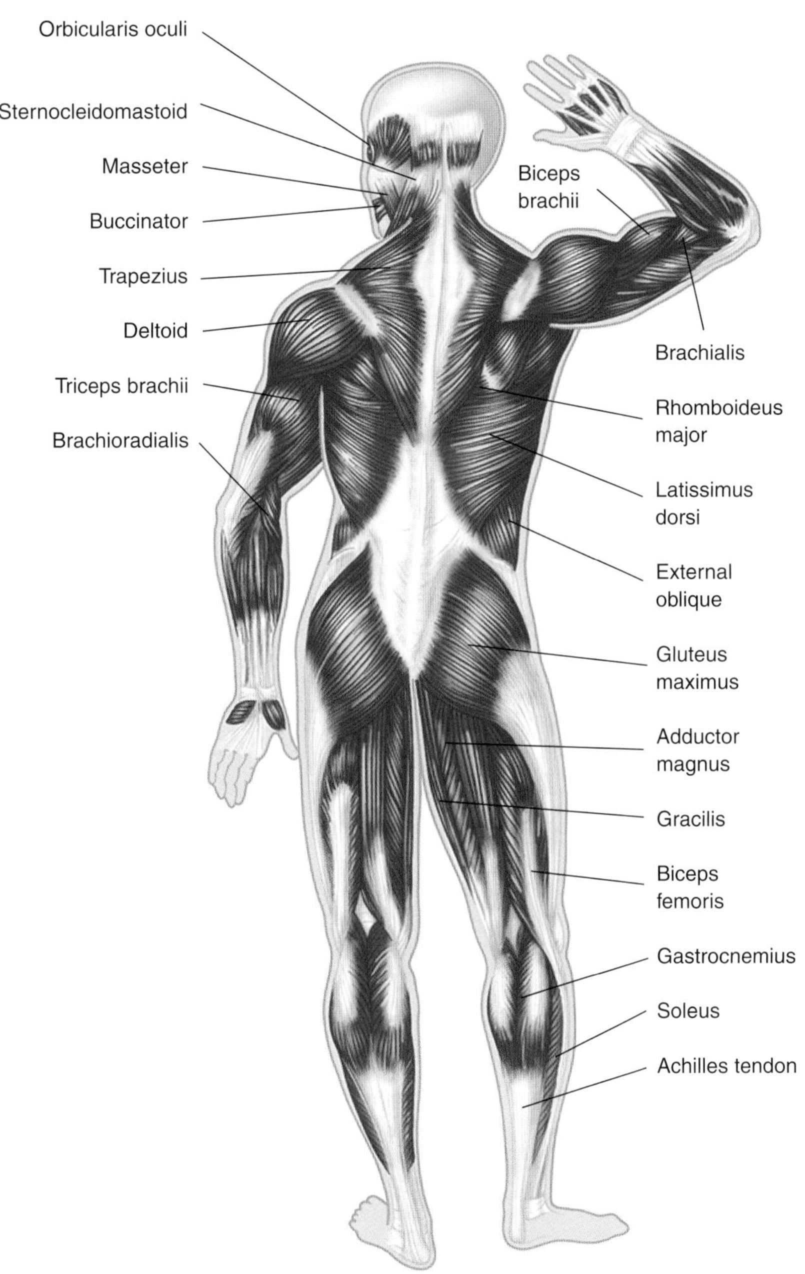

The **posterior superficial muscles.** *(Modified from* Miller-Keane Encyclopedia & Dictionary of Medicine, Nursing, & Allied Health, *ed 7, Philadelphia, 2003, Elsevier.)*

TERMINOLOGY

Meanings for terminology are found in the *Mini-Dictionary.*

Combining Form	Meaning	Terminology	Meaning
arthr/o	joint	arthroscopy	________
chondr/o	cartilage	chondroma	________
cost/o	rib	costochondritis	________
crani/o	skull	craniotomy	________
ligament/o	ligament	ligamentous	________
leiomy/o	smooth (visceral involuntary) muscle	leiomyosarcoma ________ *This type of muscle is attached to internal organs.*	
muscul/o	muscle	muscular	________
my/o	muscle	myosarcoma	________
myos/o	muscle	myositis	________
myel/o	bone marrow	myelodysplasia	________
oste/o	bone	osteomyelitis	________
pelv/o	pelvis; hip area	pelvic	________
rhabdomy/o	skeletal (striated, voluntary) muscle	rhabdomyolysis ________ *This type of muscle is attached to bones.*	
spin/o	backbones	spinal stenosis	________
spondyl/o	vertebra	spondylosis	________
vertebr/o	vertebra	intervertebral	________
ten/o	tendon	tenorrhaphy	________
tendin/o	tendon	tendinitis	________

PATHOLOGY

Definitions for additional terms in **boldface** are found in the ***Mini-Dictionary.***

Ankylosing spondylitis: Chronic, progressive **arthritis** with stiffening (**ankylosis**) of joints, primarily of the spine and hip.
Carpal tunnel syndrome: Compression of the median nerve as it passes between the ligament and the bones and tendons of the wrist.
Fracture: Breaking of a bone
Gouty arthritis: Inflammation of joints caused by excessive uric acid. Also called **gout.**
Muscular dystrophy: An inherited disorder characterized by progressive weakness and degeneration of muscle fibers.
Osteoporosis: Decrease in bone density with thinning and weakening of bone. -POROSIS means condition of containing passages or spaces.
Rhabdomyolysis: Breakdown of damaged skeletal muscle
Rheumatoid arthritis: Chronic inflammation of joints; pain, swelling, and stiffening, especially in the small joints of the hands and feet. RHEUMAT/O means flowing, descriptive of the swelling in joints.

LABORATORY TESTS AND DIAGNOSTIC PROCEDURES

Consult ***Appendix 3*** for pronunciation of terms and additional information.

Antinuclear antibody (ANA) test: Test in which a sample of plasma is tested for the presence of antibodies found in patients with systemic lupus erythematosus.
Arthrocentesis: Puncture to remove fluid from a joint.
Arthrography: X-ray imaging of a joint.
Arthroscopy: Visual examination of a joint with an arthroscope.
Bone density test: Low-energy x-rays are used to image bones in the spinal column, pelvis, and wrist to detect areas of bone deficiency. Also called bone density scanning, dual-energy x-ray absorptiometry (DEXA), or bone densitometry.
Bone scan: Procedure in which a radioactive substance is injected intravenously and its uptake in bones is measured with a special scanning device.
Calcium level: Measurement of the amount of calcium in a sample of blood (serum). This test is important in evaluating diseases of bone.
Electromyography (EMG): Recording of the electrical activity of muscle tissue. This test reveals the strength of muscles.
Erythrocyte sedimentation rate (ESR): Measurement of the rate at which red blood cells fall to the bottom of a test tube. High sedimentation rates are associated with inflammatory diseases such as **rheumatoid arthritis.**
Muscle biopsy: The removal of muscle tissue for microscopic examination.
Uric acid test: Measurement of the amount of uric acid (nitrogenous waste) in a sample of blood. High uric acid levels are associated with gouty arthritis.

TREATMENT PROCEDURES

Arthroplasty: Surgical repair of a joint. Total hip arthroplasty is the replacement of the head of the femur (thigh bone) and acetabulum (cup-shaped portion of the hip socket) with artificial parts (**prostheses**) that are cemented into the bone.

Laminectomy: Removal of a piece of backbone (lamina) to relieve pressure on nerves from a herniated disc.

Microscopic discectomy: Surgical removal of a herniated intervertebral disc with an incision that is 1 to 2 inches long and visualization of the surgical field with an operating microscope.

Vertebroplasty: Surgical repair of vertebrae. Special cement is injected into backbones to strengthen them and to relieve pain caused by compression fractures.

ABBREVIATIONS

ACL	Anterior cruciate ligament (of the knee)
ANA	Antinuclear antibody
C1-C7	Cervical vertebrae
Ca	Calcium
DEXA	Dual-energy x-ray absorptiometry
DJD	Degenerative joint disease
DOMS	Delayed-onset muscle soreness
EMG	Electromyography
ESR	Erythrocyte sedimentation rate
Fx	fracture
IM	Intramuscular
L1-L5	Lumbar vertebrae
NSAID	Nonsteroidal anti-inflammatory drug (prescribed to treat joint and muscle pain)
Ortho	Orthopedics (*or* orthopaedics)
PT	Physical therapy
ROM	Range of motion
T1-T12	Thoracic vertebrae
THR	Total hip replacement
TKR	Total knee replacement
TMJ	Temporomandibular joint

MATCHING EXERCISES

The following exercises will help you review terminology related to the musculoskeletal system. Answers begin on page 295.

A Match the term in Column I with its description in Column II.

Column I		Column II
1. cranium	_____	A. Finger bones
2. clavicle	_____	B. Thigh bone
3. humerus	_____	C. Kneecap
4. radius	_____	D. Lower arm bone on the thumb side
5. ulna	_____	E. Collarbone
6. carpals	_____	F. Tailbone
7. metacarpals	_____	G. Breastbone
8. phalanges	_____	H. Skull
9. scapula	_____	I. Ankle bones
10. sternum	_____	J. Lower arm bone (little finger side)
11. tarsals	_____	K. Upper arm bone
12. metatarsals	_____	L. Smaller of the lower leg bones
13. fibula	_____	M. Hip area
14. tibia	_____	N. Lower part of the backbone near the hip
15. patella	_____	O. Bones surrounding the chest cavity
16. sacrum	_____	P. Larger of the lower leg bones
17. coccyx	_____	Q. Hand bones
18. pelvis	_____	R. Wrist bones
19. femur	_____	S. Foot bones
20. ribs	_____	T. Shoulder bone

B Match the combining form in Column I with its meaning in Column II.

Column I		Column II
1. crani/o	_____	A. Backbone
2. arthr/o	_____	B. Cartilage
3. oste/o	_____	C. Joint
4. cost/o	_____	D. Skull
5. pelv/o	_____	E. Rib
6. my/o	_____	F. Muscle
7. ten/o	_____	G. Hip area
8. chondr/o	_____	H. Bone
9. spondyl/o	_____	I. Connects muscles to bones
10. ligament/o	_____	J. Connects bones to other bones

C Match the medical term in Column I with its meaning in Column II.

Column I		Column II
1. myelodysplasia	_____	A. Incision of the skull
2. intervertebral	_____	B. Inflammation of cartilage attached to ribs
3. osteomyelitis	_____	C. Suture of a tendon
4. arthroscopy	_____	D. Inflammation of bone and bone marrow
5. costochondritis	_____	E. Pertaining to between the backbones
6. chondroma	_____	F. Benign tumor of cartilage tissue
7. tenorrhaphy	_____	G. Abnormal growth of bone marrow cells
8. myosarcoma	_____	H. Malignant tumor of muscle tissue
9. craniotomy	_____	I. Visual examination of a joint

D Match the pathologic condition in Column I with its meaning in Column II.

Column I

1. gouty arthritis _____
2. carpal tunnel syndrome _____
3. rheumatoid arthritis _____
4. osteoporosis _____
5. ankylosing spondylitis _____
6. muscular dystrophy _____
7. rhabdomyolysis _____
8. leiomyosarcoma _____

Column II

A. Chronic, progressive arthritis with stiffening of joints between the backbones

B. Compression of the median nerve in the wrist

C. High levels of uric acid with inflammation of joints

D. Weakness and degeneration of muscle fibers; congenital condition

E. Chronic inflammation of joints, especially small bones in the hands and feet

F. Decrease in bone density with thinning and weakening of bone

G. Malignant tumor of smooth (visceral, involuntary) muscle

H. Breakdown of skeletal muscle

E Match the test or procedure in Column I with its description in Column II.

Column I		Column II
1. arthrocentesis	_____	A. Recording the strength of muscle contraction
2. serum calcium	_____	B. Measures sedimentation rate of red blood cells; indicates inflammation
3. electromyography	_____	C. Plasma is tested for antibodies that are present in patients with systemic lupus erythematosus
4. bone scan	_____	D. Removal of muscle tissue for microscopic analysis
5. ESR	_____	E. Puncture to remove fluid from a joint
6. ANA test	_____	F. Radioactive substance is injected intravenously and uptake is measured in bone tissue
7. muscle biopsy	_____	G. Measurement of an element in the blood that is necessary for normal bone formation
8. uric acid test	_____	H. X-ray imaging of a joint
9. arthroscopy	_____	I. Measurement of the amount of a substance in blood that is associated with gouty arthritis
10. arthrography	_____	J. Visual examination of a joint using an endoscope

F Match the treatment procedure in Column I with its description in Column II.

Column I		Column II
1. laminectomy	_____	A. Surgical repair of a joint
2. microscopic discectomy	_____	B. Surgical repair of a backbone
3. arthroplasty	_____	C. Removal of a herniated disc using a tiny incision and an operating microscope
4. vertebroplasty	_____	D. Surgical removal of a portion of a vertebra to allow visualization and removal of a portion of a disc

NERVOUS SYSTEM

ANATOMY

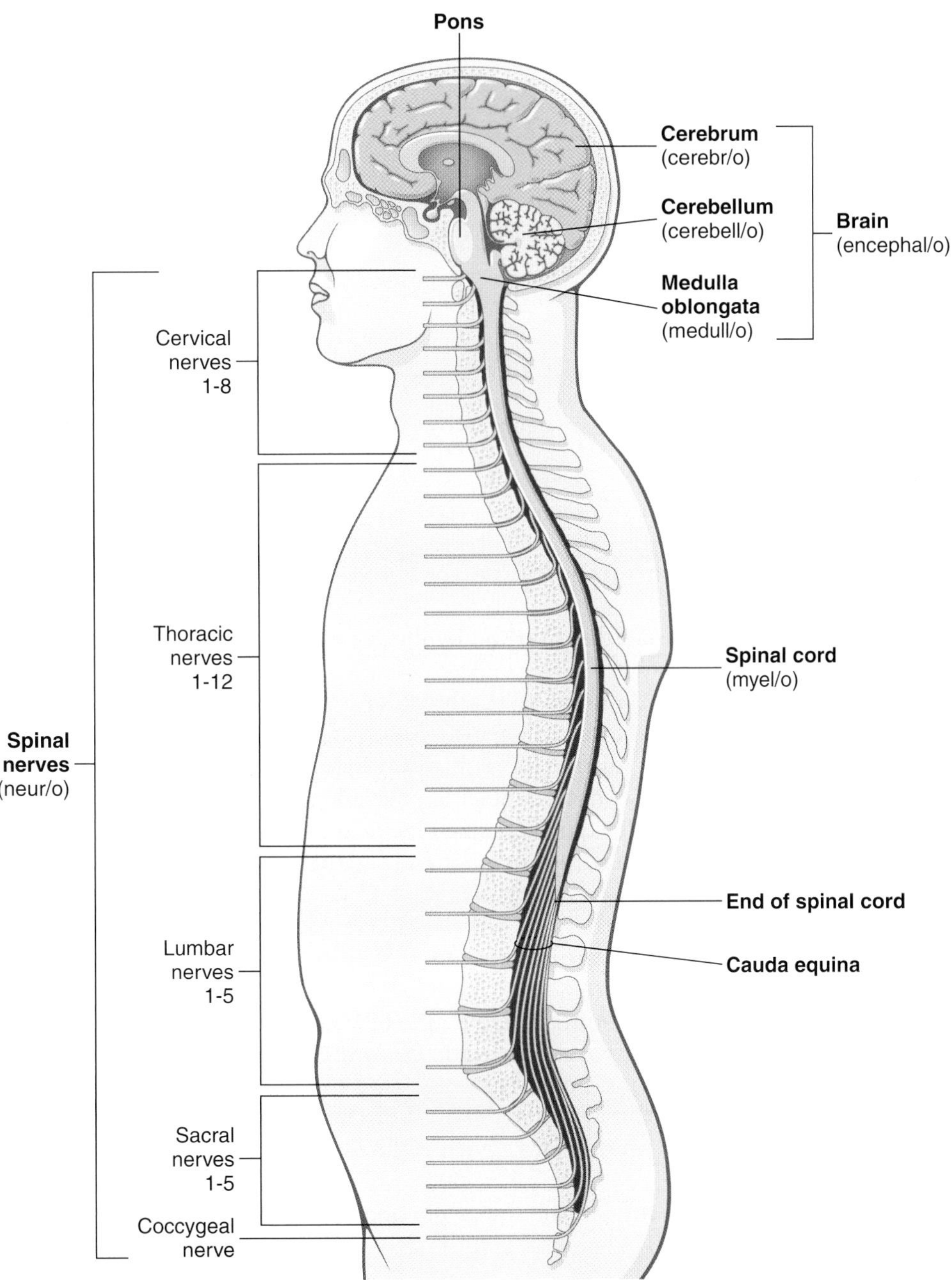

The **central nervous system** consists of the brain and the spinal cord. The **peripheral nervous system** includes the nerves that carry messages to and from the brain and spinal cord. **Spinal nerves** carry messages to and from the spinal cord, and the **cranial nerves** (not pictured) carry messages to and from the brain.

TERMINOLOGY

Meanings for terminology are found in the ***Mini-Dictionary***.

Combining Form	Meaning	Terminology	Meaning
cerebell/o	cerebellum	cerebellar	
cerebr/o	cerebrum	cerebral	
encephal/o	brain	encephalitis	
medull/o	medulla oblongata	medullary	
myel/o	spinal cord	myelitis	
neur/o	nerve	neuropathy	

PATHOLOGY

Definitions for additional terms in **boldface** are found in the ***Mini-Dictionary.***

Alzheimer disease: Brain disorder marked by deterioration of mental capacity (**irreversible dementia**).
Cerebrovascular accident: Damage to the blood vessels of the cerebrum, leading to loss of blood supply to brain tissue; a **stroke.**
Concussion: Traumatic brain injury that can cause bruising, damage to blood vessels, and injury to nerves. Loss of consciousness may occur.
Epilepsy: Chronic brain disorder characterized by recurrent **seizures.**
Glioblastoma: Malignant brain tumor arising from **glial cells.** BLAST means immature.
Hemiplegia: Paralysis (-PLEGIA) that affects the right or the left half of the body.
Meningitis: Inflammation of the **meninges** (membranes surrounding the brain and spinal cord).
Migraine: Attack of headache, usually on one side of the head, caused by changes in blood vessel size and accompanied by nausea, vomiting, and sensitivity to light (photophobia). *See page 196 for a case report related to migraines.*
Multiple sclerosis: Destruction of the **myelin sheath** on nerve cells in the central nervous system (brain and spinal cord), with replacement by plaques of sclerotic (hard) tissue.
Paraplegia: Paralysis that affects the lower portion of the body. From a Greek word meaning "to strike" (-PLEGIA) on one side (PARA-). This term was previously used to describe **hemiplegia.**
Syncope: Fainting; sudden and temporary loss of consciousness as a result of inadequate flow of blood to the brain.

LABORATORY TESTS AND DIAGNOSTIC PROCEDURES

Consult ***Appendix 3*** for pronunciation of terms and additional information.

Cerebral angiography: X-ray imaging of the blood vessels in the brain after the injection of contrast material into an artery.

Cerebrospinal fluid (CSF) analysis: Chemical tests (for sodium, chloride, protein, and glucose), cell counts, cultures, and bacterial smears on samples of CSF to detect diseases of the brain or meninges. A lumbar puncture is used to remove CSF for analysis.

Computed tomography (CT) scan: Cross-sectional x-ray images of the brain and spinal cord (with and without contrast).

Electroencephalography (EEG): Recording of the electrical activity within the brain.

Lumbar puncture (LP): Introduction of hollow needle into a space surrounding the spinal cord to withdraw cerebrospinal fluid (CSF) for analysis. Pressure of CSF is measured and contrast may be injected for imaging (myelography). Also known as a "spinal tap."

Magnetic resonance imaging (MRI): Magnetic waves and radiofrequency waves are used to create images of the brain and spinal cord.

Positron emission tomography (PET) scan: Uptake of radioactive material into the brain shows how the brain uses glucose and gives information about brain function.

TREATMENT PROCEDURES

Stereotactic radiosurgery: This is a nonsurgical type of radiation therapy used to treat abnormalities and small tumors of the brain. Also called Cyberknife® or stereotactic radiotherapy, this treatment can deliver precisely targeted radiation in fewer high-dose treatments than traditional therapy.

Transcutaneous electrical nerve stimulation (TENS): A battery-powered device delivers stimulation to nerves to relieve acute and chronic pain.

ABBREVIATIONS

AD	Alzheimer disease
CNS	Central nervous system
CSF	Cerebrospinal fluid
CVA	Cerebrovascular accident (stroke)
EEG	Electroencephalography
LP	Lumbar puncture
MS	Multiple sclerosis
TENS	Transcutaneous electrical nerve stimulation
TIA	Transient ischemic attack (temporary interference with blood supply to the brain); "mini-stroke."

MATCHING EXERCISES

The following exercises will help you review terminology related to the nervous system. Answers begin on page 295.

A Match the term in Column I with its description in Column II.

Column I		Column II
1. cerebrum	_____	A. Lower part of the brain, nearest to the spinal cord; it controls breathing and heartbeat
2. spinal cord	_____	B. Collection of nerves that are within the spinal cavity, surrounded by backbones
3. cerebellum	_____	C. Largest part of the brain; controls body movements, thought, reasoning, vision, hearing, speech
4. medulla oblongata	_____	D. Nerves that transmit messages to and from the spinal cord
5. spinal nerves	_____	E. Lower back part of the brain that controls muscular coordination and balance

B Match the combining form in Column I with its meaning in Column II.

Column I		Column II
1. cerebell/o	_____	A. Nerve
2. medull/o	_____	B. Cerebellum
3. myel/o	_____	C. Brain
4. cerebr/o	_____	D. Spinal cord
5. encephal/o	_____	E. Medulla oblongata
6. neur/o	_____	F. Cerebrum

C Match the medical term in Column I with its meaning in Column II.

Column I		Column II
1. myelitis	_____	A. Disease of nerves
2. cerebral	_____	B. Pertaining to the largest part of the brain
3. medullary	_____	C. Pertaining to the posterior portion of the brain that controls equilibrium
4. encephalitis	_____	D. Inflammation of the spinal cord
5. neuropathy	_____	E. Inflammation of the brain
6. cerebellar	_____	F. Pertaining to the lower part of the brain closest to the spinal cord

D Match the pathologic condition in Column I with its meaning in Column II.

Column I		Column II
1. cerebrovascular accident	_____	A. Inflammation of the membrane surrounding the brain and spinal cord
2. multiple sclerosis	_____	B. Brain disorder marked by deterioration in mental activity (dementia)
3. concussion	_____	C. Fainting
4. syncope	_____	D. Paralysis on one side of the body
5. epilepsy	_____	E. Damage to blood vessels in the brain; a stroke
6. meningitis	_____	F. Destruction of myelin sheath around nerve cells in the CNS
7. glioblastoma	_____	G. Blunt injury to the brain severe enough to cause loss of consciousness
8. paraplegia	_____	H. Paralysis of the lower portion of the body
9. hemiplegia	_____	I. Malignant tumor of the brain
10. Alzheimer disease	_____	J. Chronic brain disorder with seizure activity

E Match the test or procedure in Column I with its description in Column II.

Column I		Column II
1. lumbar puncture	_____	A. Uptake of radioactive material in the brain shows how the brain uses glucose
2. CSF analysis	_____	B. Chemical tests, cell counts, cultures, and smears of fluid surrounding the brain and spinal cord
3. cerebral angiography	_____	C. Record of the electrical activity in the brain
4. electroencephalogram	_____	D. Procedure to remove cerebrospinal fluid; measurement of pressure and injection of contrast
5. PET scan	_____	E. X-ray image of blood vessels in the brain after injection of contrast
6. MRI	_____	F. A battery-powered device delivers stimulation to nerves to relieve acute and chronic pain
7. stereotactic radiosurgery	_____	G. Cross-sectional x-ray images of the brain and spinal cord
8. CT scan	_____	H. Magnetic and radiofrequency waves create images of the brain and spinal cord tissue
9. TENS	_____	I. Nonsurgical type of radiation therapy used to treat abnormalities and small tumors of the brain; also called Cyberknife®

RESPIRATORY SYSTEM

ANATOMY

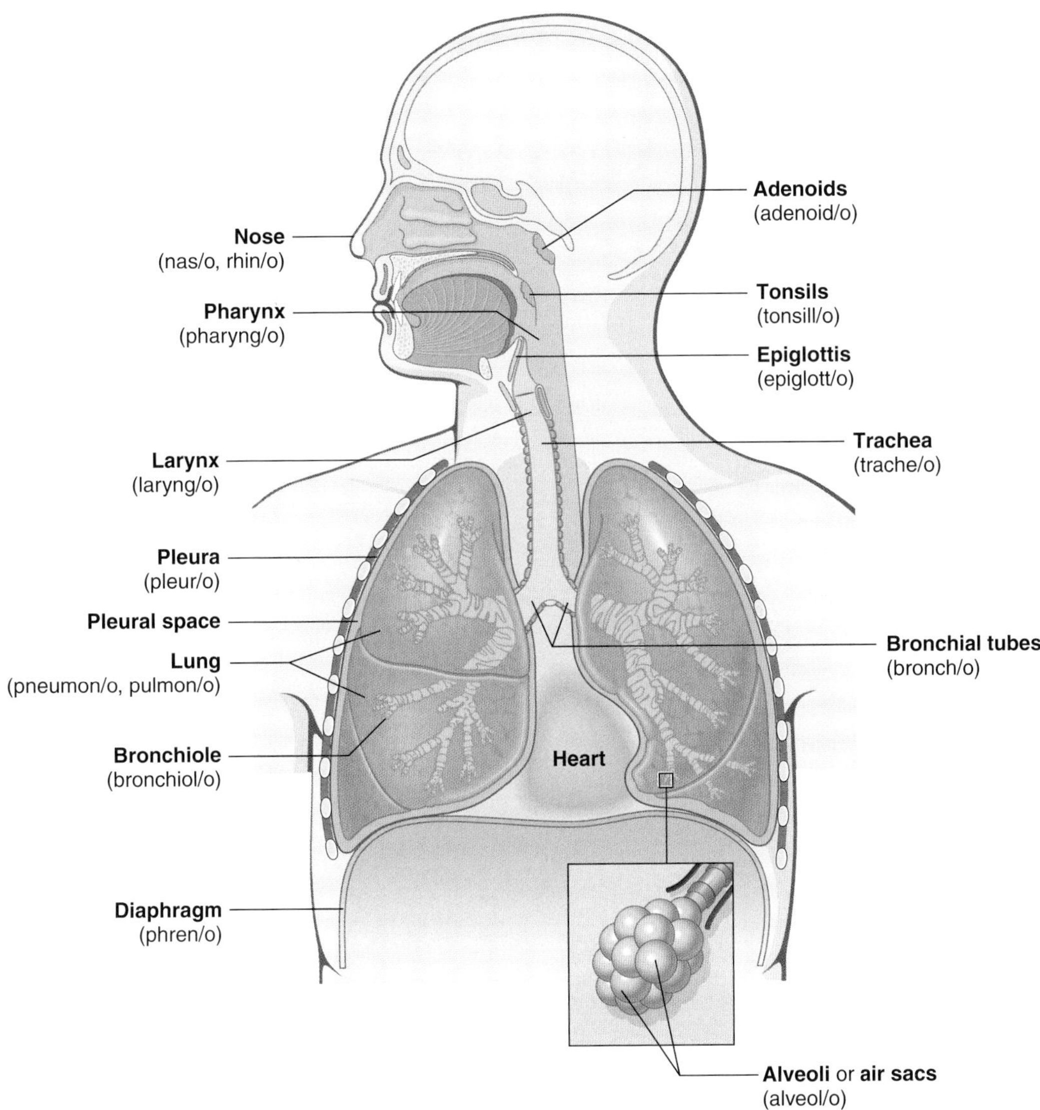

Air enters the **nose** and travels to the **pharynx** (throat). From the pharynx, air passes through the **epiglottis** and **larynx** (voice box) into the **trachea** (windpipe). The trachea splits into two tubes, the **bronchial tubes** that carry air into the lungs. The bronchial tubes divide into smaller tubes, called **bronchioles**, that end in **small alveoli**, or **air sacs**. The thin walls of these sacs allow oxygen to pass through them into tiny capillaries containing red blood cells. Red blood cells transport the oxygen to all parts of the body. In a similar manner, gaseous waste (carbon dioxide) leaves the blood by entering the alveoli and traveling out of the body through bronchioles, bronchial tubes, trachea, larynx, pharynx, and the nose. *(Modified from Chabner D-E:* The Language of Medicine, *ed 12, St. Louis, 2021, Elsevier.)*

TERMINOLOGY

Meanings for terminology are found in the ***Mini-Dictionary***.

Combining Form	Meaning	Terminology	Meaning
adenoid/o	adenoid	adenoidectomy	____________
alveol/o	alveoli (air sacs)	alveolar	____________
bronch/o	bronchial tube	bronchoscopy	____________
		bronchitis	____________
bronchiol/o	bronchiole	bronchiolitis	____________
cyan/o	blue	cyanosis	____________
epiglott/o	epiglottis	epiglottitis	____________
laryng/o	larynx	laryngeal	____________
nas/o	nose	nasal	____________
rhin/o	nose	rhinorrhea	____________
pharyng/o	pharynx	pharyngitis	____________
phren/o	diaphragm	phrenic	____________
pneumon/o	lung	pneumonectomy	____________
pulmon/o	lung	pulmonary	____________
tonsill/o	tonsils	tonsillitis	____________
trache/o	trachea	tracheitis	____________
		tracheostomy	____________

PATHOLOGY

Definitions for additional terms in **boldface** are found in the ***Mini-Dictionary.***

Asphyxia: Deficiency of oxygen in the blood and increase in carbon dioxide in blood and tissues. Major sign is a complete absence of breathing, leading to loss of consciousness or death.
Asthma: Spasm and narrowing of bronchi, leading to bronchial airway obstruction.
Atelectasis: Collapsed lung (ATEL/O means incomplete, and -ECTASIS indicates dilation or expansion).
Emphysema: Hyperinflation of air sacs with destruction of alveolar walls. Along with **chronic bronchitis,** emphysema is a type of **chronic obstructive pulmonary disease (COPD).**
Hemoptysis: Spitting up of blood.
Hemothorax: Blood from the respiratory tract in the pleural cavity (space between the **pleural membranes**).
Pneumoconiosis: Abnormal condition of dust (CONI/O) in the lungs.
Pneumonia: Abnormal condition of the lungs marked by inflammation and collection of infected material in air sacs (pus or products of the inflammatory reaction).
Tuberculosis: Infectious and inflammatory disease caused by bacteria (bacilli). The lungs and other organs are affected. Signs and symptoms are cough, weight loss, night sweats, **hemoptysis**, and pleuritic pain.

LABORATORY TESTS AND DIAGNOSTIC PROCEDURES

Consult ***Appendix 3*** reference for pronunciation of terms and additional information.

Bronchoscopy: Visual examination of the bronchial tubes with an endoscope.
Chest x-ray film: X-ray image of the chest in an AP (anteroposterior), PA (posteroanterior), or lateral (side) view.
Computed tomography (CT) scan: Cross-sectional x-ray images of the chest.
Laryngoscopy: Visual examination of the larynx via the placement of a flexible tube (laryngoscope) through the nose or mouth and into the larynx.
Magnetic resonance imaging (MRI): Magnetic waves and radiofrequency waves create images of the chest in three planes of the body.
Pulmonary angiography: X-ray images are taken of the blood vessels in the lung after injection of contrast into a blood vessel. This procedure has been largely replaced by computed tomography (CT of the lungs).
Pulmonary function test (PFT): Measurement of the ventilation (breathing capability) of the lungs. A **spirometer** measures the air taken into and breathed out of the lungs.
Sputum test: Examination of mucus coughed up to detect infection.
Tuberculin test: Agents are applied to the skin with punctures or injection and the reaction is noted. Redness and swelling result in people sensitive to the test substance and indicate previous or current infection with **tuberculosis.**
Ventilation-perfusion scan: A nuclear medicine test that uses radioactive material (radiopharmaceutical) to examine airflow (ventilation) and blood flow (perfusion).

TREATMENT PROCEDURES

Endotracheal intubation: Tube is placed through the nose or mouth into the trachea to establish an airway during surgery and for placement on a respirator (a machine that moves air into and out of the lungs).

Thoracentesis: Needle is inserted through the skin between the ribs and into the pleural space to drain a **pleural effusion.**

Thoracotomy: Incision of the chest to remove a lung (**pneumonectomy**) or a portion of a lung (**lobectomy**).

Tracheostomy: Creation of an opening into the trachea through the neck and the insertion of a tube to create an airway.

ABBREVIATIONS

ABG	Arterial blood gas
ARDS	Acute respiratory distress syndrome
CO_2	Carbon dioxide (gas expelled from the lungs)
COPD	Chronic obstructive pulmonary disease (chronic bronchitis and emphysema)
CPAP	Continuous positive airway pressure (machine used to keep airway open)
CPR	Cardiopulmonary resuscitation (technique to restore breathing and heart rate)
CXR	Chest x-ray (film or image)
O_2	Oxygen (gas entering the bloodstream through the lungs)
MDI	Metered-dose inhaler (that delivers specific amount of medication to the lungs)
PE	Pulmonary embolism (blockage of vessels in the lung by a blood clot)
PEEP	Positive end-expiratory pressure (method of mechanical ventilation)
PFT	Pulmonary function test (measurement of the breathing capability of the lung)
SOB	Shortness of breath
URI	Upper respiratory infection
VATS	Video-assisted thoracic surgery (using small incisions and an endoscope)
VQ	Ventilation-perfusion scan (also called VQ scan)

MATCHING EXERCISES

The following exercises will help you review terminology related to the respiratory system. Answers begin on page 295.

A Match the term in Column I with its description in Column II.

Column I

1. nose _____
2. epiglottis _____
3. larynx _____
4. pharynx _____
5. lung _____
6. diaphragm _____
7. trachea _____
8. bronchial tube _____
9. bronchiole _____
10. air sac _____

Column II

A. Throat

B. Windpipe

C. Muscle that separates the chest from the abdomen

D. Flap of cartilage over the "mouth" of the trachea

E. Small bronchial tube

F. Structure on the face that filters/warms air entering the body

G. Thin-walled sac through which gases can pass into and out of the bloodstream

H. One of two tubes that carry air from the windpipe to the lungs

I. Voice box

J. One of two paired organs in the chest through which oxygen enters and carbon dioxide leaves the bloodstream

B Match the combining form in Column I with its meaning in Column II.

Column I		Column II
1. pharyng/o	_____	A. Diaphragm
2. bronch/o	_____	B. Air sac
3. bronchiol/o	_____	C. Windpipe
4. nas/o *or* rhin/o	_____	D. Nose
5. laryng/o	_____	E. Throat
6. phren/o	_____	F. Voice box
7. trache/o	_____	G. Tube that carries air from the windpipe to the lung
8. epiglott/o	_____	H. Lung
9. alveol/o	_____	I. Small bronchus
10. pneumon/o	_____	J. Epiglottis

C Match the medical term in Column I with its meaning in Column II.

Column I		Column II
1. pulmonary	_____	A. Discharge from the nose
2. rhinorrhea	_____	B. Pertaining to an air sac
3. pneumonectomy	_____	C. Inflammation of the throat
4. bronchoscopy	_____	D. Pertaining to a lung
5. laryngeal	_____	E. New opening of the windpipe to the outside of the body
6. pharyngitis	_____	F. Pertaining to the nose
7. phrenic	_____	G. Visual examination of the bronchus
8. tracheostomy	_____	H. Resection of a lung
9. alveolar	_____	I. Pertaining to the voice box
10. nasal	_____	J. Pertaining to the diaphragm

D Match the pathologic condition in Column I with its meaning in Column II.

Column I		Column II
1. atelectasis	_____	A. Collapsed lung
2. hemothorax	_____	B. Condition of dust particles in the lung
3. asphyxia	_____	C. Spitting up blood
4. emphysema	_____	D. Infectious disease caused by bacilli; lungs and other organs are affected
5. asthma	_____	E. Inflammation and infection of alveoli
6. hemoptysis	_____	F. Blood in the pleural space
7. tuberculosis	_____	G. Extreme decrease in oxygen and increase in carbon dioxide in the blood
8. pneumonia	_____	H. Hyperinflation of air sacs and destruction of alveolar walls
9. pneumoconiosis	_____	I. Spasm and narrowing of bronchial tubes leading to airway obstruction

E Match the test or procedure in Column I with its description in Column II.

Column I		Column II
1. pulmonary angiography	_____	A. Radiographic image in AP, PA, or lateral view
2. laryngoscopy	_____	B. Material expelled by coughing is analyzed
3. ventilation-perfusion scans	_____	C. Visual examination of bronchial tubes
4. PFTs	_____	D. After administration of radioactive material (by injection or inhalation), images reveal distribution in lung tissue
5. chest x-ray	_____	E. Magnetic waves produce images of the chest in three planes
6. bronchoscopy	_____	F. Measurements of the ventilation capability of the lung using a spirometer
7. sputum test	_____	G. X-ray images of blood vessels in the lung
8. MRI	_____	H. Visual examination of the voice box
9. tuberculin test	_____	I. Cross-sectional x-ray images of the chest
10. chest CT scan	_____	J. Agents are applied to the skin with punctures, and reaction is noted

F Match the treatment procedure in Column I with its description in Column II.

Column I		Column II
1. tracheostomy	_____	A. Tube is placed through the nose or mouth into the windpipe to establish an airway
2. thoracentesis	_____	B. Creation of an opening into the windpipe through the neck and insertion of a tube to create an airway
3. endotracheal intubation	_____	C. Incision of the chest to remove a lung or a portion of a lung
4. thoracotomy	_____	D. Insertion of a needle through the skin between the ribs and into the pleural space to drain a pleural effusion

SKIN AND SENSE ORGANS

ANATOMY

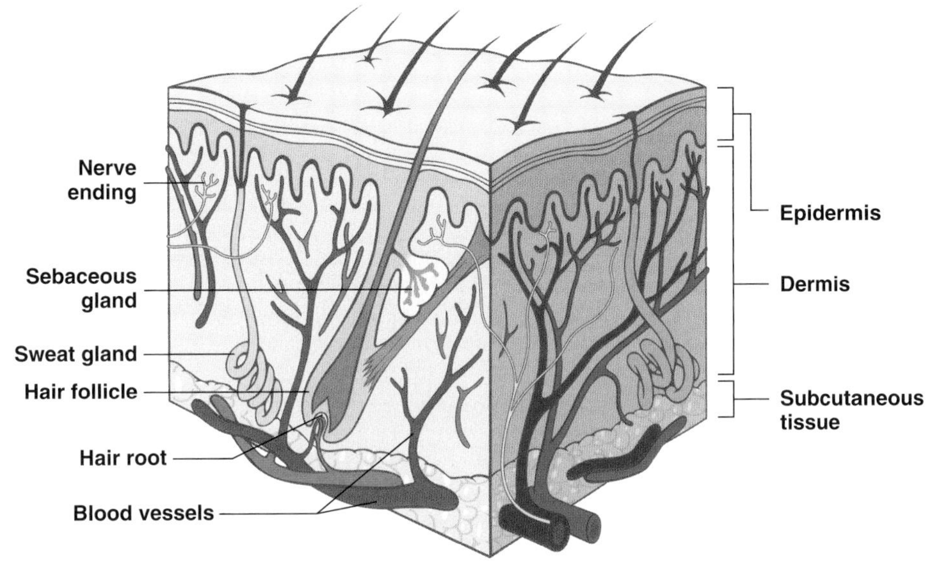

SKIN
(derm/o, dermat/o, cutane/o)

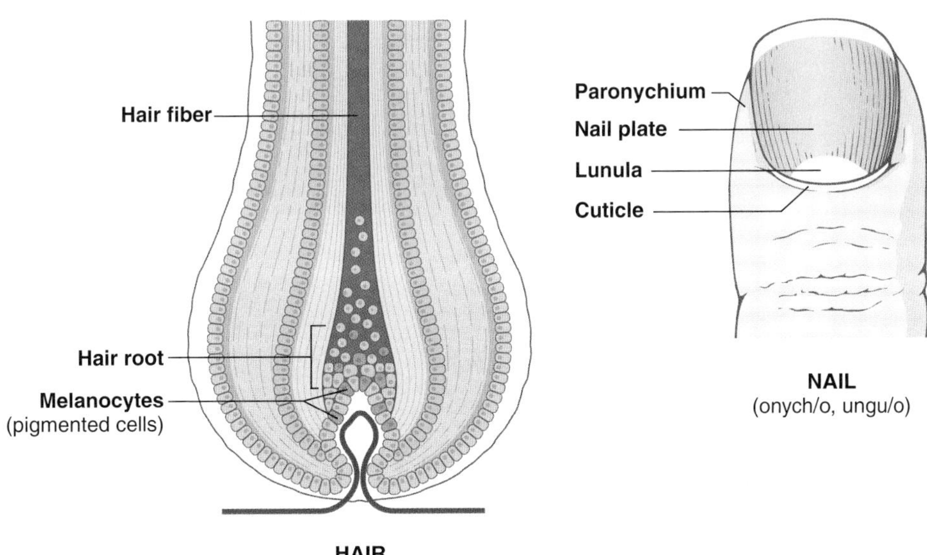

HAIR
(pil/o, trich/o)

NAIL
(onych/o, ungu/o)

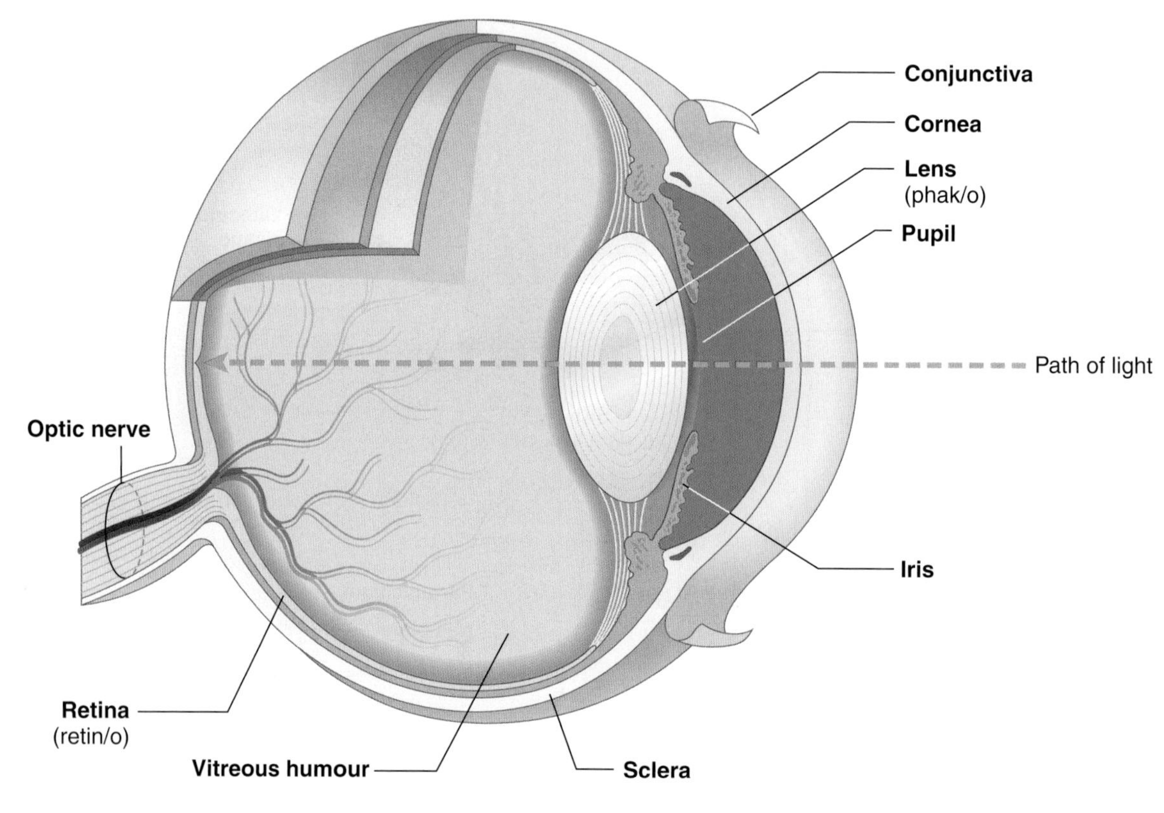

EYE
(ophthalm/o, ocul/o)

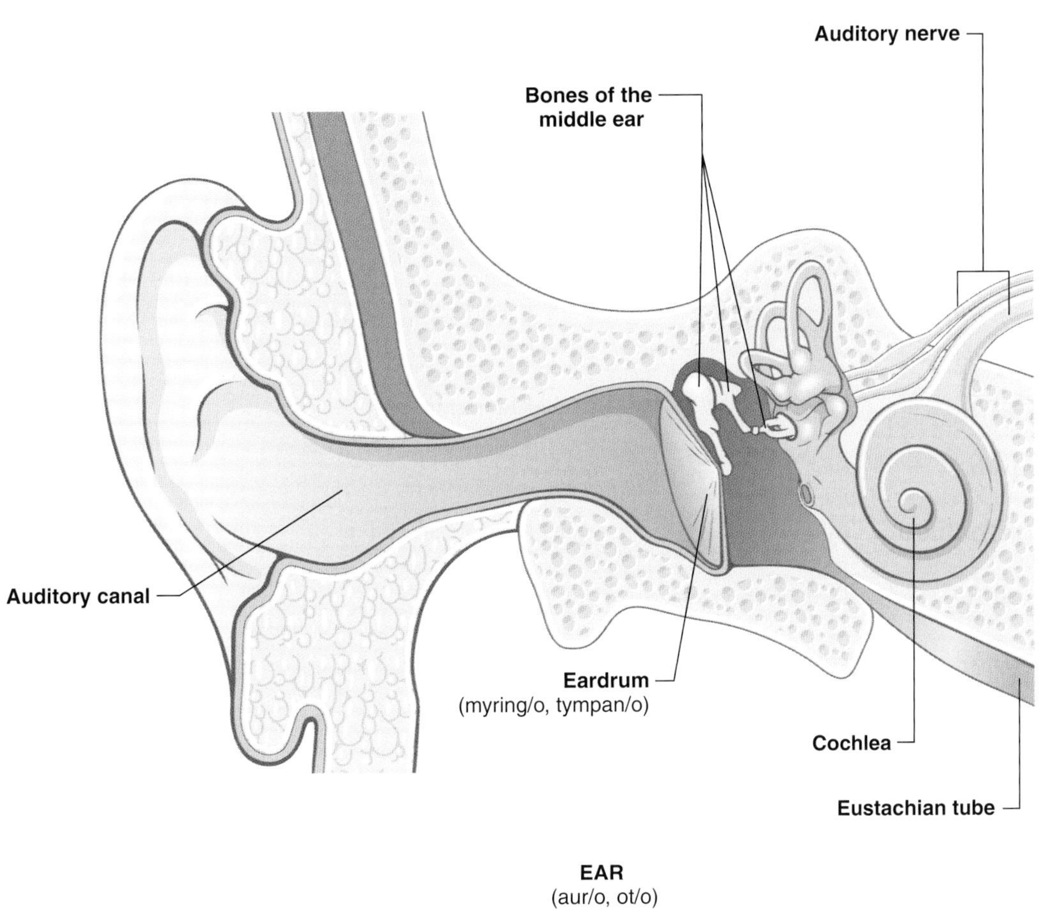

The **skin and sense organs** receive messages (touch sensations, light waves, sound waves) from the environment and send them to the brain via nerves. These messages are interpreted in the brain, making sight, hearing, and tactile (touch) perception of the environment possible. *(Modified from Chabner D-E:* The Language of Medicine, *ed 12, St. Louis, 2021, Elsevier.)*

TERMINOLOGY

Meanings for terminology are found in the ***Mini-Dictionary.***

Combining Form	Meaning	Terminology	Meaning
cutane/o	skin	subcutaneous	________
derm/o	skin	epidermis	________
dermat/o	skin	dermatology	________
onych/o	nail	onycholysis	________
ungu/o	nail	subungual	________
pil/o	hair	pilosebaceous	________
trich/o	hair	trichotillomania	________
ocul/o	eye	ocular	________
ophthalm/o	eye	ophthalmoscope	________
phak/o	lens of the eye	aphakia	________
retin/o	retina	retinopathy	________
aur/o	ear	aural discharge	________
ot/o	ear	otitis	________
myring/o	eardrum	myringotomy	________
tympan/o	eardrum	tympanoplasty	________

PATHOLOGY

Definitions for additional terms in **boldface** are found in the ***Mini-Dictionary.***

Alopecia: Absence of hair from areas where it normally grows; baldness.
Cataract: Clouding (opacity) of the lens of the eye, causing impairment of vision or blindness.
Conjunctivitis: Inflammation of the **conjunctiva.**
Glaucoma: Increase in pressure (fluid accumulation) within the chamber at the front of the eye.

Melanoma: Malignant tumor of pigmented cells (MELAN/O means black) that arises from a nevus (benign mole) in the skin.
Nevus: Pigmented lesion in or on the skin; a mole.
Stye *or* **sty:** Pus-filled (purulent) infection of glands near the eyelid (most often caused by bacteria). Also called **hordeolum.**
Tinnitus: Abnormal noise (ringing, buzzing, roaring) sound in the ears.

LABORATORY TESTS AND DIAGNOSTIC PROCEDURES

Consult ***Appendix 3*** for pronunciation of terms and additional information.

Allergy test: Procedure in which allergy-causing substances are placed on the skin and a reaction is noted. In the patch test, a patch with a suspected allergen is placed on the skin. The scratch test involves making several scratches and inserting a small amount of allergen in the scratches.
Bacterial and fungal tests: Procedures in which samples from skin lesions are taken to determine the presence of bacterial infection or fungal growth.
Fluorescein angiography: Fluorescein (a contrast substance) is injected intravenously and the movement of blood in the back of the eye is observed by ophthalmoscopy. It is used to detect diabetic or hypertensive retinopathy and also degeneration of the macular (central) area of the retina.
Ophthalmoscopy: Visual examination of the interior of the eye.
Otoscopy: Visual examination of the interior of the ear (to the eardrum).
Skin biopsy: Procedure in which samples of skin lesions are removed and sent to the pathology laboratory for microscopic examination.
Slit-lamp microscopy: Examination of the anterior eye structures (such as the cornea) using an instrument that projects intense light through a narrow opening for optimal visualization.
Tuning fork test: Procedure in which a vibration source (tuning fork) is placed in front of the opening to the ear to test air conduction of sound waves. The tuning fork is also placed on the mastoid bone behind the ear to test bone conduction of sound waves.

ABBREVIATIONS

ENT	Ears, nose, throat
HEENT	Head, eyes, ears, nose, throat
PERRLA	Pupils equal, round, reactive to light and accommodation
VA	Visual acuity (clarity of vision)
VF	Visual field

MATCHING EXERCISES

The following exercises will help you review terminology related to the skin and sense organs. Answers begin on page 296.

A Match the term in Column I with its description in Column II.

Column I		Column II
1. epidermis	_____	A. Oil-producing gland in the skin
2. sebaceous gland	_____	B. Gland in the skin that produces a watery, salt-containing fluid
3. dermis	_____	C. Innermost layer of the skin, composed of fatty tissue
4. subcutaneous tissue	_____	D. Middle layer of the skin, containing hair follicles, connective tissue, blood vessels, and glands
5. sweat gland	_____	E. Outer layer of the skin

B Match the term in Column I with its description in Column II.

Column I		Column II
1. retina	_____	A. White, outer coat of the eyeball
2. conjunctiva	_____	B. Membrane that separates the outer and middle parts of the ear
3. pupil	_____	C. Transparent structure behind the pupil that bends light rays so that they focus on the back of the eye
4. lens	_____	D. Nerve that carries messages from the inner ear to the brain
5. cornea	_____	E. Transparent layer over the front of the eye that bends light so that it is focused on the back of the eye
6. sclera	_____	F. Black center of the eye through which light enters
7. iris	_____	G. Layer of sensitive cells (rods and cones) at the back of the eye
8. eardrum	_____	H. Nerve at the back of the eye that transmits light waves to the brain
9. auditory canal	_____	I. Colored, pigmented portion of the eye
10. auditory nerve	_____	J. Passageway leading into the ear from the outside of the body
11. optic nerve	_____	K. Thin, protective membrane over the front of the eye

C Match the combining form in Column I with its meaning in Column II.

Column I		Column II
1. derm/o	_____	A. Eye
2. phak/o	_____	B. Hair
3. retin/o	_____	C. Skin
4. myring/o	_____	D. Posterior, sensitive cell layer of the eye
5. aur/o	_____	E. Nail
6. ophthalm/o	_____	F. Eardrum
7. ungu/o	_____	G. Lens of the eye
8. pil/o	_____	H. Ear

D Match the medical term in Column I with its meaning in Column II.

Column I		Column II
1. ocular	_____	A. Disease of the rod and cone layer of eye (sensitive cells at the back of the eye)
2. otitis	_____	B. Pertaining to under the nail
3. subcutaneous	_____	C. Absence of the lens of the eye
4. myringotomy	_____	D. Inflammation of the ear
5. aphakia	_____	E. Pertaining to the eye
6. epidermis	_____	F. Pertaining to under the skin
7. retinopathy	_____	G. Incision of the eardrum
8. ophthalmoscope	_____	H. Outer layer of the skin
9. tympanoplasty	_____	I. Instrument to visually examine the eye
10. subungual	_____	J. Surgical repair of the eardrum

E Match the pathologic condition in Column I with its meaning in Column II.

Column I		Column II
1. melanoma	_____	A. Clouding of the lens of the eye, causing impairment of vision
2. glaucoma	_____	B. Absence of hair from areas where it normally grows
3. conjunctivitis	_____	C. Pigmented lesion on the skin; mole
4. tinnitus	_____	D. Increase in pressure within the chamber at the front of the eye
5. cataract	_____	E. Abnormal noise (ringing, buzzing) or sound in the ears
6. nevus	_____	F. Malignant tumor of pigmented cells in the skin
7. alopecia	_____	G. Inflammation of the mucous membrane lining the inner surface of the eyelid

F Match the test or procedure in Column I with its description in Column II.

Column I		Column II
1. skin biopsy	_____	A. Samples from skin lesions are examined to detect presence of microorganisms
2. slit-lamp microscopy	_____	B. Visual examination of the interior of the eye
3. tuning fork tests	_____	C. Patch test; scratch test
4. fluorescein angiography	_____	D. Skin lesions are removed and sent to pathology laboratory for microscopic examination
5. otoscopy	_____	E. Dye is injected intravenously, and movement of blood through blood vessels in the back of the eye is observed with an ophthalmoscope
6. allergy test	_____	F. Visual examination of the ear to the eardrum
7. bacterial and fungal tests	_____	G. Microscopic examination of the anterior eye structures, such as the cornea, under intense light
8. ophthalmoscopy	_____	H. A vibration source is placed in front of the opening of the ear to test air conduction of sound waves

BODY SYSTEMS

URINARY SYSTEM

ANATOMY (FEMALE URINARY TRACT)

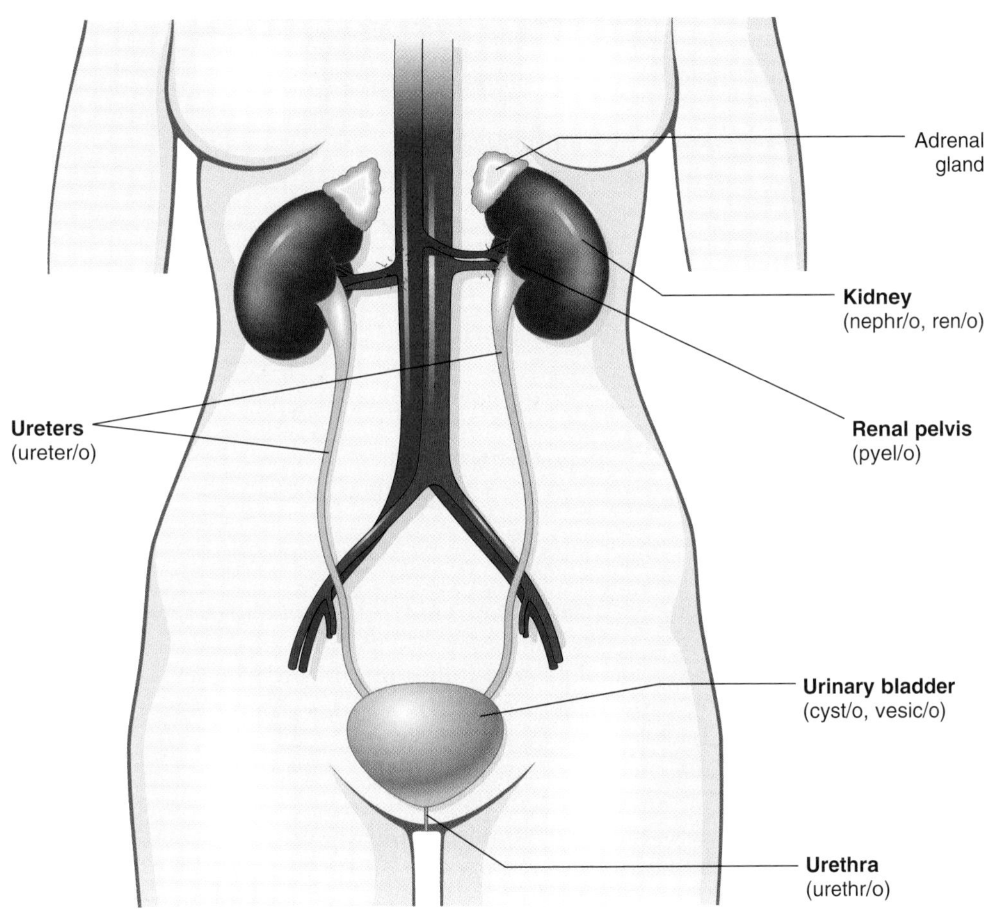

Urine is formed as waste materials, such as urea, are filtered from the blood into the tubules of the **kidney**. Urea is a nitrogenous waste product formed as proteins are used in cells. Urine passes from the kidney tubules into the central collecting section of the kidney, the **renal pelvis**. Each renal pelvis leads directly to a **ureter**, which takes the urine to the **urinary bladder**. The bladder releases urine to the **urethra**, and urine leaves the body. *(Modified from Chabner D-E:* The Language of Medicine, *ed 12, St. Louis, 2021, Elsevier.)*

TERMINOLOGY

Meanings for terminology are found in the ***Mini-Dictionary***.

Combining Form	Meaning	Terminology	Meaning
cyst/o	urinary bladder	cystoscopy	____________
vesic/o	urinary bladder	intravesical	____________
nephr/o	kidney	nephritis	____________
ren/o	kidney	renal	____________
pyel/o	renal pelvis	pyelogram	____________
ureter/o	ureter	ureterectomy	____________
urethr/o	urethra	urethritis	____________

PATHOLOGY

Definitions for additional terms in **boldface** are found in the ***Mini-Dictionary***.

Albuminuria: Abnormal condition of protein (albumin) in the urine.
Anuria: Abnormal condition of no urine production.
Dysuria: Painful urination.
Glycosuria: Abnormal condition of glucose in the urine.
Hematuria: Abnormal condition of blood in the urine.
Nephrolithiasis: Abnormal condition of stones in the kidney.
Renal failure: Condition in which the kidneys stop functioning and do not produce urine.
Uremia: Condition of high levels of **urea** (nitrogenous waste material) in the blood.

LABORATORY TESTS AND DIAGNOSTIC PROCEDURES

Consult ***Appendix 3*** for pronunciation of terms and additional information.

Blood urea nitrogen (BUN): Measures the amount of urea (nitrogenous waste) in the blood.
Cystoscopy: Visual examination of the urinary bladder with a cystoscope (endoscope).
Kidneys, ureters, bladder (KUB): X-ray images of the kidneys and urinary tract made without the use of contrast material.
Retrograde pyelogram (RP): Contrast material is injected through a catheter (a flexible, tubular instrument) into the urethra and bladder, and x-ray images are taken of the urethra, bladder, and ureters.

Voiding cystourethrogram (VCUG): X-ray films of the bladder and urethra taken after the bladder is filled with a contrast material and while the patient is expelling urine. Also called **cystogram.**

Urography: X-ray imaging of the urinary tract after injection of contrast material; pyelography.

TREATMENT PROCEDURES

Dialysis: Waste materials (**urea, creatinine,** and **uric acid**) are separated from the blood by a machine (**hemodialysis**). Alternatively, in peritoneal dialysis, an intra-abdominal catheter (a flexible tubular instrument), delivers a special fluid into the abdominal, cavity. After several hours, the fluid containing waste materials that have seeped into it from the blood is drained. *See page 195 for a case report related to hemodialysis.*

Lithotripsy: Shock waves are beamed into a patient to crush urinary tract stones. The stone fragments then pass out of the body with urine. Also called **extracorporeal shock wave lithotripsy (ESWL).** *See page 190 for a case report related to lithotripsy*.

Renal transplantation: A donor kidney is transferred to a recipient, whose kidneys have both failed.

Urinary catheterization: A catheter (a flexible tubular instrument) is passed through the urethra and into the urinary bladder for short-term or long-term drainage of urine.

ABBREVIATIONS

ARF	Acute renal failure
BUN	Blood urea nitrogen (measures kidney function)
CAPD	Continuous ambulatory peritoneal dialysis
CKD	Chronic kidney disease (rising BUN and serum creatinine levels affect many body systems)
GFR	Glomerular filtration rate (measured to document stages of kidney disease)
HD	Hemodialysis
KUB	Kidneys, ureters, bladder (series of x-ray images made without contrast)
RP	Retrograde pyelogram
UA	Urinalysis
UTI	Urinary tract infection
VCUG	Voiding cystourethrogram

MATCHING EXERCISES

The following exercises will help you review terminology related to the urinary system. Answers begin on page 296.

A Match the term in Column I with its description in Column II.

Column I		Column II
1. urinary bladder	_____	A. Tube that leads from the bladder to the outside of the body
2. kidney	_____	B. Central section of the kidney
3. renal pelvis	_____	C. Organ behind the abdomen that makes urine by filtering wastes from the blood
4. ureter	_____	D. One of two tubes that carry urine from the kidney to the urinary bladder
5. urethra	_____	E. Muscular sac that holds urine and releases it to leave the body through the urethra

B Match the combining form in Column I with its meaning in Column II.

Column I		Column II
1. ureter/o	_____	A. Urinary bladder
2. urethr/o	_____	B. Tube leading from the urinary bladder to the outside of the body
3. pyel/o	_____	C. Kidney
4. cyst/o, vesic/o	_____	D. Tube leading from the kidney to the urinary bladder
5. nephr/o, ren/o	_____	E. Renal pelvis (central collecting basin of the kidney)

C Match the medical term in Column I with its meaning in Column II.

Column I		Column II
1. pyelogram	_____	A. X-ray record of the renal pelvis
2. urethritis	_____	B. Visual examination of the urinary bladder
3. nephritis	_____	C. Resection of a ureter
4. intravesical	_____	D. Pertaining to within the urinary bladder
5. cystoscopy	_____	E. Inflammation of the kidney
6. ureterectomy	_____	F. Pertaining to the kidney
7. renal	_____	G. Inflammation of the urethra

D Match the pathologic condition in Column I with its meaning in Column II.

Column I		Column II
1. dysuria	_____	A. Kidneys stop functioning and fail to produce urine
2. hematuria	_____	B. Abnormal condition of protein in urine
3. uremia	_____	C. Blood in the urine
4. renal failure	_____	D. No urine production
5. nephrolithiasis	_____	E. High levels of urea in the bloodstream
6. albuminuria	_____	F. Sugar in the urine
7. glycosuria	_____	G. Painful urination
8. anuria	_____	H. Abnormal condition of kidney stones

E Match the test or procedure in Column I with its description in Column II.

Column I		Column II
1. KUB	_____	A. Measurement of amount of nitrogenous wastes in the blood
2. dialysis	_____	B. Visual examination of the urinary bladder
3. VCUG	_____	C. X-ray images of the kidneys and urinary tract without contrast
4. lithotripsy	_____	D. Tube is passed through the urethra into the urinary bladder for short- or long-term drainage of urine
5. renal transplantation	_____	E. Shock waves are beamed into the patient to crush stones in the kidney or ureter
6. cystoscopy	_____	F. Nitrogenous waste materials are separated from the blood by a machine
7. BUN	_____	G. After the bladder is filled with contrast, x-ray images are taken of the bladder as the patient is expelling urine
8. retrograde pyelogram	_____	H. Contrast material is injected via a catheter into the bladder, and x-ray images are taken of the ureters, bladder, and urethra
9. urinary catheterization	_____	I. A kidney from a donor is surgically implanted in a patient whose kidneys have failed

ANSWERS TO MATCHING EXERCISES

CARDIOVASCULAR SYSTEM

A 1. B 2. I 3. F 4. E 5. D 6. A 7. J 8. G 9. C 10. H

B 1. D 2. E 3. B 4. F 5. A 6. C

C 1. D 2. F 3. G 4. C 5. H 6. E 7. A 8. B 9. J 10. I

D 1. E 2. H 3. D 4. G 5. C 6. A 7. F 8. B

E 1. I 2. J 3. C 4. G 5. B 6. E 7. D 8. A 9. H 10. F

F 1. E 2. B 3. G 4. F 5. A 6. C 7. D

DIGESTIVE SYSTEM

A 1. G 2. C 3. H 4. A 5. F 6. D 7. B 8. E

B 1. C 2. H 3. A 4. F 5. D 6. B 7. G 8. E

C 1. D 2. G 3. H 4. I 5. J 6. A 7. E 8. F 9. C 10. B

D 1. C 2. F 3. G 4. H 5. D 6. I 7. J 8. E 9. A 10. B

E 1. D 2. F 3. E 4. G 5. A 6. C 7. B 8. I 9. J 10. H

F 1. G 2. I 3. A 4. D 5. C 6. H 7. J 8. F 9. E 10. B

ENDOCRINE SYSTEM

A 1. C 2. G 3. A 4. F 5. B 6. E 7. D

B 1. E 2. D 3. F 4. G 5. C 6. B 7. A

C 1. C 2. G 3. E 4. F 5. D 6. A 7. B

D 1. C 2. D 3. A 4. B 5. E

E 1. B 2. E 3. A 4. G 5. F 6. C 7. D

FEMALE REPRODUCTIVE SYSTEM

A	1. C	2. B	3. D	4. A	5. F	6. E			
B	1. D	2. E	3. B	4. A	5. C	6. F			
C	1. D	2. F	3. H	4. A	5. G	6. B	7. E	8. C	
D	1. C	2. E	3. D	4. G	5. A	6. F	7. B		
E	1. H	2. F	3. C	4. A	5. D	6. G	7. E	8. B	9. I
F	1. C	2. A	3. E	4. B	5. D				

LYMPHATIC SYSTEM

A	1. C	2. B	3. D	4. A	5. E		
B	1. C	2. D	3. E	4. A	5. B		
C	1. G	2. D	3. E	4. A	5. F	6. B	7. C
D	1. D	2. C	3. E	4. B	5. A		

MALE REPRODUCTIVE SYSTEM

A	1. C	2. B	3. D	4. A	5. E		
B	1. B	2. E	3. D	4. F	5. C	6. A	
C	1. D	2. E	3. F	4. C	5. A	6. G	7. B
D	1. E	2. F	3. C	4. D	5. B	6. A	
E	1. E	2. F	3. D	4. C	5. A	6. B	

MUSCULOSKELETAL SYSTEM

A

1. H	5. J	9. T	13. L	17. F
2. E	6. R	10. G	14. P	18. M
3. K	7. Q	11. I	15. C	19. B
4. D	8. A	12. S	16. N	20. O

B

1. D	3. H	5. G	7. I	9. A
2. C	4. E	6. F	8. B	10. J

C

1. G	3. D	5. B	7. C	9. A
2. E	4. I	6. F	8. H	

D

1. C	3. E	5. A	7. H
2. B	4. F	6. D	8. G

E

1. E	3. A	5. B	7. D	9. J
2. G	4. F	6. C	8. I	10. H

F

1. D	2. C	3. A	4. B

NERVOUS SYSTEM

A

1. C	2. B	3. E	4. A	5. D

B

1. B	2. E	3. D	4. F	5. C	6. A

C

1. D	2. B	3. F	4. E	5. A	6. C

D

1. E	3. G	5. J	7. I	9. D
2. F	4. C	6. A	8. H	10. B

E

1. D	3. E	5. A	7. I	9. F
2. B	4. C	6. H	8. G	

RESPIRATORY SYSTEM

A

1. F	3. I	5. J	7. B	9. E
2. D	4. A	6. C	8. H	10. G

B

1. E	3. I	5. F	7. C	9. B
2. G	4. D	6. A	8. J	10. H

C

1. D	3. H	5. I	7. J	9. B
2. A	4. G	6. C	8. E	10. F

D

1. A	3. G	5. I	7. D	9. B
2. F	4. H	6. C	8. E	

E

1. G	3. D	5. A	7. B	9. J
2. H	4. F	6. C	8. E	10. I

F

1. B	2. D	3. A	4. C

SKIN AND SENSE ORGANS

A	1. E	2. A	3. D	4. C	5. B	
B	1. G 2. K	3. F 4. C	5. E 6. A	7. I 8. B	9. J 10. D	11. H
C	1. C 2. G	3. D 4. F	5. H 6. A	7. E 8. B		
D	1. E 2. D	3. F 4. G	5. C 6. H	7. A 8. I	9. J 10. B	
E	1. F 2. D	3. G 4. E	5. A 6. C	7. B		
F	1. D 2. G	3. H 4. E	5. F 6. C	7. A 8. B		

URINARY SYSTEM

A	1. E	2. C	3. B	4. D	5. A
B	1. D	2. B	3. E	4. A	5. C
C	1. A 2. G	3. E 4. D	5. B 6. C	7. F	
D	1. G 2. C	3. E 4. A	5. H 6. B	7. F 8. D	
E	1. C 2. F	3. G 4. E	5. I 6. B	7. A 8. H	9. D

APPENDIX 2

Immunity and COVID-19 Vaccines

Immunity 298
Vaccines 301
COVID-19 Vaccines 302

IMMUNITY

Immunity (immun/o = protection) against foreign organisms, such as bacteria and viruses, is dependent on a well-functioning **immune system**. The immune system defends us against foreign invaders such as viruses, bacteria, or even foreign blood cells. These invaders have surface structures, usually proteins, that are recognized as foreign to the host and become **antigens.**

When antigens enter the body, a healthy immune system responds by calling out immune fighters. Antigens are recognized by **leukocytes** (white blood cells), which circulate in the bloodstream and the lymphatic system. The major disease-fighting leukocytes are:

1. **Neutrophils:** 50 percent to 70 percent of leukocytes in the bloodstream are neutrophils. They are cells that are identified by a multilobed nucleus (containing DNA or genes) and granules that become purple when a neutral stain is applied to a drop of blood (-phil means attracted to).

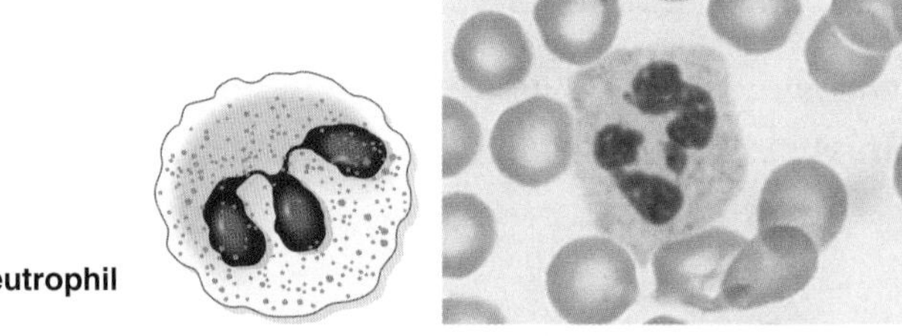

2. **Monocytes:** 3 percent to 8 percent of leukocytes are monocytes. They have one large circular nucleus and no dark-staining granules outside the nucleus. **Macrophages** are monocytes that move from the bloodstream into tissues.

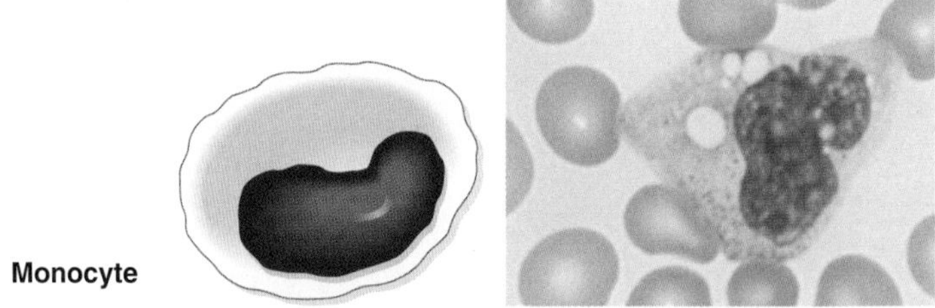

Neutrophils and monocytes, including macrophages, are phagocytes (phag/o = eat, swallow) that kill antigens by engulfing and digesting them.

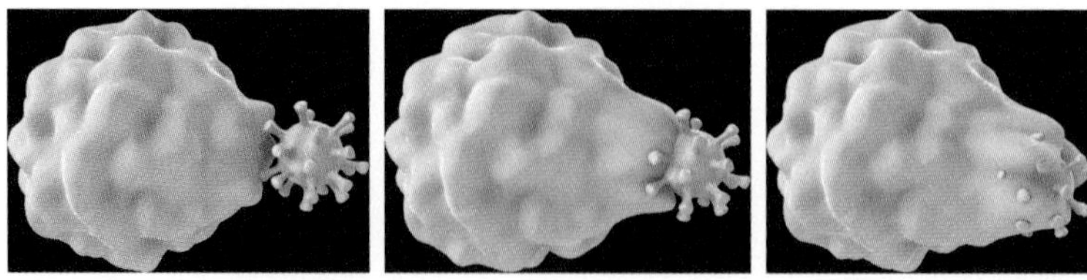

3D illustrations showing a white blood cell engulfing a virus.

3. **Lymphocytes:** 20 percent to 40 percent of WBCs are lymphocytes. These cells, like monocytes, have one distinct nucleus and few dark-staining granules outside the nucleus.

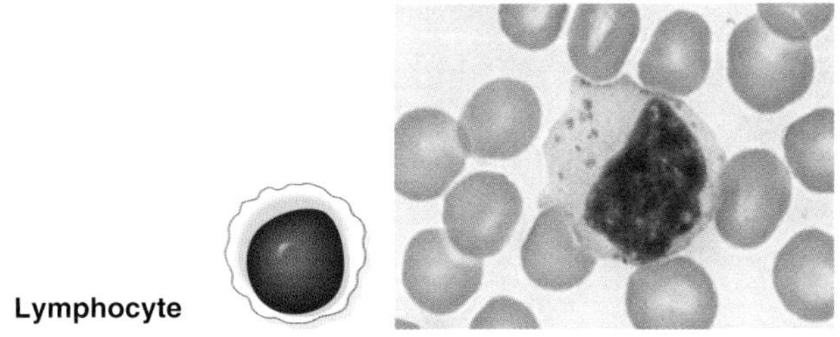

There are two major types of lymphocytes. These are **B cells** and **T cells**.

B Cells

B cell lymphocytes originate in the **bone marrow**. B cells destroy antigens and cells to which they are are attached. They do this by maturing into specialized cells called **plasma cells**, which secrete **antibodies**. Antibodies are proteins called **immunoglobulins.** Examples of immunoglobulins are IgM, IgD, IgE, IgA, and IgG.

The figure below illustrates the production of antibodies by B cells and plasma cells.

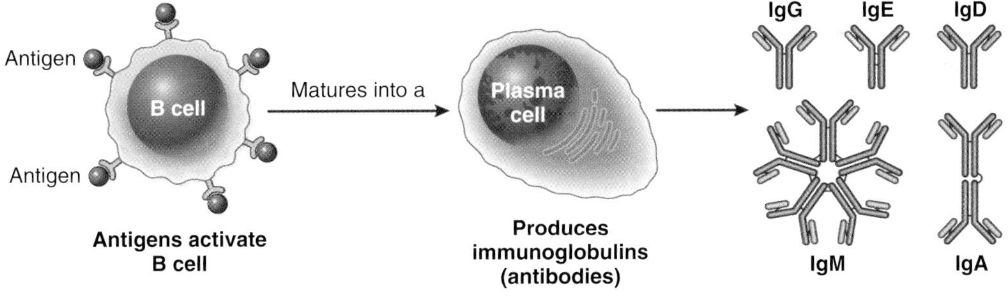

T Cells

These lymphocytes do not produce antibodies but recognize antigen antigen-bearing. The T cells attach to these foreign cells and destroy them. They also aid in stimulating B cells (plasma cells) to make antibodies.

Two types of T cells are:

Cytotoxic T cells (CD8+ cells) that kill antigen-bearing cells directly and secrete proteins called cytokines.

Helper T cells (CD4+ cells) that help B cells and cytotoxic T cells to recognize and destroy antigens.

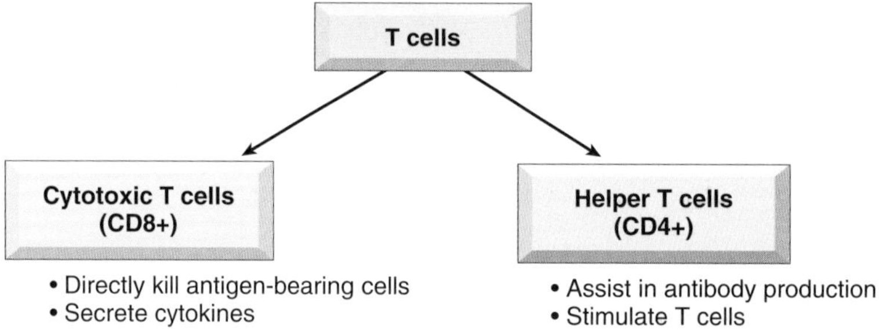

4. **Dendritic cells**
   Other fighters in the immune system are **dendritic cells**. These are cells with long projections ("dendrite" is from Greek, meaning *pertaining to a tree*). They are **antigen-presenting cells (APCs)** that digest antigens from a virus or foreign cell and present the digested antigen to B and T cell lymphocytes for attack and destruction.

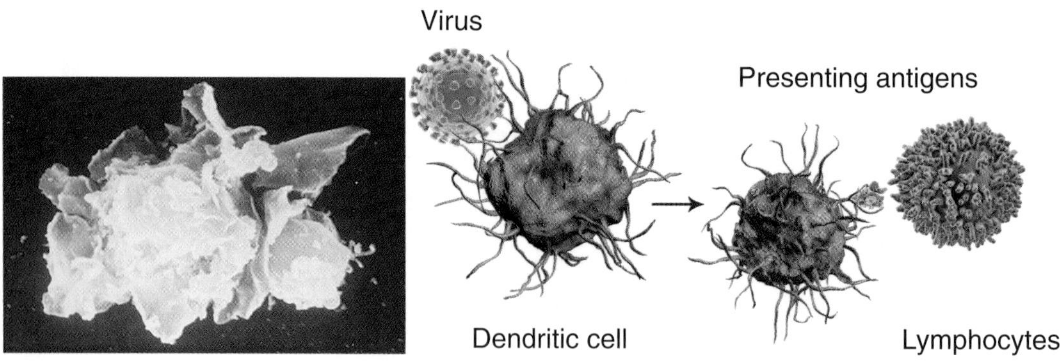

VACCINES

The idea behind vaccines is the ability of our immune system to develop immunologic memory. Immunologic memory is how B cells and T cells remember antigen exposure and know how to destroy those antigens in the future.

During vaccination, antigens are injected into the body and trigger an immune response to attack the foreign material. Lymphocytes, then, using immunologic memory, defend the body when those antigens enter the body again.

In the past, vaccines have been designed to trigger an immune response with the injection of dead or weakened virus, such as the polio, measles, or flu viruses.

Here is the sequence of events in the **viral vaccine approach**:

Viral Vaccines

1. Inject a weakened or inactivated **virus** (polio, measles, or flu) directly into the body after it is made **safe.** The inactivated virus or weakened virus doesn't make you sick but still presents a good **target or antigen**.

2. Safe viruses are engulfed by dendritic antigen-presenting cells (APCs), and viral protein pieces (antigens) are released.

3. Viral protein pieces (antigens) released by APCs activate **helper T cells** of the immune system.

4. Helper T cells signal **B cell and T cell lymphocytes** to attack the antigens. B cells make antibodies and cytotoxic T cells attack the virus directly. B cells and T cells, using **immunologic memory**, remember how to attack the virus when it may infect the body in the future.

The figure below illustrates how viral vaccines work.

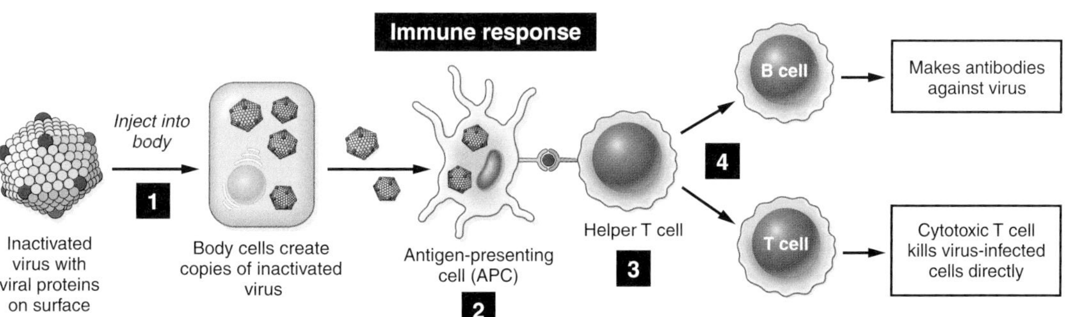

COVID-19 VACCINES

When the COVID-19 pandemic erupted, the search for a new vaccine to combat the coronavirus began. In late 2020 the first vaccines (from Pfizer and Moderna) were approved in the United States for use against the coronavirus and COVID-19. These are a new type of vaccine called **mRNA vaccines**. They are different from the earlier viral vaccines against polio, measles, and flu.

In the earlier viral vaccines, the target protein antigens were pieces of inactivated or weakened virus that trigger an immune response. However, in the mRNA vaccines against COVID-19, the **spike proteins** on the surface of the coronavirus (SARS CoV-2) are the **target antigens.**

Because of these spike proteins, as they appear under the microscope, the coronavirus looks as if it has a crown around it ("corona" means *crown*). Spike proteins on the coronavirus enable it to invade host tissues of the body by attaching, for example, to a specific site on lung tissue, causing pneumonia.

All viruses are very small infectious agents that replicate only inside the living cells of a host organism. The virus itself is composed of genetic material (DNA or RNA) surrounded by a protein coat (covering). The virus causing COVID-19 contains RNA genetic material.

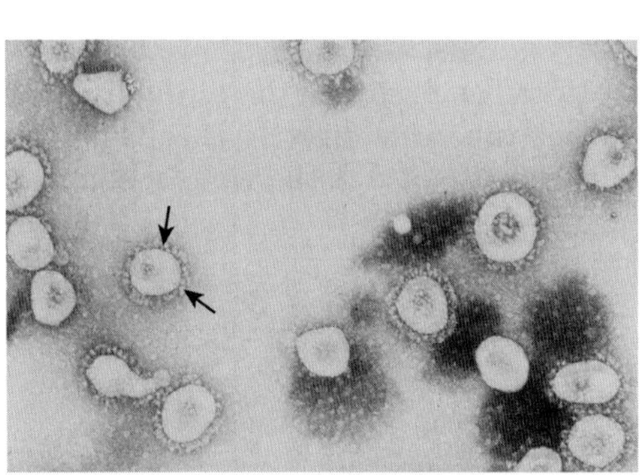
Arrows point to spike proteins surrounding the coronavirus

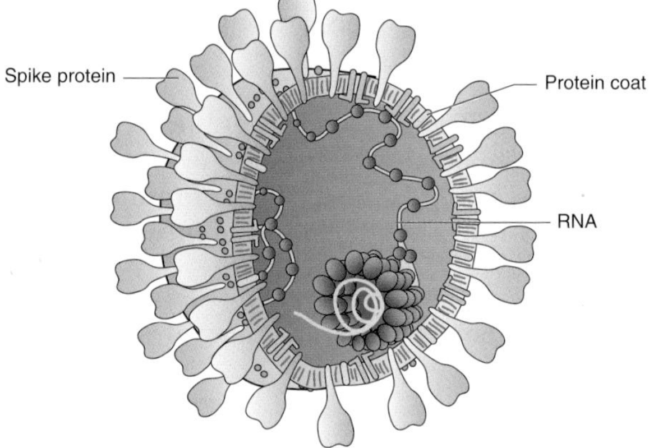

Coronavirus

When a virus infects a host cell, it gives its genetic material to the host and uses the host cell's machinery to make millions of viral copies and then release them to infect more cells. Viruses are protected from the host's immune system when they are living within host cells. However, when they travel through the bloodstream to reach new host cells, they are susceptible to attack by antibodies and T cell lymphocytes. The figure shows virus replication through a host cell.

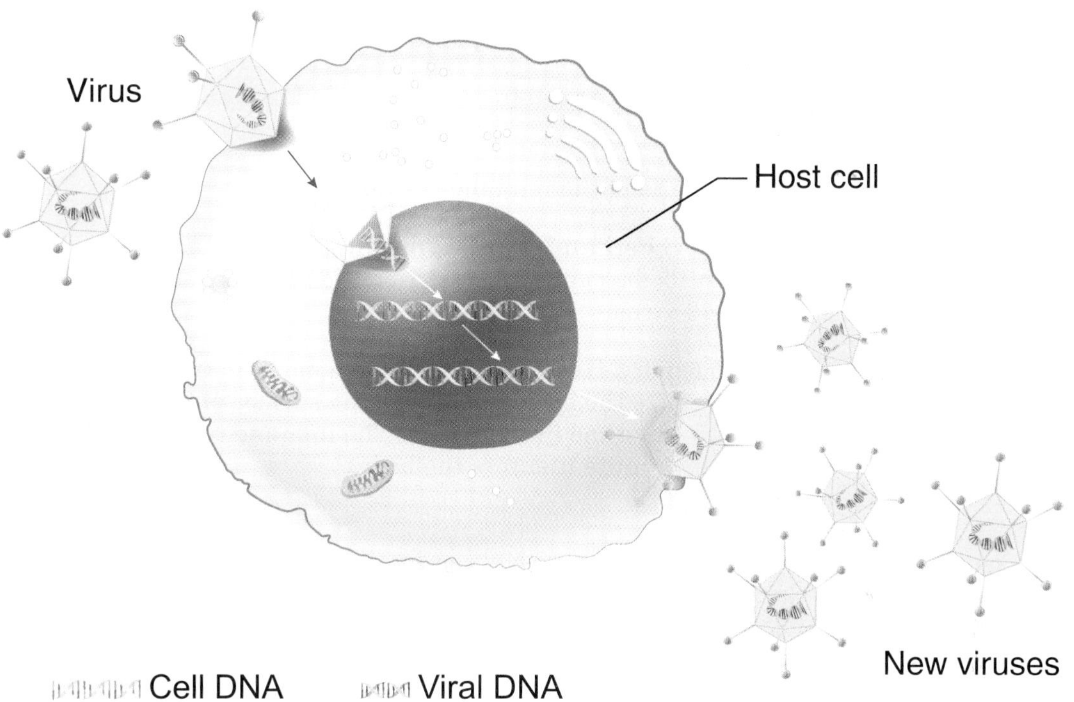

mRNA Vaccines (Pfizer and Moderna)

Here is how the new mRNA vaccines work against the coronavirus (also called SARS-CoV-2 (Severe Acute Respiratory Syndrome coronavirus 2).

1. **mRNA** is a small piece of genetic material that carries a code for making the coronavirus spike protein. The mRNA is packaged in a lipid (fat) pod so that it can get into cells easily. When injected into people, the mRNA enters muscle cells and causes those cells to manufacture **viral spike proteins,** which are harmless on their own. These viral spike protein pieces are then recognized by the immune system as a target to begin an immune response.

2. Immune response begins as spike proteins are recognized by **dendritic antigen-presenting cells (APCs).**

3. APCs activate **helper T cells** of the immune system.

4. Helper T cells then signal **B cell and T cell lymphocytes** to attack viral spike proteins. B cells make antibodies and cytotoxic T cells directly attack the spike proteins on the COVID-19 virus.

Because of immunologic memory, B cells and T cells remember how to attack the viral spike proteins. They recognize the spike protein on the surface of SARS-CoV-2 when the virus enters the body any time in the future. The immune response thus protects by killing the virus the minute it enters the body.

The figure below illustrates how the mRNA vaccine works, while the following figure, page 305, compares viral vaccines and mRNA vaccines.

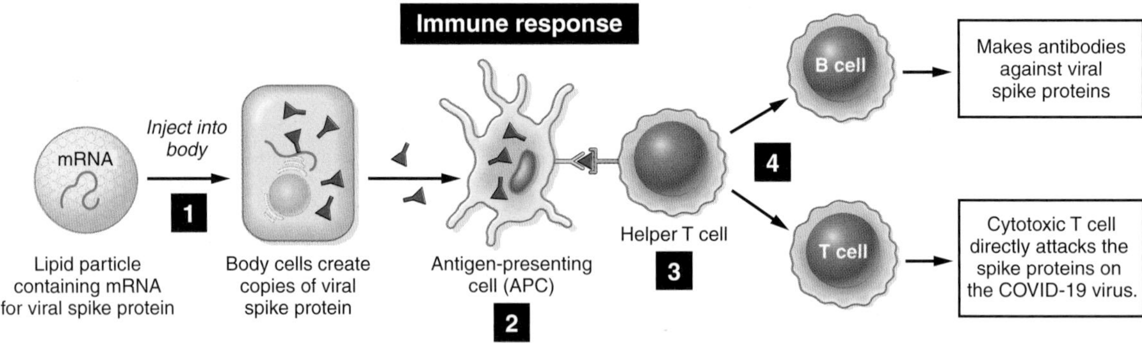

VIRAL VACCINES and mRNA VACCINES

VIRAL VACCINES

Used in polio, measles, flu, and other viral illnesses

1. **Inject the target virus** after it is made safe (inactivated or weakened).

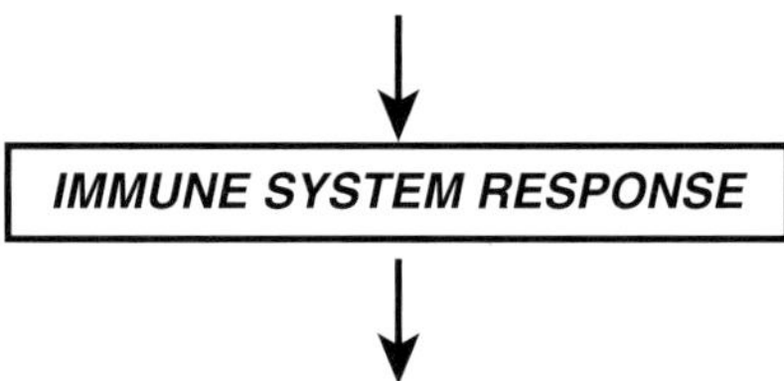

2. **Dendritic antigen-presenting cells (APCs)** engulf and break apart the safe virus (antigen).

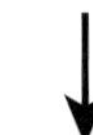

3. APCs use viral protein pieces (antigens) to activate **helper T cells.**

4. Helper T cells signal **B cell and T cell lymphocytes.** B cells create antibodies and T cells directly destroy viral-infected cells.

5. **Immunologic memory** occurs as B cells and T cells remember to attack the virus whenever it infects the body in the future.

mRNA VACCINES

Used in COVID-19

1. **Inject mRNA** (piece of genetic code) from SARS-CoV-2 into body cells. Harmless **spike proteins** are made and released from host (body) cells.

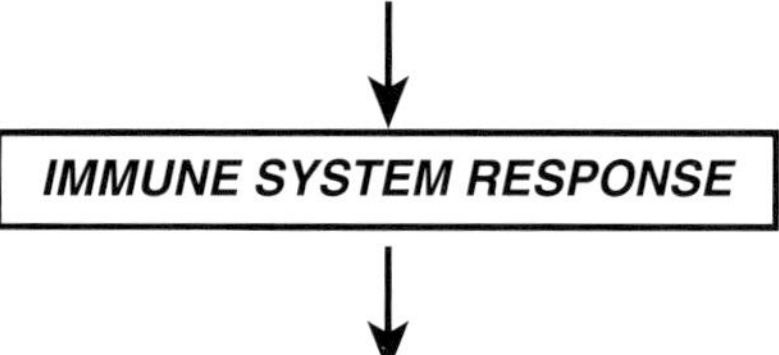

2. **Dendritic antigen-presenting cells (APCs)** recognize and pick up target spike proteins (antigens).

3. APCs use target spike protein pieces (antigens) to activate **helper T cells.**

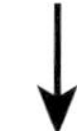

4. Helper T cells signal **B cell and T cell lymphocytes.** B cells create antibodies and T cells directly destroy spike proteins.

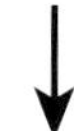

5. **Immunologic memory** occurs as B cells and T cells remember to attack the spike proteins on the COVID-19 virus whenever it infects the body.

Another vaccine that has been approved for use in the United States against COVID-19 is a viral vector vaccine from Johnson and Johnson. In the viral vector vaccine, the coronavirus SARS-CoV-2 spike proteins are injected into the body through a different virus (vector), an **adenovirus**. This different virus is genetically engineered to produce the target spike proteins that will stimulate an immune response after vaccination.

The development of mutant or variant strains of SARS-CoV-2 presents an additional concern for the control of the COVID-19 pandemic. Viruses are prone to mutation (change) as they reproduce continually in host cells. Will the current vaccines be enough to destroy these mutant or variant viral strains that spread more rapidly and cause more serious illness?

APPENDIX 3

Diagnostic Tests and Procedures

This resource contains a color-coded list of common diagnostic tests and procedures. Below is information related to the types of tests/procedures.

- **Radiology, Ultrasound, and Imaging Procedures**
  In many procedures, a *contrast* substance (sometimes referred to as a *dye*) is introduced into the bloodstream, the gastrointestinal tract, or spinal cord so that a body part can be viewed while x-ray pictures are taken. The contrast substance (often containing barium or iodine) blocks the transmission of the x-ray and appears dense on the x-ray image. It outlines the body part that it fills.
  The suffix -GRAPHY, meaning process of recording, is used in many terms describing imaging procedures. The suffix -GRAM, meaning a record, also is used and describes the actual image that is produced by this procedure.

- **Nuclear Medicine: Radionuclide Scans**
  In these diagnostic tests, radioactive material *(radionuclide* or *radioisotope)* is injected intravenously or inhaled and then detected with a scanning device in the organ in which it accumulates. X-rays, ultrasound waves, or magnetic waves are not used.

- **Clinical Procedures**
  These procedures are performed on patients to establish a correct diagnosis of an abnormal condition. In some instances, the procedure also may be used to treat the condition.

- **Laboratory Tests**
  These tests are performed on samples of a patient's blood, *plasma* (fluid portion of the blood), *serum* (plasma minus clotting proteins and produced after blood has clotted), urine, feces, *sputum* (mucus coughed up from the lungs), *cerebrospinal fluid* (fluid within the spaces around the spinal cord and brain), and skin.

In the pronunciation of each term, the syllable that gets the accent is in CAPITAL LETTERS.

Italicized terms indicate important additional terminology.

Terms in SMALL CAPITAL LETTERS are defined elsewhere in this section.

A

Abdominocentesis (ab-dom-in-o-sen-TE-sis): See PARACENTESIS.

Acid phosphatase test (AH-sid FOS-fah-tays): Measurement of the amount of an enzyme called *acid phosphatase* in serum. Enzyme levels are elevated in metastatic prostate cancer. Moderate elevations occur in bone disease and metastatic breast cancer.

Alanine transaminase (ALT) test (AL-ah-neen tranz-AM-ih-nays): Measurement of the amount of the enzyme called *alanine transaminase* in serum. The enzyme is normally present in blood but accumulates in blood with damage to liver cells. Formerly called SGPT.

Albumin test (al-BU-min): Measurement of the amount of albumin (a large protein found in blood and tissues) in both serum and urine. A decreased albumin level in serum indicates malnutrition or liver disease or may occur with extensive loss of protein in the urine or intestines, or from the skin, as in a burn. The presence of albumin in the urine (*albuminuria*) indicates malfunction of the kidney.

Alkaline phosphatase test (AL-kah-lin FOS-fah-tase): Measurement of the amount of *alkaline phosphatase* (an enzyme found in cells) in serum. Levels are elevated in liver diseases (such as hepatitis and hepatoma) and in bone disease and cancer metastatic to bone or liver. On laboratory reports, usually abbreviated as *alk phos* or *ALK PHOS.*

Allergy test (AL-er-je test): A small quantity of suspected allergic substance is applied to the skin or injected under the skin, and any reaction is noted.

Alpha-fetoprotein test (al-fah-fe-to-PRO-teen): Determination of the presence of a protein called alpha-fetoprotein in serum. The protein normally is present in the serum of the fetus, infant, and pregnant woman. In fetuses with abnormalities of the brain and spinal cord, the protein leaks into the amniotic fluid surrounding the fetus, so it is an indicator of a spinal tube defect (spina bifida) or anencephaly (lack of brain development). High levels are found in patients with cancer of the liver and other malignant diseases (testicular and ovarian cancers). Serum levels monitor the effectiveness of cancer treatment. Elevated levels are also seen in benign liver diseases such as cirrhosis and viral hepatitis. On laboratory reports, usually abbreviated *AFP.*

Amniocentesis (am-ne-o-sen-TE-sis): Puncture to remove fluid from the sac (amnion) that surrounds the fetus in the uterus. The fluid contains cells from the fetus that can be examined with a microscope for chromosomal analysis. Levels of chemicals in amniotic fluid also can detect defects in the fetus.

ANA test: See ANTINUCLEAR ANTIBODY TEST.

Angiography (an-je-OG-rah-fe) or **angiogram** (AN-je-o-gram): X-ray imaging of blood vessels. A contrast substance is injected into a blood vessel (vein or artery), and x-ray images are taken of the vessel. In *cerebral angiography,* x-ray images show blood vessels in the brain. In *coronary angiography,* x-rays detect abnormalities in vessels that bring blood to the heart. Angiograms can detect blockage by clots, cholesterol plaques, tumors, or aneurysms (ballooning or dilating of the vessel wall). Angiography is performed frequently to view arteries and is often used interchangeably with *arteriography.* It is also used to view veins *(venography)* to detect blood clots or pulmonary emboli.

Antinuclear antibody test (an-tih-NU-kle-ar AN-tih-bod-e test): A sample of plasma is tested for the presence of antibodies that are found in patients with systemic lupus erythematosus. On laboratory reports, usually abbreviated *ANA.*

Arteriography (ar-teer-e-OG-rah-fe) or **arteriogram** (ar-TEER-e-oh-gram): X-ray recording of an artery and its branches after injection of a contrast substance into an artery. *Coronary arteriography* is the visualization of arteries that travel across the outer surface of the heart and bring blood to the heart muscle.

Arthrocentesis (ar-thro-sen-TE-sis): Puncture to remove fluid from a joint. This usually is done through the skin with a *percutaneous* needle.

Arthrography (arth-ROG-rah-fe): X-ray examination of the inside of a joint with a contrast medium.

Aspartate transaminase (AST) test: Measurement of the enzyme *aspartate transaminase* in serum. The enzyme normally is present in blood but accumulates when there is damage to the heart or to liver cells. Formerly called *SGOT.*

Aspiration (as-pih-RA-shun): Withdrawal of fluid from a cavity or sac by suction through a needle or tube. The term *aspiration pneumonia* refers to an infection caused by inhalation of food or an object into the lungs.

Audiometry (aw-de-OM-eh-tre): Test using sound waves of various frequencies (e.g., 500 Hz), up to 8000 Hz, to quantify the extent and type of hearing loss. An *audiogram* is the record produced by this test.

Auscultation (aw-skul-TA-shun): Process of listening for sounds produced within the body. This is most often performed with the aid of a stethoscope to determine the condition of the heart and lungs and blood vessels or to detect the fetal heartbeat.

B

Bacterial and fungal tests (bak-TER-e-al and FUNG-al tests): Samples from skin lesions or other sites (e.g., blood, bone marrow, sputum) are cultured in a laboratory or analyzed microscopically to diagnose bacterial or fungal conditions.

Barium enema: See LOWER GASTROINTESTINAL EXAMINATION and BARIUM TESTS.

Barium swallow: See ESOPHAGOGRAPHY, BARIUM TESTS, and UPPER GASTROINTESTINAL EXAMINATION.

Barium tests (BAH-re-um tests): X-ray examinations with a liquid barium mixture that is swallowed or given by enema to outline the surface of the gastrointestinal tract. These studies may locate disorders in the esophagus *(esophagogram),* duodenum, small intestine *(small bowel follow-through),* or colon *(barium enema).* Taken before or during the examination, barium causes the intestinal tract to stand out in silhouette when viewed through a *fluoroscope* (see FLUOROSCOPY) or seen on an x-ray image. The *barium swallow* is used to examine the upper gastrointestinal tract, and the *barium enema* is for examination of the lower gastrointestinal tract. These tests are complemented by ENDOSCOPY.

Bence Jones protein test (bens jonz PRO-teen): Measurement of the Bence Jones protein in serum or urine. Bence Jones protein is a fragment of a normal serum protein, an immunoglobulin, produced in greatly excessive amounts by cancerous bone marrow cells (myeloma cells). Normally it is not found in either blood or urine, but in *multiple myeloma* (a malignant condition of bone marrow), high levels of Bence Jones protein may be detected in urine.

Bilirubin test (bil-ih-RU-bin): Measurement of the amount of bilirubin, an orange-brown pigment, in serum and urine. Bilirubin is derived from breakdown of hemoglobin, the oxygen-carrying protein in red blood cells. Its presence in high concentration in serum and urine causes *jaundice* (yellow coloration of the skin) and may indicate disease of the liver, obstruction of bile ducts, or a type of anemia due to excessive destruction of red blood cells.

Biopsy (BI-op-se): Removal of a piece of tissue from the body for subsequent examination under a microscope. The procedure is performed with a surgical knife or by needle aspiration, or *core biopsy,* or via an endoscopic approach (using a special forceps-like instrument inserted through a hollow flexible tube.) *Excisional biopsy* means that the entire tissue to be examined is removed. An *incisional biopsy* is the removal of only a small amount of tissue, and a *needle* or *core biopsy* indicates that tissue is pierced with a hollow needle and fluid and/or cells are withdrawn by aspiration for microscopic examination.

Blood chemistry profile: A comprehensive blood test that is a biochemical examination of various substances in the blood using a computerized laboratory analyzer. Tests include measurements of albumin (liver and kidney), alkaline phosphatase (liver and bone), AST (liver and heart muscle) and ALT (liver), bilirubin (liver), calcium (bones), creatinine (kidney), electrolytes (acid-base balance), globulin (liver and immune disorders), lipids (such as cholesterol and triglycerides), phosphorus (bones), and urea (kidney). Also called *sequential multiple analysis* (SMA). SMA-6, SMA-12, and SMA-18 indicate the number of blood tests performed.

Blood culture (blud KUL-chur): Test to determine whether infection is present in the bloodstream. A sample of blood is added to a special medium (food) that promotes the growth of microorganisms. The medium is then examined by a medical technologist for evidence of bacteria or other microbes.

Blood differential test (blud dih-fer-EN-shul): See WHITE BLOOD CELL (WBC) COUNT.

Blood urea nitrogen (BUN) test (blud u-RE-ah NI-tro-jen): Measurement of the amount of urea (nitrogen-containing waste material) in serum. A high level of serum urea indicates poor kidney function because it is the kidney's job to remove urea from the bloodstream and filter it into urine. On laboratory reports, usually abbreviated *BUN*. Urea is a product of the breakdown of proteins.

Bone density test (bone DEN-sih-te test): Low-energy x-rays are used for this study, which measures bone thickness and reveals areas of bone deficiency *(osteopenia)* and *osteoporosis* (bones become thinner, more fragile, and likely to break). This study is most often performed on the lower spine or hips. Also called *bone densitometry* or *DEXA* (dual-energy x-ray absorptiometry).

Bone marrow biopsy (bone MAH-ro BI-op-se): Removal of a small amount of bone marrow via a needle biopsy. The cells are then examined with a microscope. The liquid content of the marrow cavity is withdrawn by *aspiration* and examined separately from the rest of the biopsy sample. Often the hip bone (iliac crest) is used, and the biopsy is helpful in determining the number and type of blood cells in the bone marrow.

Bone scan: A radioactive substance (usually a TECHNETIUM isotope) is injected intravenously, and its uptake in bones is detected with a scanning device. Tumors in bone can be detected by increased uptake of the radioactive material in the areas of the lesions.

Brain scan: A radioactive substance is injected intravenously. It collects in any lesion that disturbs the natural barrier that exists between blood vessels and normal brain tissue (blood-brain barrier), allowing the radioactive substance to enter the brain tissue. A scanning device detects the presence of the radioactive substance and thus can identify an area of tumor, abscess, or hematoma. This procedure has largely been replaced by COMPUTED TOMOGRAPHY or MAGNETIC RESONANCE IMAGING.

Bronchoscopy (brong-KOS-ko-pe): Visual examination of the bronchial passages through a flexible tube (endoscope) inserted into the airway. The lining of the bronchial tubes can be seen, and tissue may be removed for biopsy. The tube is usually inserted through the mouth or nose but can also be directly inserted into the airway during mediastinoscopy. Sedation is required for this procedure.

BUN test: See BLOOD UREA NITROGEN TEST.

C

CA-125 test: Blood test measuring CA-125, a protein released into the bloodstream by ovarian cancer cells. Measurement of CA-125 determines response to treatment.

Calcium test (KAL-se-um): Measurement of the amount of calcium in serum, plasma, or whole blood. Low blood levels cause abnormal functioning of nerves and muscles, and high blood levels may be due to loss of calcium from bones, excessive intake of calcium, disease of the parathyroid glands, or cancer. On laboratory reports, usually given as the symbol *Ca*.

Carbon dioxide test (KAR-bon di-OK-side): Blood test that measures all forms of carbon dioxide (gas produced by cells and eliminated by the lungs) in blood. On laboratory reports, abbreviated CO_2.

DIAGNOSTIC TESTS AND PROCEDURES

Carcinoembryonic antigen test (kar-sih-no-em-bree-ON-ik AN-ti-jen): A plasma test for a protein normally found in the blood of human fetuses and produced in healthy adults in only a very small amount. High levels of this antigen may be a sign of one of a variety of cancers, especially colon or pancreatic cancer. This test monitors the response of patients to cancer treatment. On laboratory reports, usually abbreviated *CEA.*

Cardiac catheterization (KAR-de-ak kath-eh-ter-ih-ZA-shun): Procedure in which a catheter (tube) is passed via vein or artery into the chambers of the heart to measure the blood flow out of the heart and the pressures and oxygen content in the heart chambers. Contrast material is also introduced into heart chambers, and x-ray pictures are taken to show heart and heart valve structure.

Cardiac enzyme tests (CAR-dee-ak EN-zym tests): Measurements of enzymes released into the bloodstream after a heart attack. Examples are creatine kinase (CK) and troponin I and troponin T.

Catheterization (kath-eh-ter-ih-ZA-shun): Introduction of a hollow, flexible tube into a vessel or cavity of the body to withdraw or instill fluids. Catheterization also is used to measure pressure in vessels and to inject contrast material for outlining vessels or heart chambers. Male and female *Foley catheters* are used for urinary catheterization. *Cardiac catheterization* involves insertion of a catheter into a large vein or artery; from there, it is threaded through the circulation system to the heart. Contrast can be administered to visualize blood vessels for diagnosis and treatment procedures.

Cerebral angiography: See ANGIOGRAPHY.

Cerebrospinal fluid (CSF) analysis (seh-re-bro-SPI-nal FLU-id a-NAL-i-sis): Measurement of cerebrospinal fluid for pressure, protein and sugar content, blood cells, and malignant cells. The fluid also is cultured to detect microorganisms. Chemical tests are performed on specimens of the fluid removed by *lumbar puncture.* Abnormal conditions such as meningitis, tumor involving the spinal canal, and encephalitis are detected by analysis of the spinal fluid. On laboratory reports, usually abbreviated *CSF.*

Chest x-ray: An x-ray image of the chest wall, lungs, and heart. It may show infection (as in pneumonia or tuberculosis), emphysema, damage due to occupational exposure (asbestosis), lung tumors, fluid accumulation (PLEURAL EFFUSION), or heart enlargement. Also called *chest film* (or *chest x-ray film)* and *chest radiograph.*

Cholangiography (ko-lan-je-OG-rah-fe) or **cholangiogram** (ko-LAN-je-o-gram): X-ray recording or record of bile ducts. Contrast material is given by intravenous injection *(IV cholangiogram)* and collects in the gallbladder and bile ducts. Also, contrast can be introduced (through the skin) using a percutaneously placed needle inserted into an intrahepatic duct *(percutaneous transhepatic cholangiography).* X-ray images of bile ducts are obtained to identify obstructions caused by tumors or stones. This procedure has largely been replaced by COMPUTED TOMOGRAPHY and MAGNETIC RESONANCE IMAGING, and by ULTRASONOGRAPHY for stones.

Cholesterol tests (ko-LES-ter-ol): Measurement of the amount of cholesterol (substance found in animal fats and oils, egg yolks, and milk and produced by the liver) in serum. Normal values for adults are 120 to 200 mg/dL. Levels above 200 mg/dL indicate a need for further testing and efforts to reduce cholesterol level, because high levels are associated with blockage of arteries and heart disease. Blood also is tested for the presence of a lipoprotein substance that is a combination of cholesterol and protein. High levels (optimal level is 60 to 100 mg/dL) of high-density lipoprotein *(HDL)* cholesterol in the blood are beneficial because HDL cholesterol promotes the removal and excretion of excess cholesterol from the blood serum, whereas high levels of low-density lipoprotein *(LDL)* are associated with the development of atherosclerosis (optimal level is 100 mg/dL or less). The ratio of HDL to LDL is most important.

Chorionic villus sampling (kor-e-ON-ik VIL-us SAM-pling): Removal of a small piece of placental tissue for microscopic or genetic analysis to detect fetal abnormalities.

Colonoscopy (ko-lon-OS-ko-pe): Visual examination of the colon using a flexible tube (endoscope) inserted through the rectum and passed into the large bowel. Biopsy samples may be taken and benign growths, such as polyps, removed through the endoscope. The removal of a polyp is a *polypectomy* (pol-ih-PEK-to-me).

Colposcopy (kol-POS-ko-pe): Visual examination of the vagina and cervix through a special microscope inserted into the vagina. The vaginal walls are held apart with a speculum so that all tissues can be viewed.

Complete blood count (CBC): Determination of the numbers of leukocytes (white blood cells), erythrocytes (red blood cells), and platelets (clotting cells). The CBC is useful in diagnosis of anemia, infection, and blood cell disorders, such as leukemia.

Computed tomography (kom-PU-ted to-MOG-rah-fe) or **CT** and **CT scan:** X-ray examination that shows images of the body in cross section. Contrast material may be used (injected into the bloodstream) to highlight structures such as the liver, brain, or blood vessels, and barium can be swallowed to outline gastrointestinal organs. X-ray images, obtained as the x-ray tube rotates (helical CT) around the body, are processed by a computer to show "slices" of body tissues, most often within the head, chest, and abdomen.

Conization (ko-nih-ZA-shun): Removal of a cone-shaped sample of uterine cervix tissue. This sample is then examined with a microscope for evidence of cancerous growth. The special shape of the tissue sample allows the pathologist to examine the transitional zone of the cervix, where cancers are most likely to develop.

Coronary arteriography: See ARTERIOGRAPHY.

Creatine kinase test (KRE-ah-tin KI-nas): Measurement of levels of creatine kinase, a blood enzyme. Creatine kinase *(CK)* is normally found in heart muscle, brain tissue, and skeletal muscle. The presence of one form *(isoenzyme)* of creatine kinase (either CK-MB or CK2) in the blood is strongly indicative of recent myocardial infarction (heart attack) because the enzyme is released from heart muscle when the muscle is damaged or dying.

Creatinine test (kre-AT-tih-neen): Measurement of the amount of creatinine, a nitrogen-containing waste material, in serum or plasma. It is the most commonly used test for kidney function. Because creatinine normally is produced as a protein breakdown product in muscle and is excreted by the kidney in urine, an elevation in the creatinine level in the blood indicates abnormal kidney function. Elevations also are seen in patients on high-protein diets and with dehydration.

Creatinine clearance test (kre-AT-tih-neen KLEER-ans): Measurement of the rate at which creatinine is cleared (filtered) by the kidneys from the blood. A low creatinine clearance indicates that the kidneys are not functioning effectively to clear creatinine from the bloodstream and filter it into urine.

Culdocentesis (kul-do-sen-TE-sis): Puncture to remove fluid from the cul-de-sac (the space between the rectum and the uterus) through a thin, hollow needle inserted through the vagina into this space. The fluid is then analyzed for evidence of cancerous cells, infection, or blood cells.

Culture (KUL-chur): Test in which a sample of body fluids (such as urine, blood, sputum) is mixed with or applied to a sterile growth medium, and if present, bacteria, fungi, or viruses are allowed to grow for several days. Microorganisms that grow out are then identified. In *sensitivity* testing, culture plates containing a specific microorganism are prepared and antibiotic-containing discs are applied to the culture surface. After overnight incubation, the area surrounding the disc (where growth was inhibited) is measured to determine whether the antibiotic is effective against the specific organism. Stool samples may also be cultured.

Cystography (sis-TOG-rah-fe) or **cystogram** (SIS-to-gram): X-ray recording of the urinary bladder with a contrast medium so that the outline of the urinary bladder can be seen clearly. A contrast substance is injected via catheter into the urethra and urinary bladder, and x-ray images are made. A *voiding cystourethrogram* is an x-ray image of the urinary tract made while the patient is urinating.

Cystoscopy (sis-TOS-ko-pe): Visual examination of the urinary bladder through a thin tube or cystoscope (endoscope) inserted into the urethra and then passed into the bladder. This procedure is used to visualize inflammation and tumors of the bladder, to remove stones, and to perform a biopsy of suspicious areas.

D

Digital rectal examination or **DRE** (DIJ-ih-tal REK-tal eks-am-ih-NA-shun): The physician inserts a gloved finger into the patient's rectum to detect rectal cancer and as a primary method to detect prostate cancer. Stool on the removed glove is tested for occult blood, a possible sign of disease.

Digital subtraction angiography (DIJ-ih-tal sub-TRAK-shun an-je-OG-rah-fe): A unique x-ray technique for viewing blood vessels by taking two images and subtracting one from the other. Images are first obtained without contrast material and then again after contrast is injected into blood vessels. The first image is then subtracted from the second so that the final image (sharp and precise) shows only contrast-filled blood vessels and not the surrounding tissue.

Dilation and curettage or **D&C** (di-LA-shun and kur-eh-TAJ): A series of probes of increasing size are systematically inserted through the vagina into the opening of the cervix. The cervix is thus dilated (widened) so that a curette (spoon-shaped instrument) can be inserted to remove tissue from the lining of the uterus. The tissue is then examined with a microscope.

Doppler ultrasound (DOP-ler UL-trah-sownd): Technique that focuses sound waves on blood vessels and measures blood flow as echoes bounce off red blood cells. Arteries or veins in the arms, neck, legs, or abdomen are examined to detect vessels that are occluded (blocked) by clots or atherosclerosis.

E

Echocardiography (eh-ko-kar-de-OG-rah-fe) or **echocardiogram** (eh-ko-KAR-de-o- gram): Imaging of the heart by introducing high-frequency sound waves through the chest into the heart. The sound waves are reflected back from the heart, and echoes showing heart structure are displayed on a recording machine. It is a highly useful diagnostic tool in the evaluation of diseases of the valves that separate the heart chambers and diseases of the heart muscle.

Electrocardiography or **ECG/EKG** (e-lek-tro-kar-de-OG-rah-fe): Connection of electrodes (wires or "leads") to the body to record electrical impulses from the heart. The *electrocardiogram* is the actual record produced. This test is useful in discovering abnormalities in heart rhythms and for diagnosing heart disorders.

Electroencephalography or **EEG** (e-lek-tro-en-sef-ah-LOG-rah-fe): Connection of electrodes (wires or "leads") to the scalp to record electricity coming from within the brain. The *electroencephalogram* is the actual record produced. This test is useful in the diagnosis and monitoring of epilepsy and in the investigation of neurologic disorders. It also is used to evaluate patients in coma (brain inactivity) and in the study of sleep disorders.

Electrolyte panel (e-LEK-tro-lyt PAH-nul): Determination of the concentrations of *electrolytes* (chemical substances capable of conducting an electric current) in serum or whole blood. When dissolved in water, salts, such as sodium chloride, break apart into charged particles *(ions)*. The common positively charged electrolytes are *sodium* (Na^+), *potassium* (K^+), *calcium* (Ca^{2+}), and *magnesium* (Mg^{2+}). The common negatively charged electrolytes are *chloride* (Cl^-) and *bicarbonate* (HCO_3^-). These charged particles should be present at all times for proper functioning of cells. An electrolyte imbalance occurs when serum concentration is either too high or too low. Calcium imbalance can affect the bones, kidneys, gastrointestinal tract, and neuromuscular activity, and sodium imbalance will affect blood pressure, nerve functioning, and fluid levels surrounding cells. Potassium ion imbalance impairs heart and muscular activity.

Electromyography or **EMG** (e-lek-tro-mi-OG-rah-fe): Recording of the electrical activity of muscle tissue using electrodes attached to the skin or inserted into the muscle. This procedure detects neuromuscular abnormalities.

Electrophoresis: See SERUM PROTEIN ELECTROPHORESIS.

ELISA (eh-LI-zah): A laboratory assay (test) for the presence of antibodies to abnormal proteins such as tumor antigens or viruses, such as HIV. ELISA is an acronym for *e*nzyme-*l*inked *i*mmuno*s*orbent *a*ssay. It also is known as *EIA* or *enzyme immunoassay.*

Endoscopic retrograde cholangiopancreatography or **ERCP** (en-do-SKOP-ik REH-tro-grayd kol-an-je-o-pan-kre-ah-TOG-rah-fe): X-ray recording of the bile ducts, pancreas, and pancreatic duct using radiopaque contrast injected through an endoscope, passed through the mouth, esophagus, and duodenum into the bile and pancreatic ducts, and x-ray images are then obtained.

Endoscopic ultrasonography or **E-US** (en-do-SKOP-ik ul-trah-so-NOG-rah-fe): Sound waves are generated from a tube inserted through the mouth and into the esophagus. The sound waves bounce off internal structures and are detected by surface coils. This study can detect enlarged cancerous lymph nodes and tumors in the chest and upper abdomen. This procedure is used for *staging* (evaluation of size and spread) of gastric and esophageal tumors.

Endoscopy (en-DOS-ko-pe): Inspection of an organ or body cavity through a narrow, tube-like instrument (endoscope) inserted into the organ or cavity. The endoscope is placed through a natural opening (the mouth or anus) or into a surgical incision, such as through the abdominal wall. Endoscopes contain bundles of glass fibers that carry light (fiberoptic); some instruments are equipped with a small forceps-like device that withdraws a sample of tissue for microscopic study (biopsy). Examples of endoscopy are bronchoscopy, colonoscopy, esophagoscopy, gastroscopy, and laparoscopy.

Erythrocyte sedimentation rate (eh-RITH-ro-site sed-ih-men-TA-shun rate): Measurement of the rate at which red blood cells (erythrocytes) in well-mixed venous blood settle to the bottom (sediment) of a test tube. If the rate of sedimentation is markedly rapid (elevated rate), it may indicate inflammatory conditions, such as rheumatoid arthritis, or conditions that produce excessive proteins in the blood. On laboratory reports, usually abbreviated *ESR* or *sed rate.*

Esophagogastroduodenoscopy or **EGD** (eh-SOF-ah-go-GAS-tro-du-o-den-NOS-ko-pe): Visual examination of the esophagus, stomach, and first part of the small intestine using an endoscope inserted through the mouth and down the throat.

Esophagography (eh-sof-ah-GOG-rah-fe) or **esophagogram** (eh-SOF-ah-go-gram): X-ray recording or record of the esophagus performed after barium sulfate is swallowed. This test is part of a BARIUM SWALLOW and UPPER GASTROINTESTINAL EXAMINATION.

Esophagoscopy (eh-sof-ah-GOS-ko-pe): Visual examination of the esophagus performed through an endoscope inserted into the mouth and down the throat. This procedure allows detection of ulcers, tumors, or other lesions.

Estradiol assay (es-trah-DI-ol AS-a): Test for the concentration of estradiol, which is the predominant form of estrogen (female hormone) in serum, plasma, or urine.

Estrogen receptor assay (ES-tro-jen re-SEP-tor AS-a): Test performed on a breast biopsy specimen to determine whether a sample of tumor contains an estrogen receptor protein. If the protein is present (positive result) on breast cancer cells, this indicates that estrogens can stimulate growth of the tumor. Then treatment with an anti-estrogen drug would retard tumor growth. If the assay result is negative (the protein is not present), then the tumor cells would not be killed by anti-estrogen drug treatment.

Excisional biopsy (ek-SIH-zhin-al BI-op-se): See BIOPSY.

Exophthalmometry (eks-of-thal-MOM-eh-tre): Measurement of the extent of protrusion of the eyeball in *exophthalmos*. Exophthalmos may be caused by tumors behind the eye, or by an overactive thyroid gland.

F

Fluorescein angiography (flur-uh-seen an-je-OG-rah-fe): Fluorescein (a contrast substance) is injected intravenously and the movement of blood is observed by ophthalmoscopy. It is used to detect diabetes or hypertensive retinopathy and also degeneration of the macular (central) area of the retina.

Fluoroscopy (flur-OS-ko-pe): An x-ray examination that uses a fluorescent screen rather than a photographic plate to show images of the body in motion. X-rays that have passed through the body strike a screen covered with a fluorescent substance that emits yellow-green light. Internal organs are seen directly (still images are stored either on film or on a computer as digital images) and in motion. Fluoroscopy is used to guide the insertion of catheters and to direct organ biopsy, and may be enhanced with barium ingestion. CT-guided biopsy is used most often now.

Frozen section (fro-zen SEK-shun): Technique for (or method of) rapid preparation of a biopsy sample for examination during an actual surgical procedure. Tissue is taken from the operating room to the pathology laboratory and frozen. It is then thinly sliced, stained, and immediately examined with a microscope to determine whether the sample is benign or malignant and to determine the status of margins around a tumor.

G

Gallbladder ultrasound (GAWL-blah-der UL-trah-sownd): Sound waves are used to visualize gallstones. This procedure has replaced the x-ray test known as cholecystography.

Gallium scan (GAL-e-um scan): Radioactive gallium (gallium citrate) is injected into the bloodstream and is detected in the body with a scanning device that produces an image of the areas where gallium collects. Gallium accumulates in sites where cells are dividing, such as certain tumors and areas of inflammation.

- Radiology, Ultrasound, and Imaging Procedures
- Nuclear Medicine—Radionuclide Scans
- Clinical Procedures
- **Laboratory Tests**

Gastroscopy (gas-TROS-ko-pe): Visual examination of the stomach through an endoscope inserted down through the esophagus, for either diagnostic inspection or biopsy. When the upper portion of the small intestine is also visualized, the procedure is called *esophagogastroduodenoscopy (EGD)*.

Glucose test (GLU-kos test): Measurement of the amount of glucose (sugar) in serum and plasma. High levels of glucose *(hyperglycemia)* indicate the presence of diabetes mellitus. Glucose also is measured in urine, where its presence also usually indicates diabetes mellitus. The *fasting blood sugar test* is measurement of blood sugar after a patient has fasted.

Glucose tolerance test (GLU-kos TOL-er-ans test): Test to determine how the body responds to glucose. In the first part of this test, blood and urine samples are taken after the patient has fasted. Then a solution of 100 grams of glucose is given by mouth. Additional blood and urine samples are obtained a half hour after the glucose is taken and again at intervals of up to 2 hours to determine the rate of rise in and then the fall of glucose in the blood. This test will diagnose diabetes mellitus.

H

Hematocrit (he-MAT-o-krit): Measurement of the percentage blood volume occupied by red blood cells. The normal range is 40% to 50% in males and 37% to 47% in females. A low hematocrit indicates anemia. On laboratory reports, usually abbreviated *Hct* or *HCT.*

Hemoccult test (he-mo-KULT test): Examination of small sample of stool for otherwise inapparent occult (hidden) traces of blood. The sample is placed on the surface of a collection kit and reacts with a chemical (e.g., guaiac). A positive result may indicate bleeding from polyps, ulcers, or malignant tumors. This is an important screening test for colon cancer. Also called a STOOL GUAIAC TEST.

Hemoglobin assay (HE-mo-glo-bin AS-a): Measurement of the concentration of hemoglobin (protein that carries oxygen in red blood cells) in blood. The normal blood hemoglobin ranges are 13.0 to 17.0 g/dL in adult males and 12.0 to 15.0 g/dL in adult females. On laboratory reports, usually abbreviated *Hb* (or *hgb* or *Hgb).*

Holter monitoring (HOL-ter MON-ih-ter-ing): Electrocardiographic recording of heart activity over an extended period of time. The Holter monitor device is worn by the patient as normal daily activities are performed. It detects heart rhythm abnormalities. Also called *ambulatory electrocardiography.*

Human chorionic gonadotropin assay (HU-man kor-e-ON-ik go-nad-o-TRO-pin AS-a): Measurement of the concentration of human chorionic gonadotropin (a hormone secreted by cells of the fetal placenta) in urine. It is detected in urine within days after fertilization of egg and sperm cells and provides the basis of the most commonly used pregnancy test. It also is elevated in patients with certain tumors. On laboratory reports, usually abbreviated *HCG* or *hCG.*

Hysterosalpingography (his-ter-o-sal-ping-OG-rah-fe) or **hysterosalpingogram** (his-ter-o-sal-PING-o-gram): X-ray recording (imaging) or record of the uterus and fallopian tubes. Contrast material is inserted through the vagina into the uterus and fallopian tubes, and x-ray images are obtained to detect blockage or tumor.

Hysteroscopy (his-ter-OS-ko-pe): Visual examination of the uterus using an endoscope passed through the uterine neck or cervix into the uterus.

I

Immunoassay (im-u-no-AS-a): A method of testing blood and urine for the concentration of various chemicals, such as hormones, drugs, or proteins. The technique makes use of the immunological reaction between antigens and antibodies. An *assay* is a determination of the amount of any particular substance in fluid or tissue.

Immunoglobulin test (im-u-no-GLOB-u-lin test): Measurement (in serum) of proteins (antibodies) that bind to and destroy foreign substances (antigens). Immunoglobulins are made by cells of the immune system.

Immunohistochemistry (im-u-no-his-to-KEM-is-tre): An antibody tagged with a fluorescent label or dye is spread over a tissue biopsy specimen and used to detect the presence of a particular antigen produced by the tissue or a tumor or infection.

Incisional biopsy (in-SIZH-un-al BI-op-se): See BIOPSY.

Intravenous pyelography: See UROGRAPHY.

K

Kidneys, ureters, bladder (KID-neez, UR-eh-terz, BLAH-der) or **KUB:** X-ray images of the kidney, ureters, and urinary bladder, made without contrast material.

L

Laparoscopic sleeve gastrectomy (lap-ah-ro-SKOP-ik sleeve gas-TREK-to-me): Minimally invasive weight-loss procedure performed by removing about 80% of the stomach. The remaining stomach is a small, tubular sleeve (pouch) that reduces the amount of food consumed and helps decrease appetite.

Laparoscopy (lap-ah-ROS-ko-pe): Examination of the abdominal cavity through an endoscope inserted into the abdomen. After the patient receives a local anesthetic, a laparoscope is placed through an incision in the abdominal wall. This procedure gives the physician a view of the abdominal cavity, the surface of the liver and spleen, and the pelvic region. Laparoscopy can be used to remove some organs (such as the gallbladder, appendix, and ovary) and tumors and for fallopian tube ligation to prevent pregnancy.

Laryngoscopy (lah-rin-GOS-ko-pe): Visual examination of the voice box (larynx) through an endoscope inserted down the trachea (airway). The laryngoscope transmits a magnified image of the larynx through a system of lenses and mirrors. The procedure can reveal tumors and explain changes in the voice. Sputum samples and tissue biopsy specimens are obtained by using brushes or forceps attached to the laryngoscope.

Lipid tests (LIP-id tests): Lipids are fatty substances such as cholesterol and triglycerides. See CHOLESTEROL and TRIGLYCERIDE.

Lipoprotein tests (li-po-PRO-teen tests): See CHOLESTEROL.

Liver function tests (LIV-er FUNG-shun tests): See ALKALINE PHOSPHATASE, BILIRUBIN, ALT, and AST.

Lower gastrointestinal examination (LO-wer gas-tro-in-TES-tin-al ek-zam-ih-NA-shun): X-ray pictures of the colon taken after a liquid contrast substance called barium sulfate is inserted through a plastic tube (enema) into the rectum and large intestine (colon). If a tumor is present in the colon, it may appear as an obstruction or irregularity. Also known as a BARIUM ENEMA.

Lumbar puncture or **LP** (LUM-bar PUNK-shur): Introduction of a hollow needle into a space surrounding the spinal cord to withdraw fluid for analysis. Contrast material may be injected for imaging. Medicines may be introduced for treating disease involving the central nervous system.

M

Magnetic resonance imaging or **MRI** (mag-NET-ik REZ-o-nans IM-ah-jing): A powerful magnetic field is created surrounding the whole patient, or only the head, and water molecules are aligned and then relaxed, generating electromagnetic currents that provide a detailed picture of organs and blood vessels. A computer produces images of body structures at successive depths (as with CT slices). This procedure is particularly useful for imaging tumors of the brain and spinal cord and abnormalities of the lungs and abdominal and pelvic organs. No x-rays are used, and the study may be performed with intravenous contrast material (gadolinium), depending on the purpose of the evaluation. In *magnetic resonance angiography (MRA* or *MR angiography),* blood vessels are examined in key areas of the body such as the brain, kidneys, pelvis, legs, lungs, and heart.

Mammography (mah-MOG-rah-fe) or **mammogram** (MAM-o-gram): X-ray recording or record of the breast. X-rays of low voltage are beamed at the breast, and images are produced. Mammography detects abnormalities in breast tissue, such as breast cancer. In *stereotactic breast biopsy,* a hollow needle is passed through the skin into a suspicious lesion with the help of mammographic imaging. Breast *tomosynthesis,* also called 3D mammography, creates three-dimensional images of the breast and aids in detection of early breast disease.

Mediastinoscopy (me-de-ah-stih-NOS-ko-pe): Procedure for viewing structures in the mediastinum through an endoscope inserted into this space (in the chest between the lungs and in front of the heart). A *mediastinoscope* is introduced through a small incision in the neck while the patient is under anesthesia. This procedure is used to biopsy lymph nodes and suspected tumors within the mediastinum.

MUGA scan (MUH-gah scan): Test that uses radioactive technetium to measure the rate of cardiac output of blood by a *mu*ltiple-*g*ated *a*cquisition (MUGA) technique. Also called *technetium-99m ventriculography.*

Muscle biopsy (MUH-sl BI-op-se): A sample of muscle tissue is removed and analyzed microscopically.

Myelography (mi-eh-LOG-rah-fe) or **myelogram** (MI-eh-lo-gram): X-ray recording of the spinal cord after injection of contrast. This procedure has been largely replaced by MRI for detecting tumors or ruptured "slipped" discs between vertebrae (backbones).

N

Nasogastric intubation (na-zo-GAS-trik in-tu-BA-shun): Insertion of a tube through the nose into the stomach to withdraw fluid for analysis or to give nutrition directly into the stomach.

Needle biopsy (NE-dl BI-op-se): See BIOPSY.

O

Occult blood test: See HEMOCCULT TEST.

Ophthalmoscopy (of-thal-MOS-ko-pe): Visual examination of the eye. A physician uses an *ophthalmoscope* to look directly into the eye, evaluating the optic nerve, retina, and blood vessels in the back of the eye and the lens in the front of the eye for cataracts. In *fluorescein angiography,* a contrast substance is injected intravenously, and movement of the dye through blood vessels in the back of the eye is observed with ophthalmoscopy.

Otoscopy (o-TOS-ko-pe): Visual examination of the interior of the ear. A physician uses an *otoscope* inserted into the ear canal to check for obstructions (e.g., wax), infection, fluid, and eardrum perforation or scarring.

Palpation (pal-PA-shun): Examination by touch. This is a technique of manual physical examination by which a doctor feels underlying tissues and organs through the skin.

Pap smear (pap smeer): Insertion of a cotton swab or wooden spatula into the vagina to obtain a sample of cells from the outer surface of the cervix (neck of the uterus). The cells are then smeared on a glass slide, preserved, and sent to the laboratory for microscopic examination. This test for cervical cancer was developed by and named after the late Dr. George Papanicolaou. Results are graded and reported as negative (no abnormalities) or as ranging from mildly abnormal (presence of ASC or abnormal squamous cells) to high-grade squamous intraepithelial lesion (HSIL).

Paracentesis (pah-rah-sen-TE-sis): Puncture of the membrane surrounding the abdomen (peritoneum) to remove fluid from the abdominal cavity. Fluid is drained for analysis and to prevent its accumulation in the abdomen. Also known as *abdominocentesis*

PCR test: Blood test to find and analyze DNA and RNA in viruses, diagnose genetic diseases, and do DNA fingerprinting. Multiple copies of DNA or RNA are made. PCR stands for *p*olymerase *c*hain *r*eaction and can detect very small amounts of RNA or DNA.

Pelvic exam (PEL-vik ek-ZAM): Physician inserts fingers into the vagina while keeping the other hand over the abdomen to palpate the uterus and ovaries. This examination checks the uterus and ovaries for enlargement, cysts, tumors, or abnormal bleeding. It is also known as an internal exam or a bimanual exam.

Percussion (per-KUSH-un): The technique of striking a part of the body with short, sharp taps of the fingers to determine the size, density, and position of the underlying parts by the sound obtained. Percussion is commonly used over the lungs to detect fluid, atelectasis (collapsed lung), and infection, and on the abdomen to examine the liver.

Phlebotomy (fleh-BOT-o-me): Puncture of a vein to remove samples of blood for analysis. Also called *venipuncture.*

PKU test: Test that determines whether the urine of a newborn baby contains substances called *phenylketones.* If these ketones are present, the baby is diagnosed with a condition called *phenylketonuria (PKU).* PKU affects infants who lack a specific enzyme. When the enzyme is missing, high levels of *phenylalanine* (an amino acid) accumulate in the blood, affecting the infant's brain and causing intellectual disability. This situation is prevented by placing the infant on a special diet that prevents accumulation of phenylalanine in the bloodstream.

Platelet count (PLAYT-let kownt): Determination of the number of clotting cells (platelets) in a sample of blood.

Positron emission tomography or **PET scan** (POZ-ih-tron e-MISH-un to-MOG-rah-fe scan): A radioactive substance (usually an isotope incorporated into a sugar molecule) that releases radioactive particles called positrons is injected and travels to specialized areas of the body. Because of the way in which the positrons are released, cross-sectional color pictures can be made showing the location of the radioactive substance. The most common use for PET scans is to detect cancer and examine the effects of cancer therapy by showing biochemical changes in tumors. Tumors pick up the radioactive substance (isotope) and appear as "hot spots" (areas of high glucose uptake) on the film. Also, PET scans can be performed on the heart to assess blood flow to heart muscle and to evaluate patients for coronary artery disease. PET scans of the brain are used to evaluate patients with memory disorders, seizure disorders, and brain tumors. Metabolically active parts of the brain appear as hot spots. *PET-CT* scans combine PET and CT imaging technology to aid in the localization of "hot" areas.

Potassium test (po-TAS-e-um test): Measurement of the concentration of potassium in serum. Potassium is an important chemical for regulating electrical currents and maintaining the cell membrane charge. Muscle and nerve function depends on movement of potassium and other electrolytes across the cell membrane. On laboratory reports, usually given as the symbol K^+. See also ELECTROLYTES.

Pregnancy test (PREG-nan-se test): Measurement in blood or urine of *human chorionic gonadotropin,* or hCG, a hormone secreted by the placenta early in pregnancy.

Proctosigmoidoscopy (prok-to-sig-moy-DOS-ko-pe): Examination of the first 10 to 12 inches of the rectum and colon using an endoscope inserted through the anus. When the sigmoid colon is visualized with a longer (20-inch) flexible endoscope, the procedure is called *sigmoidoscopy.* The procedure detects polyps, malignant tumors, and sources of bleeding.

Progesterone receptor assay (pro-JES-teh-rone re-SEP-tor AS-a): Test to determine whether a sample of tumor contains a progesterone receptor protein. A positive test result identifies that a breast cancer tumor would be responsive to antihormone therapy.

Prostate-specific antigen (PSA) test (PROS-tat speh-SIH-fic AN-tih-jen): Blood test that measures the amount of an antigen elevated in patients with prostatic cancer and in some with an inflamed prostate gland. On laboratory reports, usually abbreviated *PSA.*

Protein electrophoresis: See SERUM PROTEIN ELECTROPHORESIS TEST.

Prothrombin time (pro-THROM-bin time): Measurement of the activity of factors in the blood that participate in clotting. Deficiency of any of these factors can lead to a prolonged prothrombin time and difficulty in blood clotting. The test is important as a monitor for patients taking anticoagulants, substances that block the activity of blood clotting factors but increase the risk of bleeding.

Pulmonary angiography (PUL-mo-nair-e an-je-OG-rah-fe): X-ray images of blood vessels of the lung are obtained after injection of contrast. This procedure has been largely replaced by COMPUTED TOMOGRAPHY of the lung.

Pulmonary function test (PUL-mo-nair-e FUNG-shun test): Measurement of the volume and flow rate (ventilation) of air taken into and exhaled from the lungs by means of an instrument called a *spirometer.* Test results may be abnormal in patients with asthma, chronic bronchitis, emphysema, or occupational exposures to asbestos, chemicals, and dusts.

Pulmonary perfusion scan (PUL-mo-nair-e per-FU-shun scan): Radioactive particles are injected intravenously and travel rapidly to areas of the lung that are adequately filled with blood. Regions of obstructed blood flow caused by tumor, blood clot, swelling, and inflammation can be seen as nonradioactive areas on the scan.

Pulmonary ventilation scan (PUL-mo-nair-e ven-tih-LA-shun scan): Radioactive gas is inhaled, and a special camera detects its presence in the lungs. The scan is used to detect lung segments that fail to fill with the radioactive gas. Lack of filling is usually due to diseases that obstruct the bronchial tubes and air sacs. This scan is also used in the evaluation of lung function before surgery.

Pyelography or pyelogram: See UROGRAPHY.

R

Red blood cell (RBC) count: Test in which the number of erythrocytes in a sample of blood is counted. A low RBC count may indicate anemia. A high count can indicate *polycythemia vera.*

Rheumatoid factor assay (ROO-mah-toyd FAK-tor AS-a): Detection of the abnormal protein *rheumatoid factor* in the serum. This factor is found in patients with rheumatoid arthritis and some other autoimmune diseases.

S

Semen analysis (SE-men ah-NAL-ih-sis): Microscopic examination of sperm cells to detect number, viability, and motility of sperm cells.

Serum enzyme tests (SE-rum EN-zym tests): see CARDIAC ENZYME TESTS.

Serum protein electrophoresis test (SE-rum PRO-teen e-lek-tro-for-E-sis test): A procedure that separates proteins through their migration in an electric current. The material tested, such as serum, containing various proteins, is placed on gel or in liquid, and under the influence of an electric current, the proteins separate (-PHORESIS means separation) so that they can be identified and measured. The procedure is also known as *protein electrophoresis.*

Sigmoidoscopy (sig-moy-DOS-ko-pe): See PROCTOSIGMOIDOSCOPY.

Skin biopsy (skin BI-op-se): Procedure in which samples of skin lesions are removed and sent to the pathology laboratory for microscopic examination.

Skin tests: Tests in which substances are applied to the skin or injected under the skin and the reaction of immune cells in the skin is observed. These tests detect the patient's sensitivity to substances such as dust or pollen. They also can indicate whether the person has been exposed to the bacteria that cause tuberculosis or diphtheria.

Slit-lamp microscopy (slit-lamp mi-KROS-ko-pe): Examination of the anterior eye structures (such as the cornea) using an instrument that projects intense light through a narrow opening for optimal visualization.

SMA: See BLOOD CHEMISTRY PROFILE.

Small bowel follow-through: See BARIUM TESTS and UPPER GASTROINTESTINAL EXAMINATION.

Sodium level test: Measurement of the concentration of sodium (Na^+) in serum. Sodium is one of the most important elements in the body. It is the chief *electrolyte* in fluid outside cells, and it exchanges with potassium within cells during muscle contraction or nerve conduction. Excess sodium is excreted by the kidneys, and sodium is thus involved in water (fluid) balance and acid-base chemical balance during muscle contraction or nerve conduction.

Sonography: See ULTRASONOGRAPHY.

Sputum test (SPU-tum test): Examination of mucus coughed up from the patient's lungs to detect tumor or infection. The sputum is examined microscopically, analyzed chemically, and cultured for the presence of microorganisms.

Stool culture (stool KUL-chur): Stool (feces) is placed in a growth medium (culture) and analyzed microscopically for evidence of microorganisms (bacteria).

Stool guaiac test (stool GWI-ak test): See HEMOCCULT TEST.

Stress test: Electrocardiography performed during exercise. With intense exercise, the ECG may become abnormal as a result of poor blood flow through blocked arteries. This study may reveal hidden heart disease or confirm the cause of cardiac signs and symptoms.

Technetium Tc-99m sestamibi scan (tek-NE-she-um Tc-99m ses-tah-MIH-be scan): Sestamibi, tagged with technetium-99, is injected, and the radioactivity is not taken up in areas of decreased blood flow (ischemia). This procedure can be used with an *exercise tolerance test (ETT-MIBI)* to help define areas of poor blood flow to the heart muscle.

Thallium-201 scintigraphy (THAL-e-um-201 sin-TIH-grah-fe): Thallium-201 is injected into a vein, and images of blood flow through the heart muscle are recorded. Cold spots correlate with areas of myocardial infarction. *Sestamibi scans* also are used to assess the status of blood flow through heart muscle during an *exercise tolerance test (ETT-MIBI)*. It also is useful in localizing disease of the parathyroid glands.

Thoracentesis (thor-ah-sen-TE-sis): Insertion of a needle into the chest to remove fluid from the space surrounding the lungs (pleural cavity). After injection of a local anesthetic, a hollow needle is placed through the skin and muscles of the back and into the space between the lungs and chest wall. Fluid is then withdrawn by applying suction. Excess fluid *(pleural effusion)* may be a sign of infection, heart failure, or malignant disease. This procedure is used to diagnose conditions, to drain a pleural effusion, or to re-expand a collapsed lung *(atelectasis)*.

Thoracoscopy (thor-ah-KOS-ko-pe): Visual examination of the surface of the lungs using an endoscope inserted through an incision in the chest. *VATS* is *video-assisted thoracoscopy* (or *thorascopy)*.

Thyroid function tests (THI-royd FUNG-shun tests): Tests that measure the levels of thyroid hormones, such as *thyroxine* (T4) and *triiodothyronine* (T3), in serum. *Thyroid-stimulating hormone* (TSH), which is produced by the pituitary gland and stimulates the release of T4 and T3 from the thyroid gland, is also measured in serum. These tests diagnose hypothyroidism and hyperthyroidism, and are helpful in monitoring response to thyroid treatment.

Thyroid scan and uptake (THI-royd scan and UP-take): In a thyroid scan, radioactive iodine (the radiotracer) is injected intravenously or swallowed and then collects in the thyroid gland. A scanning device (probe) detects the radiotracer in the gland tissue, producing an image that shows the size, shape, and position of the thyroid. The thyroid uptake test, or *radioactive iodine uptake* (RAIU) test, evaluates the function of the thyroid. Radioactive iodine is swallowed, and a probe is placed over the thyroid gland to detect increased or decreased activity, as shown by the thyroid's ability to absorb the radiotracer. This test also can be used to detect areas of poor uptake (cold nodules), which may be cancerous.

Tomography (to-MOG-rah-fe) or **tomogram** (TO-mo-gram): X-ray recording or record that shows an organ in depth. Several pictures ("slices") are taken of an organ by moving the x-ray tube and film in sequence to blur out certain regions and bring others into sharper focus. Tomograms of the kidney and lung are examples.

Triglycerides test (tri-GLIS-er-ides test): Determination of the amount of triglycerides (fatty substances) in the serum. Elevated triglyceride levels (normal is 150 to 200 mg/dL) are considered to be an important risk factor for the development of heart disease.

Troponin test (tro-PO-nin): Measurement of levels of proteins *troponin I* and *troponin T* in blood is used to indicate the presence and degree of myocardial injury, as from a heart attack.

Tuning fork tests (TOO-ning fork tests): Procedure in which a vibration source (tuning fork) is placed in front of the opening to the ear to test air conduction of sound waves. The tuning fork is also placed on the mastoid bone behind the ear to test bone conduction of sound waves.

Tuberculin test (too-BUR-ku-lin tests): Agents are applied to the skin with punctures or injection and the reaction is noted. Redness and swelling result in people sensitive to the test substance and indicate previous or current infection with tuberculosis.

U

Ultrasonography (ul-trah-so-NOG-rah-fe) or **ultrasound imaging** (UL-trah-sownd IM-a-jing): Images are produced by beaming high-frequency sound waves (not x-rays) into the body and capturing the echoes that bounce off organs. These echoes are then processed to produce an image showing the difference between fluid and solid masses and the general position of organs. Because ultrasound images are captured in real time, they can show structure and movement of internal organs, as well as blood flowing through blood vessels. Ultrasonography is particularly useful for detecting gallstones, fibroid tumors of the uterus and ovarian tumors and cysts *(pelvic ultrasonography),* enlargement of the heart or defects in heart valves *(echocardiography),* blood flow through major arteries and veins *(Doppler ultrasound),* and enlargement of lymph nodes in the abdomen and chest. Also called *sonography.*

Upper gastrointestinal examination (UP-er gas-tro-in-TES-tin-al ek-zam-ih-NA-shun): X-ray pictures are taken of the esophagus (BARIUM SWALLOW), duodenum, and small intestine after a liquid contrast substance (barium sulfate) is swallowed. In a *small bowel follow-through,* pictures are taken at increasing time intervals to follow the progress of barium through the small intestine. Identification of obstructions or ulcers is possible.

Uric acid test (UR-ik AS-id test): Measurement of the amount of uric acid (a nitrogen-containing waste material from breakdown of DNA and RNA) in the serum. High serum levels are associated with a type of arthritis called *gout.* In gout, uric acid accumulates as crystals in joints and in tissues. High levels of uric acid may also cause kidney stones.

Urinalysis (u-rih-NAL-ih-sis): Examination of urine as an aid in the diagnosis of disease. Routine urinalysis involves the observation of unusual color or odor; determination of specific gravity (amount of materials dissolved in urine); chemical tests (for protein, sugar, acetone); and microscopic examination for bacteria, blood cells, and sediment. Urinalysis is used to detect abnormal functioning of the kidneys and bladder, infections, and diabetes mellitus. On laboratory reports, usually abbreviated *UA.*

Urography (u-ROG-rah-fe) or **urogram** (U-ro-gram): X-ray recording (imaging) of the kidney and urinary tract. If x-ray pictures are taken after contrast material is injected intravenously, the procedure is called *intravenous urography (descending* or *excretion urography)* or *intravenous pyelography* (*IVP*). If x-ray pictures are taken after introduction of contrast directly into the bladder through the urethra, the study is called a *cystogram.* If contrast flows up the ureters into the kidneys, the procedure is called *retrograde urography* or *retrograde pyelography.* PYEL/O means renal pelvis (the collecting chamber of the kidney).

V

Venography (ve-NOG-rah-fe): X-ray examination of veins performed after contrast material is injected into veins. It is used to detect *deep vein thrombosis, pulmonary emboli,* or *venous insufficiency.*

Ventilation-perfusion scan or **V/Q scan:** Nuclear medicine test that uses radioactive materials (radiopharmaceuticals) to examine air flow (ventilation) and blood flow (perfusion) in the lungs. The purpose of this scan is to find evidence of a blood clot (pulmonary embolism) in the lungs. Scans are performed together. If ventilation occurs in a segment that is not perfused, the mismatch implies a pulmonary embolism. When the scans match, abnormalities may reflect pneumonia or other lung disease.

Viral load test for HIV: Measures the number of viral particles in the blood. It is used to determine the effectiveness of antiviral treatment.

Voiding cystourethrogram (voy-ding sis-to-u-RE-thro-gram) or **VCUG:** X-ray films of the bladder and urethra taken after the bladder is filled with a contrast material and while the patient is expelling urine.

W

Western blot (WES-tern blot): Test used to detect infection by *HIV* (the AIDS virus). It is more specific than the ELISA. A patient's serum is mixed with purified proteins from HIV, and the reaction is examined. If the patient has made antibodies to HIV, those antibodies react with the purified HIV proteins, and the test result is positive.

White blood cell (WBC) count: Determination of the number of leukocytes in the blood. Higher-than-normal counts can indicate the presence of infection or leukemia. A *differential* (differential count) is the percentages of different types of white blood cells (neutrophils, eosinophils, basophils, lymphocytes, and monocytes) in a sample of blood. It gives more specific information about leukocytes and aids in the diagnosis of infection, allergic diseases, disorders of the immune system, and various forms of leukemia.

APPENDIX 4

Abbreviations, Acronyms, Symbols, Eponyms, and Plurals

Abbreviations....330
Acronyms....341
Symbols....342
Eponyms....343
Plurals....347

ABBREVIATIONS

A

AAA abdominal aortic aneurysm
AB abortion
Ab antibody
ABC aspiration, biopsy, cytology
abd abdomen
ABG arterial blood gas
a.c., ac before meals *(ante cibum)*
ACE angiotensin-converting enzyme (ACE inhibitors treat hypertension)
ACL anterior cruciate ligament (of knee)
ACS acute coronary syndrome (myocardial infarction, unstable angina)
ACTH adrenocorticotropic hormone (secreted by the pituitary gland)
AD Alzheimer disease
ADD attention deficit disorder
ADH antidiuretic hormone (secreted by the pituitary gland)
ADHD attention deficit/hyperactivity disorder
ad lib freely as desired *(ad libitum)*
AED automated external defibrillator
AICD automatic implantable cardioverter-defibrillator
AIDS acquired immunodeficiency syndrome
alb albumin (protein)
ALL acute lymphocytic leukemia
alk phos alkaline phosphatase (enzyme elevated in liver disease)
ALS amyotrophic lateral sclerosis (Lou Gehrig disease)
ALT alanine transaminase (enzyme elevated in liver disease); formerly called SGPT
AMI acute myocardial infarction
AML acute myelocytic (myelogenous) leukemia
ANA antinuclear antibody; test for rheumatoid arthritis
AP *or* A/P anteroposterior (front to back)
A&P auscultation and percussion
aq water *(aqua)*
ARDS acute respiratory distress syndrome
AS aortic stenosis
ASD atrial septal defect
ASHD arteriosclerotic heart disease
AST aspartate transaminase (elevated in liver and heart disease); formerly called SGOT
AV arteriovenous; atrioventricular
A&W alive and well

B

BE barium enema
B cells white blood cells (lymphocytes) produced in bone marrow
b.i.d., bid twice a day *(bis in die)*
BM bowel movement; bone marrow
BMT bone marrow transplant

BP, B/P blood pressure
BPH benign prostatic hypertrophy (hyperplasia)
bronch bronchoscopy
bs blood sugar; bowel sounds; breath sounds
BSE breast self-examination
BSO bilateral salpingo-oophorectomy
BUN blood urea nitrogen (test of kidney function)
BW birth weight
Bx, bx biopsy

C

$\bar{c}$ with *(cum)*
C1, C2 first cervical vertebra, second cervical vertebra
CA cancer; carcinoma; cardiac arrest; chronologic age
Ca calcium
CABG coronary artery bypass graft
CAD coronary artery disease
CAPD continuous ambulatory peritoneal dialysis
cap capsule
cath catheter; catheterization
CBC complete blood count
cc cubic centimeter (1 cc equals 1/1000 liter, or 1 mL)
CC chief complaint
CCU coronary care unit; critical care unit
CF cystic fibrosis
chemo chemotherapy
CHF congestive heart failure
chol cholesterol
CIN cervical intraepithelial neoplasia
CIS carcinoma in situ
CKD chronic kidney disease
cm centimeter (1 cm is 1/100 meter)
CLL chronic lymphocytic leukemia
CML chronic myelocytic (myelogenous) leukemia
CMP comprehensive metabolic panel
CNS central nervous system (brain and spinal cord)
c/o complains of
CO_2 carbon dioxide
COPD chronic obstructive pulmonary disease
COVID-19 coronavirus disease 2019
CP cerebral palsy; chest pain
CPAP continuous positive airway pressure (provided by machine to aid breathing in patients with sleep apnea)
CPD cephalopelvic disproportion
CPR cardiopulmonary resuscitation
C&S, C+S culture and sensitivity (testing)
C-section, CS cesarean section
CSF cerebrospinal fluid
CT scan computed tomography scan (x-ray images in cross-sectional view)
CTE chronic traumatic encephalopathy

CVA	cerebrovascular accident (stroke)
c/w	compare with; consistent with
CX, CXR	chest x-ray (image)
Cx	cervix
cysto	cystoscopy

D

D&C	dilation (dilatation) and curettage (of the uterine lining)
DES	diethylstilbestrol (estrogen causing defects in children whose mothers took the drug during pregnancy)
DEXA (DXA)	dual-energy x-ray absorptiometry
DIC	disseminated intravascular coagulation
diff.	differential (percentages of types of white blood cells)
DJD	degenerative joint disease
DKA	diabetic ketoacidosis
DM	diabetes mellitus
DNA	deoxyribonucleic acid
DNR	do not resuscitate
DO	doctor of osteopathic medicine
DOB	date of birth
DOE	dyspnea on exertion
DOMS	delayed-onset muscle soreness
DRE	digital rectal examination
DT	delirium tremens (caused by alcohol withdrawal)
DTR	deep tendon reflex
DUB	dysfunctional uterine bleeding
DVT	deep vein thrombosis
Dx	diagnosis

E

EBV	Epstein-Barr virus (cause of mononucleosis)
ECC	emergency cardiac care
ECG	electrocardiography
ECHO	echocardiography
ECMO	extracorporeal membrane oxygenator
ECT	electroconvulsive therapy
ED	emergency department; erectile dysfunction
EDD	expected date of delivery
EEG	electroencephalography
EENT	eyes, ears, nose, throat
EGD	esophagogastroduodenoscopy
eGFR	estimated glomerular filtration rate
EKG	electrocardiography (*ECG* is preferred)
ELISA	enzyme-linked immunosorbent assay (e.g., used as an AIDS test)
EMG	electromyography
ENT	ears, nose, throat
eos.	eosinophils (type of white blood cell)
ER	emergency room; estrogen receptor
ERCP	endoscopic retrograde cholangiopancreatography

ESR	erythrocyte sedimentation rate; see *sed rate*
ESRD	end-stage renal disease
ESWL	extracorporeal shock wave lithotripsy
ET	endotracheal
ETOH	ethyl alcohol (ethanol)
ETT	exercise tolerance test; endotracheal tube

F

FBS	fasting blood sugar
FDA	U.S. Food and Drug Administration
FDG-PET	fluorodeoxyglucose positron emission tomography (nuclear medicine test)
Fe	iron
FEV	forced expiratory volume
FH	family history
FHR	fetal heart rate
FSH	follicle-stimulating hormone (secreted by the pituitary gland)
F/U, f/u	follow-up
FUO	fever of unknown (undetermined) origin
Fx	fracture

G

G	gravida (a pregnant woman)
g, gm	gram
Ga	gallium (element used in nuclear medicine diagnostic tests)
GB	gallbladder
GC	gonococcus (bacterial cause of gonorrhea; another name for *Neisseria gonorrhoeae*)
Gd	gadolinium (widely used MRI contrast agent)
GERD	gastroesophageal reflux disease
GH	growth hormone (secreted by the pituitary gland)
GI	gastrointestinal
Grav. 1, 2, 3	gravida—a woman who has had a first, second, or third pregnancy of any duration
GFR	glomerular filtration rate
gt, gtt	drop, drops
GTT	glucose tolerance test
GU	genitourinary
GVHD	graft-versus-host disease
Gy	gray (unit of irradiation)
GYN, gyn	gynecology

H

H	hydrogen
h, hr	hour
HAART	highly active antiretroviral therapy (for AIDS)

Hb, hgb, Hgb	hemoglobin
HbA1c	glycosylated hemoglobin (measured to test for diabetes)
HBV	hepatitis B virus
HCC	hepatocellular carcinoma
HCG, hCG	human chorionic gonadotropin (secreted during pregnancy)
Hct, HCT	hematocrit
HCV	hepatitis C virus
HD	hemodialysis (performed by artificial kidney machine); heart disease
HDL	high-density lipoprotein (associated with decreased incidence of coronary artery disease)
HEENT	head, ears, eyes, nose, throat
Hg	mercury
Hgb, hgb, Hb	hemoglobin
HIPAA	Health Insurance Portability and Accountability Act (of 1996)
HIV	human immunodeficiency virus
h/o	history of
H_2O	water
H&P	history and physical (examination)
HPV	human papillomavirus
HRT	hormone replacement therapy
h.s.	at bedtime *(hora somni);* write out so as not to confuse with hs (half strength)
HSG	hysterosalpingography
HSV-1, HSV-2	herpes simplex virus type 1, type 2
HTN	hypertension (high blood pressure)
Hx	history

I

I	iodine
I-131	iodine-131 (radioactive iodine)
I&D	incision and drainage
IBD	inflammatory bowel disease (ulcerative colitis and Crohn disease)
IBS	irritable bowel syndrome (of unknown etiology)
ICD	implantable cardioverter-defibrillator
ICU	intensive care unit
ID	infectious disease
IgA, IgD, IgE, IgG, IgM	immunoglobulins (antibodies)
IM	intramuscular; infectious mononucleosis
INH	isoniazid (drug to treat tuberculosis)
INR	international normalized ratio (system for reporting results of blood coagulation tests)
I&O	intake and output (measurement of patient's fluids)
IOL	intraocular lens (implant)
IUD	intrauterine device (contraceptive)
IV	intravenous
IVF	*in vitro* fertilization
IVP	intravenous pyelography; intravenous push

K

K	potassium
kg	kilogram (1 kg is 1000 grams)
KS	Kaposi sarcoma (malignant lesion associated with AIDS)
KUB	kidneys, ureters, bladder (x-ray study without contrast)

L

L, l	left; liter; lower
L1, L2	first lumbar vertebra, second lumbar vertebra
LA	left atrium
LAD	left anterior descending artery (of the heart); lymphadenopathy
lat	lateral
LBP	low back pain; low blood pressure
LDH	lactate dehydrogenase (elevations associated with heart attacks)
LDL	low-density lipoprotein (high levels associated with heart disease)
LE	lupus erythematosus
LEEP	loop electrocautery excision procedure
LES	lower esophageal sphincter
LFTs	liver function tests
LLQ	left lower quadrant (of the abdomen)
LMP	last menstrual period
LP	lumbar puncture
LPN	licensed practical nurse
LTB	laryngotracheal bronchitis (croup)
LUQ	left upper quadrant (of the abdomen)
LV	left ventricle
LVAD	left ventricular assist device (bridge to cardiac transplantation)
L&W	living and well
lymphs	lymphocytes
lytes	electrolytes

M

m	meter; milli (one thousandth)
MAC	monitored anesthesia care
MCH	mean corpuscular hemoglobin (amount in each red blood cell)
MCHC	mean corpuscular hemoglobin concentration (amount per unit of blood)
MCV	mean corpuscular volume (size of individual red blood cell)
MD, M.D.	doctor of medicine; muscular dystrophy
MDI	metered-dose inhaler
MDS	myelodysplastic syndrome (a bone marrow disorder)
mets	metastases
mg	milligram (1 mg is 1/1000 gram)
Mg	magnesium
MH	marital history; mental health
MI	myocardial infarction (heart attack)
mL	milliliter (1 mL is 1/1000 liter)
mm	millimeter (1 mm is 1/1000 meter)
mm Hg	millimeters of mercury (units for measurement of blood pressure)
mono	monocytes (type of white blood cell)

MRA	magnetic resonance angiography
MRI	magnetic resonance imaging
MRSA	methicillin-resistant *Staphylococcus aureus*
MS	mental status; mitral stenosis; multiple sclerosis
MSW	medical social worker
MTD	maximum tolerated dose
MVP	mitral valve prolapse
myop	myopia (nearsightedness)

N

N	nitrogen
Na	sodium
NB	newborn
NED	no evidence of disease
NG tube	nasogastric tube
NICU	neonatal intensive care unit
NKA	no known allergies
NPO	nothing by mouth *(nil per os)*
NSAID	nonsteroidal anti-inflammatory drug
NSR	normal sinus rhythm (of the heart)
NT	not tender (to touch)
NTP	normal temperature and pressure
N+V	nausea and vomiting

O

O_2	oxygen
OA	osteoarthritis
OB	obstetrics
OD	doctor of optometry
OR	operating room
ORIF	open reduction plus internal fixation (to set a broken bone)
ORTH, ortho.	orthopedics *or* orthopaedics
os	mouth
OSA	obstructive sleep apnea
OT	occupational therapy
OV	office visit

P

$\bar{p}$	after; following
P	phosphorus; plan; posterior; pressure; pulse; pupil
PA	posteroanterior (back to front); pulmonary artery
PAC	premature atrial contraction
PaCO2	arterial pressure of carbon dioxide in the blood; may also be written "arterial PCO2"
PACS	picture archival communications system
palp	palpable; palpation (examine by touch)

PaO2	arterial pressure of oxygen in the blood; may also be written "arterial PO2"
Pap smear	Papanicolaou smear (preparation of cells from the cervix and vagina for microscopic examination)
para	paracentesis (abdominocentesis)
Para 1, 2, 3	Woman who has produced one, two, or three viable offspring; unipara, bipara, tripara
p.c., pc	after meals *(post cibum)*
PCI	percutaneous coronary intervention
PCP	Pneumocystis pneumonia (opportunistic infection seen in patients with AIDS)
PE	physical examination; pulmonary embolus
PEEP	positive end-expiratory pressure
per	by
PERRLA	pupils equal, round, reactive to light and accommodation
PET	positron emission tomography
PE tube	pressure-equalizing tube (ventilating tube for the eardrum)
PFT	pulmonary function test
pH	hydrogen ion concentration (measurement of acidity or alkalinity of a solution)
PH	past history
PI	present illness
PID	pelvic inflammatory disease
PKU	phenylketonuria (disease due to lack of an enzyme in infants)
PM; pm	afternoon *(post meridiem)*; postmortem
PMH	past medical history
PMS	premenstrual syndrome
PND	paroxysmal nocturnal dyspnea; postnasal drip
p/o	postoperative
p.o., po	by mouth *(per os)*
polys	polymorphonuclear leukocytes (neutrophils)
poplit	popliteal (behind the knee)
post-op	after operation
PP	after meals *(postprandial)*; after birth *(postpartum)*
PPD	purified protein derivative (skin test for tuberculosis)
pre-op	before operation (preoperative)
prep	prepare for
p.r.n., prn	as needed *(pro re nata)*
procto	proctoscopy (visual examination of the anus and rectum)
pro time	prothrombin time (test of blood clotting)
PSA	prostate-specific antigen (screening test for prostate cancer)
pt	patient
PT	physical therapy; prothrombin time
PTA	prior to admission (to hospital)
PTCA	percutaneous transluminal coronary angioplasty (balloon angioplasty)
PTH	parathyroid hormone
PTR	patient to return
PTSD	post-traumatic stress disorder
PTT	partial thromboplastin time (test of blood clotting)
PVC	premature ventricular contraction (abnormal heart rhythm)
PVD	peripheral vascular disease

PVT paroxysmal ventricular tachycardia
PWB partial weight bearing
Px prognosis

Q

q every *(quaque)*
q.d. each (every) day *(quaque die);* better to write out "each day," because can be misread as q.i.d.
q.h. each (every) hour *(quaque hora)*
q2h each (every) two hours *(quaque secunda hora)*
q.i.d. four times a day *(quater in die)*
q.n. each (every) night *(quaque nox)*
q.n.s. quantity not sufficient *(quantum non sufficit)*
q.s. quantity sufficient *(quantum sufficit)*
qt quart

R

R, r respiration; right
RA rheumatoid arthritis; right atrium
rad radiation absorbed dose
RBC, rbc red blood cell (count)
REM rapid eye movement
RIA radioimmunoassay (minute quantities are measured)
RLQ right lower quadrant (of the abdomen)
R/O, r/o rule out
ROM range of motion
ROS review of systems; reactive species
RP retrograde pyelography (urography)
RR recovery room; respiration rate
RRR regular rate and rhythm (of the heart)
RT radiation therapy; radiologic technologist; respiratory therapist
RUQ right upper quadrant (of the abdomen)
RV right ventricle (of the heart)
Rx treatment; therapy; prescription (*recipe,* "to take")

S

$\bar{s}$ without *(sine)*
S1, S2 first sacral vertebra, second sacral vertebra
S-A node sinoatrial node (pacemaker of the heart)
SAD seasonal affective disorder
SARS severe acute respiratory syndrome
SARS-CoV-2 severe acute respiratory syndrome coronavirus-2
SBFT small bowel follow-through (x-ray study of the small intestine with contrast)
sed rate erythrocyte sedimentation rate (time it takes red blood cells to settle out of blood)
segs segmented white blood cells (granulocytes)
SERM selective estrogen receptor modulator (tamoxifen is an example)

s.gl.	without glasses
SGOT	see *AST*
SGPT	see *ALT*
SH	serum hepatitis; social history
sig.	"let it be labeled" (directions or medical instructions)
SIDS	sudden infant death syndrome
SIRS	systemic inflammatory response syndrome (severe bacteremia)
SLE	systemic lupus erythematosus
SMA-12	blood chemistry profile including 12 different studies or assays (*s*equential *m*ultiple *a*nalysis)
SOAP	subjective data (symptoms perceived by the patient), objective data (exam findings), assessment (evaluation of condition), plan (goals for treatment)
SOB	shortness of breath
S/P, s/p	status post (previous disease condition)
SPECT	single-photon emission computed tomography
sp. gr.	specific gravity
SSRI	selective serotonin reuptake inhibitor (antidepressant drug)
staph	staphylococci (bacteria)
STAT, stat	immediately *(statim)*
STD	sexually transmitted disease (older name for STI)
STI	sexually transmitted infection
strep	streptococci (bacteria)
sub-Q	subcutaneous (under the skin)
Sx	signs and symptoms
Sz	seizure

T

T	temperature; time
T1, T2	first thoracic vertebra, second thoracic vertebra
T3	triiodothyronine (thyroid gland hormone)
T4	thyroxine (thyroid gland hormone)
T&A	tonsillectomy and adenoidectomy
tab	tablet
TAB	therapeutic abortion
TAH-BSO	total abdominal hysterectomy–bilateral salpingo-oophorectomy
TB	tuberculosis
T cells	lymphocytes originating in the thymus gland
TEE	transesophageal echocardiography
TENS	transcutaneous electrical nerve stimulator
TFT	thyroid function test
THR	total hip replacement
TIA	transient ischemic attack
t.i.d., tid	three times a day *(tris in die)*
TKR	total knee replacement
TLC	total lung capacity
TM	tympanic membrane
TMJ	temporomandibular joint
TNM	tumor-node-metastasis (staging system for cancer)
TPN	total parenteral nutrition (administration of IV solution to maintain nutrition)

TPR	temperature, pulse, respiration
TSH	thyroid-stimulating hormone (secreted by the pituitary gland)
TTE	transthoracic echocardiography
TUR, TURP	transurethral resection of the prostate gland
TVH	total vaginal hysterectomy
Tx	treatment

U

UA, U/A	urinalysis
UE	upper extremity
UGI	upper gastrointestinal
umb	navel (umbilical cord region)
ung	ointment
U/O	urine output
URI	upper respiratory infection
U/S, u/s	ultrasound (imaging examination)
UTI	urinary tract infection
UV	ultraviolet

V

VA	visual acuity
VATS	video-assisted thoracoscopy or video-assisted thoracic surgery
VC	vital capacity (of lungs)
VCUG	voiding cystourethrogram
VEGF	vascular endothelial growth factor
VF	visual field; ventricular fibrillation
Vfib	ventricular fibrillation
VS, V/S	vital signs; versus
VSD	ventricular septal defect
VSS	vital signs stable
V tach, VT	ventricular tachycardia (abnormal heart rhythm)

W

WBC, wbc	white blood cell (count)
W/C	wheelchair
wd	wound
WDWN	well-developed and well-nourished
WNL	within normal limits
WT, wt	weight
w/u	workup

X

XRT	radiation therapy

Y

y, yr	year(s)
y/o	year(s) old

ACRONYMS*

An *acronym* is the name for an abbreviation that forms a pronounceable "word."

ACE (ace)	angiotensin-converting enzyme
AIDS (aydz)	acquired immune deficiency syndrome
Apgar (apgahr)	appearance, pulse, grimace, activity, respiration (letters spell out name of originator of scoring system, Virginia Apgar)
ARDS (ardz)	acute respiratory distress syndrome
BUN (bun)	blood urea nitrogen
CABG (cabbage)	coronary artery bypass graft (grafting)
CAT (cat)	computerized axial tomography (older name for CT)
CPAP (seepap)	continuous positive airway pressure
CRISPR (krisper)	clustered regularly interspaced short palindromic repeats
DEXA (deksah)	dual energy x-ray absorptometry
ELISA (eliza)	enzyme-linked immunosorbent assay
GERD (gird)	gastroesophageal reflux disease
HAART (heart)	highly active antiretroviral therapy
HIPAA (hippah)	Health Insurance Portability and Accountability Act of 1996
LASER (layzer)	light amplification by stimulated emission of radiation
LASIK (laysick)	laser-assisted in situ keratomileusis
LEEP (leap)	loop electrocautery excision procedure
MAC (mack)	monitored anesthesia care
MICU (mickyou)	medical intensive care unit
MIS (miss)	minimally invasive surgery
MODS (modz)	multiorgan dysfunction syndrome
MUGA (muh-guh)	multiple-gated acquisition (scan)
NICU (nickyou)	neonatal intensive care unit
NSAID (ensayd)	nonsteroidal anti-inflammatory drug
PACS (packs)	picture archival communications system
PALS (pals)	pediatric advanced life support
PANDAS (pandaz)	pediatric autoimmune neuropsychiatric disorder(s) associated with streptococcal infection(s)
PEEP (peep)	positive end-expiratory pressure
PEG (peg)	percutaneous endoscopic gastrostomy
PERRLA (perlah)	pupils equal, round, reactive to light and accommodation
PET (pet)	positron emission tomography
PICC (pick)	peripherally inserted central catheter
PICU (pickyou)	pediatric intensive care unit
PIP (pip)	proximal interphalangeal (joint)
pixel (picksul)	picture element
PUVA (poovah)	psoralen ultraviolet A
REM (rem)	rapid eye movement
SAD (sad)	seasonal affective disorder
SARS (sarz)	severe acute respiratory syndrome
SERM (serm)	selective estrogen receptor modulator
SICU (sickyou)	surgical intensive care unit
SIDS (sidz)	sudden infant death syndrome

*Modified from Chabner D-E: *The Language of Medicine,* ed 12, Philadelphia, 2021, Elsevier.

SIRS (sirz)	**s**ystemic **i**nflammatory **r**esponse **s**yndrome
SMAC (smack)	**s**equential **m**ultiple **a**nalyzer **c**omputer (for blood testing)
SOAP (soap)	**s**ubjective, **o**bjective, **a**ssessment, **p**lan (formatted approach to nursing care)
SPECT (spekt)	**s**ingle-**p**hoton **e**mission **c**omputed **t**omography
SPORE (spore)	**s**pecialized **p**rogram **o**f **r**esearch **e**xcellence
TENS (tenz)	**t**ranscutaneous **e**lectrical **n**erve **s**timulation
TRUS (truss)	**t**rans**r**ectal **u**ltra**s**ound
TURP (turp)	**t**rans**u**rethral **r**esection of the **p**rostate
VATS (vatz)	**v**ideo-**a**ssisted **t**horaco**s**copy
voxel (vocksul)	**vo**lume **el**ement (of CT scan)

SYMBOLS*

=	equals
≠	does not equal
+	positive
−	negative
↑	above, increase
↓	below, decrease
♀	female
♂	male
→	to (in the direction of)
>	is greater than
<	is less than
1°	first-degree (burn, heart block); primary
2°	second-degree (burn, heart block); secondary
ʒ	dram
%	percent
°	degree; hour
:	ratio (“is to”)
±	plus or minus (either positive or negative)
′	foot
″	inch
∴	therefore
@	at, each
c̄	with *(cum)*
s̄	without *(sine)*
#	pound; number
≈	approximately, about
Δ	change, change in
p	short arm of a chromosome
q	long arm of a chromosome

*Modified from Chabner D-E: *The Language of Medicine,* ed 12, Philadelphia, 2021, Elsevier.

EPONYMS

Achilles tendon
(Achilles, Greek mythologic hero)

This tendon connects the calf muscles to the heel. It lies at the only part of Achilles' body that was still vulnerable after his mother dipped him as an infant into the river Styx, when she held him by the heel.

Alzheimer disease
(Alois Alzheimer, German neurologist, 1864-1915)

Progressive mental deterioration marked by confusion, memory failure, and disorientation.

Apgar score
(Virginia Apgar, American anesthesiologist, 1909-1974)

Evaluation of an infant's physical condition, usually performed 1 minute and then 5 minutes after birth. Highest score is 10. An Apgar rating of 9/10 is a score of 9 at 1 minute and 10 at 5 minutes.

Asperger syndrome
(Hans Asperger, Austrian psychiatrist, 1906-1980)

Developmental disorder characterized by impairment of social interactions (resembling autism) but lacking in delays in language development and mental functioning.

Bell palsy
(Charles Bell, Scottish surgeon, 1774-1842)

Unilateral (one-sided) paralysis of the facial nerve.

Barlow syndrome
(John Barlow, South African cardiologist, born 1924)

Mitral valve prolapse.

Barrett esophagus
(Norman Barrett, Australian thoracic surgeon, 1903-1979)

Abnormal changes in the lining of the esophagus, resulting from acid reflux from the stomach.

Burkitt lymphoma
(Denis Burkitt, English surgeon in Africa, 1911-1993)

Malignant tumor of lymph nodes; chiefly seen in central Africa. The Epstein-Barr virus is associated with this lymphoma.

Cheyne-Stokes respiration
(John Cheyne, Scottish physician, 1777-1836; William Stokes, Irish physician, 1804-1878)

Abnormal pattern of breathing with alternating periods of stoppage of breathing and deep, rapid breathing.

Colles fracture
(Abraham Colles, Irish surgeon, 1773-1843)

Break (fracture) of the radius (bone near the wrist).

Crohn disease
(Burrill B. Crohn, American physician, 1884-1983)

Chronic inflammatory bowel disease of unknown origin; usually affecting the ileum (last part of the small intestine), colon, or any part of the gastrointestinal tract.

Cushing syndrome (Harvey W. Cushing, American surgeon, 1869-1939)	Disorder resulting from chronic, excessive production of cortisol from the adrenal cortex. It can also result from administration of glucocorticoids (cortisone) in large doses for long periods of time.
Duchenne muscular dystrophy (Guillaume Benjamin Amand Duchenne, French neurologist, 1806-1875)	Abnormal, inherited condition that infants are born with; marked by progressive hardening of muscles in the leg and hips (pelvis).
Epstein-Barr virus (Michael A. Epstein, English pathologist, born 1921; Yvonne M. Barr, English virologist, born 1932)	The herpesvirus that causes infectious mononucleosis and is associated with malignant conditions such as nose and throat cancer, Burkitt lymphoma, and Hodgkin lymphoma.
eustachian tube (Bartolomeo Eustachio, Italian anatomist, 1524-1574)	A tube that joins the throat and the middle ear cavity.
Ewing sarcoma (James Ewing, American pathologist, 1866-1943)	Malignant tumor that develops from bone marrow, usually in long bones or the hip (pelvis).
fallopian tube (Gabriele Falloppio, Italian anatomist, 1523-1562)	One of a pair of tubes or ducts leading from the ovary to the upper portion of the uterus.
Foley catheter (Frederic Foley, American physician, 1891-1966)	Rubber tube that is placed in the urethra to provide drainage of urine.
Giardia (Alfred Giardia, French biologist, 1846-1908)	One-celled organism (protozoan) that causes gastrointestinal infection with diarrhea, abdominal cramps, and weight loss. Cause of infection usually is fecally contaminated water.
Hodgkin lymphoma (Thomas Hodgkin, English physician, 1798-1866)	Malignant tumor of the lymph nodes.
Horner syndrome (Johann Friedrich Horner, Swiss ophthalmologist, 1831-1886)	Partial ptosis (prolapse or drooping) of the upper eyelid, along with other signs of damage to nerves controlling the eye muscles and face.
Huntington disease (George S. Huntington, American physician, 1851-1916)	Rare, hereditary condition marked by chronic, progressively worsening dance-like movements (chorea) and mental deterioration, resulting in dementia.

Kaposi sarcoma
(Moricz Kaposi, Austrian dermatologist, 1837-1902)

Malignant neoplasm of cells that line blood and lymph vessels. Soft brownish or purple papules appear on the skin. The tumor can metastasize to lymph nodes and internal organs. It often is associated with AIDS.

Marfan syndrome
(Bernard-Jean A. Marfan, French pediatrician, 1858-1942)

Hereditary condition that affects bones, muscles, the cardiovascular system (leading to aneurysms) and eyes (lens dislocation). Affected people have long, "spidery" extremities, underdeveloped muscles, and easily movable joints.

Ménière disease
(Prosper Ménière, French physician, 1799-1862)

Chronic disease of the inner ear with recurrent episodes of dizziness (vertigo), hearing loss, and ringing in the ears (tinnitus).

Neisseria gonorrhoeae
(Albert L. S. Neisser, Polish dermatologist, 1855-1916)

A type of bacterium that causes gonorrhea (sexually transmitted infection).

Paget disease
(James Paget, English surgeon, 1814-1899)

Disease of bone, often affecting middle-aged or elderly people; marked by bone destruction and poor bone repair.

Pap test
(George Papanicolaou, Greek physician in the United States, 1883-1962)

Method of examining stained cells obtained from the cervix and vagina. It is a common way to detect cervical cancer.

Parkinson disease
(James Parkinson, English physician, 1755-1824)

Slowly progressive degenerative neurological disorder marked by tremors, mask-like facial appearance, shuffling gait (manner of walking), and muscle rigidity and weakness.

Raynaud phenomenon
(Maurice Raynaud, French physician, 1834-1881)

Intermittent attacks of loss of blood flow (ischemia) in the extremities of the body (fingers, toes, ears, and nose). Episodes most often are caused by exposure to cold.

Reye syndrome
(R. Douglas Reye, Austrian pathologist, 1912-1978)

Acute brain disease (encephalopathy) and disease of internal organs following an acute viral infection.

Rinne test
(Heinrich A. Rinne, German otologist, 1819-1868)

Hearing test using a vibrating tuning fork placed against a bone behind the patient's ear (mastoid bone).

Rorschach test (Herman Rorschach, Swiss psychiatrist, 1884-1922)	Personality test based on a patient's interpretation of 10 inkblots.
Salmonella (Daniel E. Salmon, American pathologist, 1850-1914)	Type of bacterium (rod-shaped) that causes typhoid fever and types of gastroenteritis (inflammation of stomach and intestines).
Shigella (Kiyoshi Shiga, Japanese bacteriologist, 1870-1957)	Type of bacterium that causes severe infectious gastroenteritis (inflammation of stomach and intestines) and dysentery (diarrhea, abdominal pain, and fever).
Sjögren syndrome (Heinrik S.C. Sjögren, Swedish ophthalmologist, 1899-1986)	Abnormal dryness of the mouth, eyes, and mucous membranes, caused by deficient fluid production. It is a disorder of the immune system.
Snellen test (Herman Snellen, Dutch ophthalmologist, 1834-1908)	Test of visual clarity (acuity) using a special chart. Letters, numbers, or symbols are arranged on the chart in decreasing size from top to bottom.
Tay-Sachs disease (Warren Tay, English ophthalmologist, 1843-1927; Bernard Sachs, American neurologist, 1858-1944)	Inherited disorder of nerve degeneration caused by deficiency of an enzyme. Most affected children die between the ages of 2 and 4 years.
Tourette syndrome (George Gilles de la Tourette, French neurologist, 1857-1927)	Condition marked by abnormal facial grimaces, inappropriate speech, involuntary movements (tics) of eyes, arms, and shoulders.
von Willebrand disease (Erick A. von Willebrand, Finnish physician, 1870-1949)	Inherited blood disorder marked by abnormally slow blood clotting; caused by deficiency in a blood clotting factor (factor VIII).
Weber tuning fork test (Hermann D. Weber, English physician, 1823-1918)	Test of hearing by placing the stem of vibrating tuning fork in the center of the person's forehead.
Whipple procedure (Allen O. Whipple, American surgeon, 1881-1963)	Surgical procedure to remove a portion of the pancreas and the stomach and the entire first part of the small intestine (duodenum). Used in the treatment of pancreatic cancer and other conditions.
Wilms tumor (Max Wilms, German surgeon, 1867-1918)	Malignant tumor of the kidney occurring in young children.

PLURALS

The rules commonly used to form plurals of medical terms are as follows:

1. For words ending in **a**, retain the **a** and add **e.**
   Examples:

Singular	Plural
bulla	bullae
bursa	bursae
vertebra	vertebrae

2. For words ending in **is**, drop the **is** and add **es.**
   Examples:

Singular	Plural
anastomosis	anastomoses
epiphysis	epiphyses
metastasis	metastases
prosthesis	prostheses
pubis	pubes

3. For words ending in **ex** and **ix**, drop the **ex** or **ix** and add **ices.**
   Examples:

Singular	Plural
apex	apices
varix	varices

4. For words ending in **on**, drop the **on** and add **a.**
   Examples:

Singular	Plural
ganglion	ganglia
spermatozoon	spermatozoa

5. For words ending in **um**, drop the **um** and add **a.**
   Examples:

Singular	Plural
bacterium	bacteria
diverticulum	diverticula
ovum	ova

6. For words ending in **us**, drop the **us** and add **i.**
   Examples:

Singular	Plural
bronchus	bronchi
calculus	calculi
nucleus	nuclei

Two exceptions to this rule are vir<u>uses</u> and sin<u>uses</u>.

7. Additional rules are used to form plurals in other word families.
   Examples:

Singular	Plural
anomal<u>y</u>	anomal<u>ies</u>
biops<u>y</u>	biops<u>ies</u>
fem<u>ur</u>	fem<u>ora</u>
foram<u>en</u>	foram<u>ina</u>
ir<u>is</u>	ir<u>ides</u>
phala<u>nx</u>	phala<u>nges</u>
thora<u>x</u>	thora<u>ces</u>

APPENDIX 5

Quick Drug Reference

Top 50 Prescribed Medications*

Rank	Generic Name	Brand Name	Use
1.	Atorvastatin	Lipitor®	Lowers cholesterol levels
2.	Levothyroxine	Synthroid®	Thyroid hormone to treat low thyroid condition
3.	Lisinopril	Prinivil®	Treats high blood pressure; ACE inhibitor
4.	Metformin	Glucophage®	Antidiabetic; reduces blood sugar in type 2 diabetes
5.	Metoprolol	Lopressor®	Treats abnormal heart rhythms and high blood pressure; beta blocker
6.	Amlodipine	Norvasc®	Calcium channel blocker; treats high blood pressure
7.	Albuterol	ProAir® HFA	Asthma inhaler
8.	Omeprazole	Prilosec®	Treats acid reflux in treatment of GERD
9.	Losartan potassium	Cozaar®	A2RB; treats high blood pressure
10.	Gabapentin	Neurontin®	Treats seizures (epilepsy) and nerve pain
11.	Hydrochlorothiazide	Esidrix®	Diuretic; increases urine production (water pill)
12.	Sertraline	Zoloft®	SSRI; antidepressant
13.	Simvastatin	Zocor®	Lowers cholesterol levels
14.	Montelukast	Singulair®	Reduces wheezing and shortness of breath (asthma attacks)
15.	Hydrocodone/APAP	Vicodin®	Pain relief
16.	Pantoprazole sodium	Protonix®	Treats acid reflux in treatment of GERD
17.	Furosemide	Lasix®	Diuretic; increases urine production (water pill)
18.	Fluticasone	Flonase®	Nasal spray for allergy relief
19.	Escitalopram	Lexapro®	Antidepressant
20.	Fluoxetine hydrochloride	Prozac®	SSRI; antidepressant
21.	Rosuvastatin	Crestor®	Lowers cholesterol levels
22.	Bupropion	Aplenzin®	Antidepressant; smoking cessation
23.	Amoxicillin	Amoxil®	Antibiotic; treats bacterial infection
24.	Dextroamphetamine	Adderall®	Stimulant medication to treat ADHD
25.	Trazodone	Desyrel®	Antidepressant
26.	Duloxetine	Cymbalta®	Antidepressant
27.	Prednisone	Cortan®	Corticosteroid drug to reduce inflammation
28.	Tamsulosin	Flomax®	Relieves symptoms of enlarged prostate (BPH)

Rank	Generic Name	Brand Name	Use
29.	Ibuprofen	Advil®	NSAID; reduces inflammation and pain
30.	Citalopram	Celexa®	Antidepressant
31.	Meloxicam	Mobic®	NSAID; reduces inflammation and pain
32.	Pravastin sodium	Pravachol®	Statin; metabolic agent
33.	Carvedilol	Coreg®	Treats heart failure (CHF)
34.	Potassium	K-Tab®	Treats low levels of potassium (important electrolyte)
35.	Tramadol	Ultram®	Pain relief
36.	Clopidogrel	Plavix®	Antiplatelet; prevents platelets from clumping together and forming blood clots
37.	Insulin glargine	Basaglar®	Insulin; antidiabetic
38.	Aspirin	Bayer®	Analgesic; reduces pain
39.	Atenolol	Tenormin®	Treats abnormal heart rhythms and high blood pressure; beta blocker
40.	Venlafaxine	Effexor®	Antidepressant
41.	Alprazolam	Xanax®	Antianxiety
42.	Ethinyl estradiol; norethindrone	Alyacen®	Hormone medication to prevent pregnancy
43.	Allopurinol	Lopurin®	Treats gout
44.	Cyclobenzaprine	Flexeril®	Muscle relaxant
45.	Clonazepam	Klonopin®	Antianxiety
46.	Zolpidem	Ambien®	Sedative (sleep) medicine treats insomnia
47.	Azithromycin	Zithromax®	Antibiotic; treats bacterial infections
48.	Warfarin	Coumadin®	Blood thinner; treats blood clots (anticoagulant)
49.	Methylphenidate	Concerta®	Stimulant medication to treat ADHD
50.	Apixaban	Eliquis®	Blood thinner; treats blood clots (anticoagulant)

Abbreviations:
A2RB = Angiotensin 2 Receptor Blocker
ACE = Angiotensin-Converting Enzyme
ADHD = Attention-Deficit Hyperactivity Disorder
APAP = Acetaminophen
CHF = Congestive Heart Failure
GERD = Gastroesophageal Reflux Disease
HFA = Hydrofluoroalkane—type of inhaler
NSAID: Nonsteroidal Anti-inflammatory Drug
SSRI = Selective Serotonin Reuptake Inhibitor

***Source:** from www.clinCalc.com Top 200 Drugs of 2019 as sourced from United State government AHRQ survey in annual Medical Expenditure Panel Survey (MEPS); and www.pharmacy-tech.test.com/ top 200 drugs for drug uses

APPENDIX 6

Allied Health Careers

Title/Description	Education Requirements	Certification or Licensure Requirements	National Association or Additional Information
Audiologist Works with people who have hearing problems by using testing devices to measure hearing loss.	Clinical doctoral degree—Doctor of Audiology (AuD) graduate degree, including 9 to 12 months of clinical experience.	In addition to complying with state license requirements (which may include requirement for teaching certification for a particular practice setting), ASHA administers the Certification of Clinical Competency in Audiology (CCC- A).	American Speech-Language-Hearing Association (ASHA) 2200 Research Boulevard Rockville, MD 20850 (800) 498-2071 American Academy of Audiology (AAA) 11730 Plaza America Dr., Suite 300 Reston, VA 20190 800-AAA-2336
Blood bank technologist Collects, types, and prepares blood and its components for transfusions and laboratory tests.	Baccalaureate degree in clinical laboratory science or other physical science degree, plus a 12-month program in blood bank technology. Some programs also offer master's degrees.	Certification through Board of Registry of the American Society of Clinical Pathologists (ASCP).	American Association of Blood Banks (AABB) 4550 Montgomery Avenue Suite 700, North Tower Bethesda, MD 20814 (301) 907-6977
Chiropractor Treats health problems associated with the muscular, nervous, and skeletal systems, especially the spine.	College degree plus 4 years of resident instruction in a college of chiropractics.	Must pass the National State Board Exam.	American Chiropractic Association (ACA) Public Information Department 1701 Clarendon Blvd., Suite 200 Arlington, VA 22209 (703) 276-8800
Clinical laboratory scientist (CLS) (also called Medical laboratory Scientist or MLS).	Baccalaureate degree including completion of accredited medical laboratory science program and certification exam.	Certification through American Society for Clinical Pathology Board of Certification and American Medical Technologist Association	American Society for Clinical Pathology (ASCP) 33 West Monroe Street, Suite 1600 Chicago, IL 60603 (312) 541-4999

Title/Description	Education Requirements	Certification or Licensure Requirements	National Association or Additional Information
Clinical laboratory technologist (CLT) (also see *Medical laboratory technologist [MLT]*) Performs tests to examine and analyze body fluids, tissues and cells.	2-year associate's degree or 12-month certificate program and certification exam.	Certification available through the following: American Society for Clinical Pathology Board, American Medical Technologists Association, and the National Credentialing Agency for Laboratory Personnel.	American Medical Technologists Association (AMT) 10700 West Higgins Road, Suite 150 Rosemont, IL 60018 (847) 823-5169 American Society for Clinical Pathology (ASCP) 33 West Monroe Street, Suite 1600 Chicago, IL 60603 (312) 541-4999
Dental assistant Assists a dentist with dental procedures.	Typically, 9- to 11-month program at a community college, vocational school, or career school. It is also possible to work as a dental assistant without attending a program and learn on the job.	In most states, certification is optional. Person is eligible to take exam if a graduate of an accredited dental assisting program or has 2 years of work experience. Exam for Certified Dental Assistant (CDA) is administered by the American Dental Assistants Association.	American Dental Assistants Association (ADAA) 140 N. Bloomingdale Road Bloomingdale, IL 60108-1017 (630) 994-4247 (877) 874-3785
Dental hygienist Provides preventive dental care and teaches the practice of good oral hygiene.	2-year associate's degree or 4-year baccalaureate degree.	State requirements vary. In most states, the person must graduate from an accredited dental hygiene program, pass the state-authorized licensure exam, and pass the comprehensive written exam. On passing the exam, the dental hygienist becomes a Registered Dental Hygienist (RDH).	American Dental Hygienists Association (ADHA) 444 N. Michigan Ave., Suite 400 Chicago, IL 60611 (312) 440-8900
Dental laboratory technician Prepares materials (crowns, bridges) for use by a dentist.	A 2-year program at a community, vocational, or technical college, either an associate's degree or certificate. The person also can work as a dental laboratory technician with on-the-job training.	In most states, certification to become a Certified Dental Technician (CDT) is optional.	National Board of Certification in Dental Laboratory Technology (NBCDLT) 325 John Knox Road, #L103 Tallahassee, FL 32303 (800) 684-5310 (850) 205-5627

Title/Description	Education Requirements	Certification or Licensure Requirements	National Association or Additional Information
Diagnostic medical sonographer Performs diagnostic ultrasound procedures.	From 1 to 4 years for certificate, associate's degree, or baccalaureate degree.	Optional certification exam through American Registry of Diagnostic Medical Sonographers (ARDMS), with the designation Registered Diagnostic Medical Sonographer (RDMS).	Society of Diagnostic Medical Sonography (SDMS) 2745 Dallas Pkwy., Suite 350 Plano, TX 75093 (214) 473-8057
Dietitian/ Nutritionist Plans nutrition programs and supervises the preparation and serving of meals.	2-year component within a baccalaureate or master's degree program, plus internship of 6–12 months.	National certification exam to become a Certified Registered Dietitian (RD) or Registered Dietitian Nutritionist (RDN) through the Commission on Dietetic Registration (CDR). Most states require licensure or certification.	Academy of Nutrition and Dietetics (formerly the American Dietetic Association) 120 S. Riverside Plaza, Suite 2190 Chicago, IL 60606 (312) 899-0400, ext. 5500 (800) 877-1600
ECG technician (cardiovascular technician) Operates an electrocardiograph to record ECGs and for Holter monitoring and stress tests.	Training often done on the job in 8- to 16-week programs. Longer programs are also available.	Optional	Alliance of Cardiovascular Professionals (ACP) P.O. Box 2007 Midlothian, VA 23113 (804) 639-9213
Emergency medical technician 1. Emergency Medical Responder 2. Emergency Medical Technician-Basic (EMT-B) 3. Emergency Medical Technician-Advanced 4. Emergency Medical Technician-Paramedic (EMT-P) Gives immediate care and transports sick or injured to medical facilities.	Four levels: *Emergency Medical Responder:* state-approved EMR course, approximately 40 hours *EMT Basic*: 120-150 hours *EMT Advanced*: 200 to 400 hours *EMT Paramedic*: 1000+ hours	Administered by the National Registry of Emergency Medical Technicians (NREMT) for each level from Emergency Medical Responders to Paramedics.	National Association of Emergency Medical Technicians (NAEMT) P.O. Box 1400 Clinton, MS 39060 132 A East Northside Drive Clinton, MS 39056 (800) 34-NAEMT

Title/Description	Education Requirements	Certification or Licensure Requirements	National Association or Additional Information
Health information management professional 1. Health information technician (HIT) 2. Health information administrator (HIA) Designs, manages, and administers the use of health care data and information.	Two levels: *Health Information Technician (HIT):* 2-year associate's degree *Health Information Administrator (HIA):* 4-year baccalaureate degree	On completion of the education program, a test is required through the national association (AHIMA) to become a Registered Health Information Technician (RHIT) or Registered Health Information Administrator (RHIA).	American Health Information Management Association (AHIMA) 233 N. Michigan Ave., Suite 2150 Chicago, IL 60601 (312) 233-1100
Home health aide Cares for elderly, disabled, and ill persons in their own homes, helping them live there instead of in an institution.	Often on-the-job training or technical/career college.	National Association for Home Care & Hospice offers optional certification in Private Duty Home Care.	National Association for Home Care & Hospice (NAHCH) 228 Seventh Street, SE Washington, DC 20003 (202) 547-7424
Licensed practical nurse (LPN) or Licensed Vocational nurse (LVN) Cares for sick, injured, convalescing, and handicapped persons, under the direct supervision of physicians and registered nurses; provides basic bedside care.	Approximately 1-year state-approved program, with 28 to 36 semester hours.	Must pass the National Council Licensure Examination for Practical Nurses (NCLEX-PN).	National Federation for Licensed Practical Nurses (NFLPN) 1418 Aversboro Road Garner, NC 27529 (919) 779-0046
Medical assistant Helps physicians examine and treat patients and performs tasks to keep offices running smoothly.	Associate's degree, certificate, and diploma programs available. Medical assistants can focus on either administrative or clinical duties or both.	Optional certifications available. Exam to become a Certified Medical Assistant (CMA) through the AAMA or a Registered Medical Assistant (RMA) through American Medical Technologists Association	American Association of Medical Assistants (AAMA) 20 N. Wacker Dr., Suite 1575 Chicago, IL 60606 (800) 228-2262 American Medical Technologists Association (AMT) 10799 West Higgins Rd. Ste 150 Rosemont, IL 60018 (847) 823-5169

Title/Description	Education Requirements	Certification or Licensure Requirements	National Association or Additional Information
Medical laboratory scientist (MLS) (also see Clinical laboratory Scientist or CLS).	Baccalaureate degree including completion of accredited medical laboratory science program and certification exam.	Certification through American Society for Clinical Pathology Board of Certification and American Medical Technologist Association	American Society for Clinical Pathology (ASCP) 33 West Monroe Street, Ste 1600 Chicago, IL 60603 (312) 541-4999
Medical laboratory technologist (also see *Clinical laboratory technologist [CLT]*) Performs routine tests and laboratory procedures.	A 2-year associate's degree or a 12-month certificate program.	Certification available through the following: Board of Registry of the American Society for Clinical Pathology, the American Medical Technologists Association, the National Credentialing Agency for Laboratory Personnel, and the Board of Registry of the American Association of Bioanalysts.	American Medical Technologists Association (AMT) 10700 West Higgins Road, Suite 150 Rosemont, IL 60018 (847) 823-5169 American Society for Clinical Pathology (ASCP) 33 West Monroe Street, Suite 1600 Chicago, IL 60603 (312) 541-4999
Nuclear medicine technologist Performs radioactive tests and procedures under the supervision of a nuclear medicine physician, who interprets the results.	Professional portion of the program is 1-2 years within an associate's or baccalaureate degree program.	On completion of an accredited program, certification exam is available through the Nuclear Medicine Technology Certification Board.	Society of Nuclear Medicine & Molecular Imaging—SNMMI Technologist Section (SNMTS) 1850 Samuel Morse Dr. Reston, VA 20190 (703) 708-9000 American Society of Radiologic Technologists (ASRT) 15000 Central Ave. SE Albuquerque, NM 87123
Nurse anesthetist Aids in the delivery of anesthesia during surgery.	RN with baccalaureate degree plus 24-month anesthesiology training course (leading to a master's degree).	Required exam by the Council on Certification for Nurse Anesthetists, to become a Certified Registered Nurse Anesthetist (CRNA).	American Association of Nurse Anesthesiology (AANA) 222 S. Prospect Ave. Park Ridge, IL 60068 (847) 692-7050 Additional information: National League for Nursing

Title/Description	Education Requirements	Certification or Licensure Requirements	National Association or Additional Information
Nursing aide (nursing assistant, orderly, hospital attendant) Helps care for ill, injured, or disabled patients confined to nursing, hospital, or residential care facilities.	Often on-the-job training or technical/career college.	Optional certification is available through state nursing registries for Certified Nursing Assistant (CNA).	National Association of Health Care Assistants (NAHCA) 6079 CL 299 Carl Junction, MO (417) 623-6049
Occupational therapist (OT) Helps people with mentally, physically, developmentally, or emotionally disabling conditions to develop, recover, or maintain daily living and working skills.	Two levels: Master's or doctoral degree programs	National certification exam through National Board for Certification of Occupational Therapy (NBCOT). All states also regulate occupational therapists. Upon passing the exam, the occupational therapist becomes an Occupational Therapist Registered (OTR).	American Occupational Therapy Association (AOTA) 6116 Executive Boulevard, Suite 200 North Bethesda, MD 20852 (301) 652-6611
Occupational therapy assistant (OTA) Under the direction of an occupational therapist, the OTA works with patients to restore or enhance activities of daily living.	*OTA-A*—Occupational therapy assistant, associate's degree *OTA-B*—Occupational therapy assistant, baccalaureate degree	National certification exam for OTA administered by: National Board for Certification of Occupational Therapy (NBCOT). Many states also regulate occupational therapy assistants.	American Occupational Therapy Association (AOTA) 6116 Executive Boulevard, Suite 200 North Bethesda, MD 20852 (301) 652-6611
Ophthalmic professional 1. Ophthalmic assistant 2. Ophthalmic technician/ technologist Helps ophthalmologists provide medical eye care.	Two levels: *Assistant*: less than 1 year *Technician/ technologist*: 1-2 years	After 1 year on the job, the person may test to become a Certified Ophthalmic Medical Assistant (COMA) through the Joint Commission on Allied Health Professionals in Ophthalmology (JCAHPO).	Association of Technical Personnel in Ophthalmology (ATPO) 446 East High St, Suite 10 Lexington, KY 40507 (859) 977-7453
Pharmacy technician Under the direction of licensed pharmacists, dispenses, distributes, and administers medications prescribed.	Usually 15 weeks (minimum 600 hours) of training required; can be on the job or through a career, technical, or community college.	Optional through the AAPT and Pharmacy Technician Certification Board, to become a Certified Pharmacy Technologist (CPhT).	American Association of Pharmacy Technicians (AAPT) P.O. Box 391043 Omaha, NE 68139 (336) 252-8761

Title/Description	Education Requirements	Certification or Licensure Requirements	National Association or Additional Information
Phlebotomist Draws and tests blood under the supervision of a medical technologist or laboratory manager.	Minimum 100 hours of clinical instruction.	Optional certification available through the following: American Medical Technologists Association, National Credentialing Agency for Laboratory Personnel, and Board of Registry of the American Association of Bioanalysts.	American Medical Technologists Association (AMT) 10700 West Higgins Road, Suite 150 Rosemont, IL 60018 (847) 823-5169 American Society of Phlebotomy Technicians (ASPT) P.O. Box 1831 Hickory, NC 28603 (828) 327-3000 National Phlebotomy Association (NPA) 1809 Brightseat Road Landover, MD 20785 (301) 386-4200
Physical therapist (PT) Improves mobility, relieves pain, and prevents or limits permanent physical disabilities of patients experiencing injuries or disease.	Doctoral degree programs granting a doctorate in physical therapy (DPT).	On completion of accredited program, national exam is required. Other requirements vary by state.	American Physical Therapy Association (APTA) 3030 Potomac Ave., Suite 100 Alexandria, VA 22305-3085 (800) 999-2782
Physical therapy assistant (PTA) Under the direction of a physical therapist, works with patients to improve mobility.	Most programs are associate's degree programs, one year of which is for technical courses and clinical experience.	Most states require physical therapy assistants to be licensed, registered, or certified.	American Physical Therapy Association (APTA) 3030 Potomac Ave., Suite 100 Alexandria, VA 22305-3085 (800) 999-2782
Physician assistant (PA) Medical providers who diagnose and treat patients; may act as patient's principal healthcare professional, typically in coordination with a physician.	Master's degree level; commonly a 25- to 27-month program in addition to a baccalaureate degree.	All states require passage of national exam through National Commission on Certification of Physician Assistants (NCCPA). To practice, PAs must also meet any additional state criteria and have a sponsoring physician.	American Association of Physician Assistants (AAPA) 2318 Mill Road, Ste. 1300 Alexandria, VA 22314 (703) 836-2272 National Commission on Certification of Physician Assistants (NCCPA) 12000 Findley Road, Suite 100 Duluth, GA 30097 (678) 417-8100

Title/Description	Education Requirements	Certification or Licensure Requirements	National Association or Additional Information
Radiation therapist Prepares cancer patients for treatment and examinations, and administers medications (this career is a specialty within imaging technology—see next entry).	After becoming a radiographer, 1 to 2 years of training.	Certification through American Registry of Radiologic Technologists (ARRT).	American Society of Radiologic Technologists (ASRT) 15000 Central Ave. SE Albuquerque, NM 87123 (505) 298-4500 American Registry of Radiologic Technologists (ARRT) 1255 Northland Drive St. Paul, MN 55120 (651) 687-0048
Radiologic Technologist/ Radiographer Produces x-ray images of parts of the body for use in diagnosing medical problems.	2- to 4-year training program resulting in degree or certificate.	Certification through American Registry of Radiologic Technologists (ARRT).	American Society of Radiologic Technologists (ASRT) 15000 Central Ave. SE Albuquerque, NM 87123 (505) 298-4500 American Registry of Radiologic Technologists (ARRT) 1255 Northland Drive St. Paul, MN 55120 (651) 687-0048
Registered nurse (RN) Cares for sick and injured people by assessing and recording symptoms, assisting physicians during treatments and examinations, and administering medications.	ADN—community college or technical school, 2 years Diploma—hospital-based, often 3 years BSN—baccalaureate degree program, 4 years	All registered nurses must pass the NCLEX-RN, administered by the National Council of Licensure Examinations for RN.	American Nurses Association (ANA) 8515 Georgia Avenue, Suite 400 Silver Spring, MD 20910 (800) 284-2378 National League for Nursing (NLN) The Watergate 2600 Virginia Avenue, NW, 8th Floor Washington, DC 20037 (800) 669-1656

Title/Description	Education Requirements	Certification or Licensure Requirements	National Association or Additional Information
Respiratory therapist Evaluates, treats, and cares for patients with breathing disorders.	*Entry level*: 2-year associate's degree program. *Advanced level*: 2- to 4-year program with baccalaureate or graduate degree.	Certification through National Board for Respiratory Care for Certified Respiratory Therapist (CRT).	American Association for Respiratory Care (AARC) 9425 N. MacArthur Blvd., Suite 100 Irving, TX 75063 (972) 243-2272
Speech-language pathologist Assesses and treats persons with speech, language, voice, and fluency disorders.	2-year master's degree plus typically 9 to 12 months of clinical experience.	Comply with state requirements for licensure, standards, and teaching certificates; requirements vary by state. Exam administered by ASHA for Certification of Clinical Competency in Speech-Language Pathology (CCC-SLP).	American Speech-Language-Hearing Association (ASHA) 2200 Research Boulevard Rockville, MD 20850 (301) 296-5700
Surgical technologist (CST) Assists in operations under the supervision of surgeons or registered nurses.	12- to 24-month associate's degree or certificate program.	Requirements for certification by exam vary by state through National Board for Surgical Technologists and Surgical Assistants for Certified Surgical Technician (CST).	Association of Surgical Technologists (AST) 6 West Dry Creek Circle Littleton, CO 80120 (800) 637-7433

GLOSSARY 1

Mini-Dictionary

Pronunciation of each term is given with its meaning. The syllable that gets the accent is in CAPITAL LETTERS. Terms in SMALL CAPITAL LETTERS are defined elsewhere in this glossary.

A

Abdomen (AB-do-men): Space below the chest that contains organs such as the stomach, liver, intestines, and gallbladder. The abdomen lies between the diaphragm and the pelvis.

Abdominal (ab-DOM-ih-nal): Pertaining to the abdomen.

Abdominal cavity (ab-DOM-ih-nal KAV-ih-te): See ABDOMEN.

Ablation (ab-LA-shun): Removal of abnormal tissue by surgical or mechanical means.

Abnormal (ab-NOR-mal): Pertaining to being away (AB-) from the norm; irregular.

Acquired immunodeficiency syndrome (ah-KWYRD im-u-no-deh-FISH-en-se SIN-drohm) or AIDS: Suppression or deficiency of the immune response caused by exposure to the HUMAN IMMUNODEFICIENCY VIRUS (HIV).

Acromegaly (ak-ro-MEG-ah-le): Enlargement of extremities as a result of thickening of the bones and soft tissues; it is caused by excessive secretion of growth hormone from the pituitary gland (after completion of puberty).

Acute (uh-KYOOT): Sharp, sudden, and intense for a short period of time.

Acute myocardial ischemia (uh-KYOOT mi-o-KAR-de-al is-KE-me-ah): Sudden decrease in blood flow to the heart muscle.

Adenectomy (ad-eh-NEK-to-me): Removal of a gland.

Adenitis (ad-eh-NI-tis): Inflammation of a gland.

Adenocarcinoma (ah-deh-no-kar-sih-NO-mah): Cancerous tumor derived from glandular cells.

Adenoidectomy (ah-deh-noyd-EK-to-me): Removal of the adenoids.

Adenoids (AD-eh-noydz): Lymphatic tissue in the upper part of the throat near the nasal passageways.

Adenoma (ah-deh-NO-mah): Tumor (benign) of a gland. Benign means not cancerous.

Adenopathy (ah-deh-NOP-ah-the): Disease of glands. Often this term refers to enlargement of lymph nodes (which are not true glands, but collections of lymphatic tissue).

Adnexa uteri (ad-NEKS-ah U-ter-i): Accessory structures of the uterus (ovaries and fallopian tubes).

Adrenal cortex (ah-DRE-nal KOR-teks): Outermost part of the adrenal gland. The adrenal cortex secretes steroid hormones such as GLUCOCORTICOIDS (cortisone).

Adrenal glands (ah-DRE-nal glanz): Two endocrine glands, each above a kidney. The adrenal glands produce hormones such as adrenaline (epinephrine) and hydrocortisone (cortisol).

Adrenalectomy (ah-dre-nal-EK-to-me): Removal (excision) of adrenal glands.

Adrenaline (ah-DREN-ah-lin): Hormone secreted by the adrenal glands. It is released into the bloodstream in response to stress, such as from fear or physical injury. Also called EPINEPHRINE.

Adrenocorticotropic hormone (ah-dre-no-kor-tih-ko-TROP-ic HOR-mone): Hormone secreted by the pituitary gland. It stimulates the adrenal gland (cortex or outer region) to secrete the hormone cortisone. Also called ACTH.

Adrenopathy (ah-dreh-NOP-a-the): Disease of ADRENAL GLANDS.

AIDS: See ACQUIRED IMMUNODEFICIENCY SYNDROME.

Air sacs (ayr saks): Thin-walled sacs within the lung. Inhaled oxygen passes into the blood from the sacs, and carbon dioxide passes out from the blood into the sacs to be exhaled; ALVEOLI.

Albumin (al-BU-min): A large-molecule protein found in blood and tissues.

Albuminuria (al-bu-min-U-re-ah): Albumin (protein) in the urine; it indicates a malfunction of the kidney.

Alkaline phosphatase (AL-kah-line PHOS-fah-tays): An enzyme present in blood and body tissues, such as bone and liver. Elevated in diseases such as those of bone and liver. Also called alk phos.

Allergist (AL-er-jist): Medical doctor specializing in identifying and treating abnormal sensitivity to substances such as pollen, dust, foods, and drugs.

Alopecia (ah-lo-PE-shah): Loss of hair; baldness.

ALT: Alanine transferase, an enzyme normally found in blood and tissues, especially the liver. ALT is elevated in liver disease. (Formerly called SGPT.)

Alveolar (al-VE-o-lar): Pertaining to air sacs (alveoli) within the lungs.

Alveoli (al-VE-o-li): Thin-walled sacs within the lung. Inhaled oxygen passes into the blood from the sacs, and carbon dioxide passes out from the blood into the sacs to be exhaled (*singular*: ALVEOLUS).

Alveolus (al-ve-O-lus): An air sac within the lung (*plural:* ALVEOLI).

Alzheimer disease (ALTZ-hi-mer di-ZEEZ): Deterioration of mental capacity (irreversible dementia) marked by intellectual deterioration, disorganization of personality, and difficulties in carrying out tasks of daily living.

Amenorrhea (a-men-o-RE-ah): Absence of menstrual flow.

Amniocentesis (am-ne-o-sen-TE-sis): Puncture to remove fluid from the amnion (sac surrounding the developing fetus).

Anal (A-nal): Pertaining to the anus (opening of the rectum to the outside of the body).

Analgesic (an-al-JE-zik): Medication that reduces or eliminates pain.

Analysis (ah-NAL-ih-sis): Separating a substance into its component parts.

Anastomosis (ah-nah-sto-MO-sis): New surgical connection between two previously unconnected bowel parts, vessels, or ducts.

Androgen (AN-dro-jen): Hormone that controls the development of masculine characteristics. An example is TESTOSTERONE.

Anemia (ah-NE-me-ah): Deficiency of hemoglobin and/or in number of red blood cells. This results in reduced delivery of oxygen to body cells. Literally, *anemia* means lacking (AN-) in blood (-EMIA).

Anemic (ah-NE-mik): Pertaining to ANEMIA.

Anesthesiologist (an-es-the-ze-OL-o-jist): Medical doctor specializing in administering agents capable of bringing about loss of sensation and consciousness.

Anesthesiology (an-es-the-ze-OL-o-je): Study of how to administer agents capable of bringing about loss of sensation and consciousness.

Aneurysm (AN-u-rizm): Localized widening of the wall of an artery, of a vein, or of the heart. From the Greek *aneurysma*, meaning "widening."

Angina (an-JI-nah): Sharp pain in the chest resulting from a decrease in blood supply to heart muscle. Also called angina pectoris (PECT/O means chest).

Angiography (an-je-OG-rah-fe): X-ray recording of blood vessels after contrast is injected.

Angioplasty (AN-je-o-plas-te): Surgical repair of a blood vessel. A tube (catheter) is placed in a clogged artery and a balloon at the end of the tube is inflated to flatten the clogged material against the wall of the artery. This enlarges the opening of the artery so that more blood can pass through. Also called balloon angioplasty.

Angiotensin (an-je-o-TEN-sin): Hormone that is a powerful vasoconstrictor and raises blood pressure.

Ankylosing spondylitis (ang-kih-LO-sing spon-dih-LI-tis): Chronic inflammation of the vertebrae (backbones) with stiffening of spinal and hip joint so that movement becomes increasingly painful.

Ankylosis (ang-kih-LO-sis): Stiffening and immobility of a joint caused by injury, disease, or a surgical procedure.

Anomaly (ah-NOM-ah-le): Irregularity; a deviation from the normal. A congenital anomaly (irregularity) is present at birth.
Antenatal (an-teh-NA-tal): Before birth.
Antepartum (an-teh-PAR-tum): Before birth.
Anterior (an-TE-re-or): Located in the front (of the body or of a structure).
Antiandrogen (an-tih-AN-dro-jen): Substance that inhibits the effects of androgens (male hormones).
Antiarrhythmic (an-te-ah-RITH-mik): Pertaining to a drug that works against or prevents abnormal heartbeats (arrhythmias).
Antibiotic (an-tih-bi-OT-ik): A chemical substance produced by various microorganisms or fungi (immature plants) that inhibits or destroys bacteria or other small organisms. Examples of antibiotics are penicillin and streptomycin. They are used in the treatment of infectious diseases.
Antibody (AN-tih-bod-e): A substance that works against (ANTI-) germs ("bodies" of infection). Antibodies are produced by white blood cells when germs (antigens) enter the bloodstream.
Anticoagulant (an-tih-ko-AG-u-lant): Drug that prevents clotting (coagulation). Anticoagulants are given when there is danger of clot formation in blood vessels, as may happen after a heart attack.
Anticonvulsant (an-tih-kon-VUL-sant): Drug that prevents or relieves convulsions (involuntary muscular contractions).
Antidepressant (an-tih-de-PRES-ant): Drug used to prevent or treat depression.
Antidiabetic (an-tih-di-ah-BET-ik): Drug that prevents or relieves symptoms of diabetes.
Antiestrogen (an-tih-ES-tro-jen): Substance that inhibits the effects of estrogens (female hormones).
Antifungal (an-tih-FUNG-al): Drug that destroys or inhibits the growth of fungi (organisms such as yeasts, molds, and mushrooms).
Antigen (AN-tih-jen): Foreign protein (such as on a bacterium or virus) that stimulates white blood cells to make antibodies. Antigens are then destroyed by the antibodies.
Antihistamine (an-tih-HIS-tah-meen): Drug used to counteract the effects of histamine production in allergic reactions and colds.
Antihypertensive (an-te-hi-per-TEN-siv): Drug that reduces high blood pressure.
Antitubercular (an-tih-too-BER-ku-lar): Agent or drug used to treat tuberculosis.
Antiviral (an-tih-VI-ral): Agent that inhibits and prevents the growth and reproduction of viruses.
Anuria (an-U-re-ah): Abnormal condition of no urine production.
Anus (A-nus): Opening of the rectum to the surface of the body; solid wastes (feces) leave the body through the anus.
Aorta (a-OR-tah): Largest artery that leads from the lower left chamber of the heart to arteries all over the body.
Aortic stenosis (a-OR-tik steh-NO-sis): Narrowing of the aorta.
Apex (A-peks): Pointed end of an organ (*plural:* apices [A-pih-seez]).
Aphakia (ah-FA-ke-ah): Absence of the lens of the eye.
Aphasia (ah-FA-ze-ah): Absence or impairment of communication through speech.
Apnea (AP-ne-ah): Not (A-) able to breathe (-PNEA); temporary stoppage of breathing. In sleep apnea, during sleep, a person is momentarily unable to contract respiratory muscles and maintain air flow through the nose and mouth.
Appendectomy (ap-en-DEK-to-me): Removal of the appendix.
Appendicitis (ap-en-dih-SI-tis): Inflammation of the appendix.
Appendix (ah-PEN-dikz): Small sac that hangs from the juncture of the small and large intestines in the right lower quadrant of the abdomen. Its function is unknown.

Arachnoid membrane (ah-RAK-noyd MEM-brayn): The middle membrane of the MENINGES (coverings around the brain and spinal cord).
Areola (ah-RE-o-lah): Dark, pigmented area around the nipple of the breast.
Arrhythmia (a-RITH-me-ah): Abnormal heart rhythm.
Arteriography (ar-teer-e-OG-rah-fe): Process of recording (x-ray) of arteries after injecting contrast material.
Arteriole (ar-TEER-e-ole): Small artery.
Arteriolitis (ar-teer-e-o-LI-tis): Inflammation of small arteries (arterioles).
Arteriosclerosis (ar-teer-e-o-skleh-RO-sis): Hardening of arteries. The most common form is *atherosclerosis*, which is hardening of arteries caused by collection of fatty, cholesterol-like deposits (plaque) in arteries.
Arteriovenous fistula (ar-teer-e-o-VE-nus FIST-u-lah): An abnormal communication between an artery and a vein. It can also be created surgically to provide access for hemodialysis.
Artery (AR-ter-e): Largest (in diameter) blood vessel. Arteries carry blood away from the heart.
Arthralgia (ar-THRAL-jah): Pain in a joint.
Arthritis (ar-THRI-tis): Inflammation of a joint.
Arthrocentesis (ar-thro-sen-TE-sis): Puncture to remove fluid from a joint for diagnosis or treatment.
Arthrogram (AR-thro-gram): X-ray record of a joint.
Arthropathy (ar-THROP-ah-the): Disease of joints.
Arthroplasty (AR-thro-plas-te): Surgical repair of a joint, especially to restore mobility in osteoarthritis or rheumatoid arthritis.
Arthroscope (AR-thro-skope): Instrument used to examine (inside of) a joint.
Arthroscopy (ar-THROS-ko-pe): Process of visual examination of a joint.
Arthrosis (ar-THRO-sis): Abnormal condition of a joint.
Ascites (ah-SI-teez): Abnormal collection of fluid in the abdomen.
Asphyxia (as-FIK-se-ah): Deficiency of oxygen in the blood and increase in carbon dioxide in blood and tissues. Major sign is a complete absence of breathing, leading to loss of consciousness or death.
Aspiration (as-per-A-shun): Withdrawal of fluid from a cavity or sac.
AST: Aspartate transferase, an enzyme normally present in blood and tissues such as heart and liver. (Formerly called SGOT.)
Asthma (AZ-mah): Difficult breathing caused by a spasm of the bronchial tubes or a swelling of their mucous membrane lining.
Asymptomatic (a-simp-to-MAT-ik): Without symptoms.
Atelectasis (ah-teh-LEK-tah-sis): Collapsed lung or part of a lung (ATEL-, meaning incomplete; -ECTASIS, meaning widening or dilation).
Atherosclerosis (ah-theh-ro-skle-RO-sis): See ARTERIOSCLEROSIS.
Atrium (A-tre-um): Upper chamber of the heart (*plural:* atria).
Atrophy (AT-ro-fe): Decrease in size of cells within an organ.
Auditory canal (AW-dih-tor-e kah-NAL): Passageway leading into the ear from the outside of the body.
Auditory nerve (AW-dih-tor-e nurv): Nerve that transmits sound waves from the inner ear to the brain, making hearing possible.
Aura (AW-rah): A strange sensation coming before more definite symptoms of illness. An aura often precedes a migraine headache or an epileptic seizure, warning the patient that an attack is beginning.
Aural discharge (AW-rahl DIS-charj): Fluid or material that is expelled from the ear.

Autopsy (AW-top-se): Examination of a dead body to determine the cause of death. Also called a POSTMORTEM exam or NECROPSY. Literally, it means "to see" (-OPSY) with "one's own" (AUT-) eyes.
Axial (AKS-e-al): Pertaining to an axis (an imaginary line through the center of a body or about which a structure revolves). Axial (transverse plane) views are seen in CT and MRI scans.
Axillary (AKS-ih-lar-e): Pertaining to the armpit or underarm.

B

Bactericidal (bak-tih-re-SI-dal): Pertaining to an agent that destroys bacteria.
Bacteriostatic (bak-tih-re-o-STAT-ik): Pertaining to an agent that inhibits bacterial growth.
Bacterium (bak-TIH-re-um): Type of one-celled organism whose genetic material (DNA) is not organized within a nucleus (*plural:* bacteria).
Balanitis (bah-lah-NI-tis): Inflammation of the penis.
Bariatric surgery (bah-re-AH-trik SUR-jer-e): Surgery on part of the gastrointestinal tract for obesity. BARI/O means weight, and IATR/O means treatment.
Barium (BAH-re-um): Substance used as a radiopaque (x-rays cannot pass through it) contrast medium for x-ray examination of the digestive tract.
Barium enema (BAH-re-um EN-eh-mah): X-ray study of the lower digestive tract performed by instilling a solution of barium into the rectum, which highlights structures seen on the x-ray images.
Barium swallow (BAH-re-um SWAH-lo): X-ray study of the upper digestive tract performed by having the patient swallow a solution of barium, which highlights structures seen on the x-ray images.
Benign (be-NIN): Not cancerous; a tumor that does not spread and is limited in growth. Benign is the opposite of malignant.
Benign prostatic hyperplasia (be-NIN pro-STAH-tik hi-per-PLA-ze-ah): Nonmalignant enlargement of the prostate gland. Also called benign prostatic hypertrophy (hi-PER-tro-fe).
Benzodiazepine (ben-zo-di-AZ-eh-pin): Drug used to relieve anxiety, relax muscles, and produce sedation.
Beta blocker (BA-tah BLOK-er): Drug that is used for the treatment of high blood pressure (hypertension), chest pain (angina), and abnormal rhythms of the heart (arrhythmias).
Bilateral (bi-LAT-er-al): Pertaining to two (both) sides.
Bile (bile): A yellow or orange fluid produced by the liver. It breaks up large fat globules and helps in the digestion of fats.
Bile duct (bile dukt): Tube that carries bile from the liver and gallbladder to the intestine.
Bilirubin (bil-ih-RU-bin): A red blood cell pigment excreted with bile from the liver into the intestine.
Biology (bi-OL-o-je): Study of life.
Biopsy (BI-op-se): Living tissue is removed and viewed under a microscope. In a *core (needle) biopsy*, a small sample of tissue is removed using a hollow needle. It is typically performed under imaging guidance such as ULTRASOUND or CT SCAN.
Bladder (BLAD-er): See URINARY BLADDER.
Bone (bone): Hard, rigid type of connective tissue that makes up most of the skeleton. It is composed of calcium salts.
Bone marrow (bone MAH-ro): Soft, sponge-like material in the inner part of bones. Blood cells are made in the bone marrow.

Bones of the middle ear: Three small bones (ossicles) that transmit sound vibrations to the inner ear; malleus, incus, and stapes.
Bradycardia (bra-de-KAR-de-ah): Slow heartbeat.
Brain (brayn): Organ in the head that controls the activities of the body.
Breast (brest): One of two glandular organs on the front of the chest. The breasts produce milk after childbirth.
Bronchial tube (BRONG-ke-al toob): One of two tubes that carry air from the windpipe to the lungs. Also called a bronchus (*plural:* bronchi).
Bronchiole (BRONG-ke-ol): Small bronchial tube.
Bronchiolitis (brong-ke-o-LI-tis): Inflammation of bronchioles.
Bronchitis (brong-KI-tis): Inflammation of bronchial tubes.
Bronchoscope (BRONG-ko-skope): Instrument used to visually examine bronchial tubes.
Bronchoscopy (brong-KOS-ko-pe): Visual examination of bronchial tubes by passing an endoscope through the trachea (windpipe) into the bronchi.
Bronchus (BRONG-kus): See BRONCHIAL TUBE.
Bursa (BUR-sah): Sac of fluid near a joint (*plural:* bursae [BUR-se]).
Bursitis (bur-SI-tis): Inflammation of a bursa.

C

Calcaneus (kal-KA-ne-us): Heel bone.
Calcification (cal-sih-fih-KA-shun): Accumulation of calcium salts in tissues.
Calcium channel blocker (KAL-se-um CHAN-el BLOK-er): Drug that dilates arteries by inhibiting the flow of calcium into muscle cells that line arteries. It is used to treat hypertension (high blood pressure) and angina (chest pain caused by insufficient oxygen to heart muscle).
Calculus (KAL-ku-lus): Stone (*plural:* calculi [KAL-ku-li]).
Callus (KAL-us): Bony deposit formed between and around the broken ends of a fractured bone. Also, a painless thickening of skin cells in areas of external pressure or friction.
Capillary (KAP-ih-lar-e): Smallest blood vessel (*plural:* capillaries).
Carbon dioxide (KAR-bon di-OK-side): Odorless, colorless gas formed in tissues and eliminated by the lungs.
Carcinoma (kar-sih-NO-mah): Cancerous tumor. Carcinomas form from epithelial cells that line the internal organs and cover the outside of the body.
Cardiac (KAR-de-ak): Pertaining to the heart.
Cardiac catheter ablation (KAR-de-ak KATH-eh-ter ab-LA-shun): Procedure to correct an ARRHYTHMIA by advancing a flexible tube (catheter) through blood vessels into the heart. High-frequency electrical impulses then destroy the abnormal tissue that is causing the arrhythmia.
Cardiologist (kar-de-OL-o-jist): Physician specializing in the study of the heart and heart disease.
Cardiology (kar-de-OL-o-je): Study of the heart.
Cardiomegaly (kar-de-o-MEG-ah-le): Enlargement of the heart.
Cardiomyopathy (kar-de-o-mi-OP-ah-the): Disease of heart muscle.
Cardiovascular surgeon (kar-de-o-VAS-ku-lar SUR-jun): Specialist in operating on the heart and blood vessels.
Cardioversion (KAR-de-o-ver-zhun): Brief discharges of electricity passing across the chest to stop a cardiac ARRHYTHMIA. Also called DEFIBRILLATION.
Carpals (KAR-palz): Wrist bones.
Carpal tunnel syndrome (KAR-pal TUN-el SYN-drohm): Group of symptoms resulting from compression of the median nerve in the wrist. Symptoms include tingling, pain, and burning sensations in the hand and wrist.

Cartilage (KAR-tih-laj): Flexible, fibrous connective tissue, found as part of the nose, ears, voice box, and windpipe and chiefly attached to bones at joints.
Cataract (KAT-ah-rakt): Clouding of the lens of the eye.
Cathartic (ka-THAR-tik): Pertaining to a substance that causes the release of feces from the large intestine.
Catheter (KATH-eh-ter): Flexible or rigid hollow tube used to drain fluids from the body or inject fluids into the body. Catheters are also used to help keep passageways open.
CAT scan (kat skan): Computerized axial tomography. See CT SCAN.
Cauda equina (KAW-dah eh-KWI-nah): Bundle of nerve fibers and nerve roots extending from the end of the spinal cord (L3) to the sacral and coccygeal nerves. *Cauda equina* is Latin for "horse's tail," which describes its appearance.
Caudal (KAW-dal): Pertaining to the tail or the lower portion of the body.
Cauterization (kaw-tur-e-ZA-shun): Heat is used to destroy abnormal tissue; the procedure may be used, for example, in the lining of the cervix (lower neck-like region of the uterus).
Cautery (KAW-tur-e): Instrument or agent used to destroy tissue by burning.
Cell (sel): Smallest unit or part of an organ.
Cellulitis (sel-u-LI-tis): Inflammation of soft tissue under the skin; it is marked by swelling, redness, and pain, and is caused by bacterial infection.
Cephalgia (seh-FAL-jah): Headache. Shortened form of *cephalalgia*.
Cephalic (seh-FAL-ik): Pertaining to the head. *Cephalic presentation* refers to a fetal position in which the head of the fetus appears at the uterine cervix as the infant is born.
Cephalosporin (sef-ah-lo-SPOR-in): Antibiotic similar to penicillin and used to treat infections of the respiratory tract, ear, urinary tract, bones, and blood.
Cerebellar (ser-eh-BEL-ar): Pertaining to the CEREBELLUM.
Cerebellum (ser-eh-BEL-um): Lower, back part of the brain that coordinates muscle movement and balance.
Cerebral (seh-RE-bral or SER-eh-bral): Pertaining to the CEREBRUM.
Cerebrospinal fluid (seh-RE-bro SPI-nal FLOO-id): Fluid surrounding the brain and spinal cord.
Cerebrovascular accident (seh-re-bro-VAS-ku-lar AK-sih-dent): Blood is prevented from reaching areas of the cerebrum, and brain cells die; also called a STROKE.
Cerebrum (seh-RE-brum): Largest part of the brain. It controls thought processes, hearing, speech, vision, and body movements.
Cervical (SER-vih-kal): Pertaining to the neck of the body or the neck (cervix) of the uterus.
Cervical region (SER-vih-kal RE-jun): Seven backbones in the area of the neck.
Cervical vertebra (SER-vih-kal VER-teh-brah): Backbone in the neck.
Cervix (SER-viks): Lower, neck-like portion of the uterus opening into the vagina.
Cesarean section (seh-ZAR-re-an SEK-shun): Incision of the uterus to remove the fetus at birth.
Chlamydial infection (klah-MID-e-al in-FEK-shun): A bacterial infection commonly transmitted by sexual contact.
Chemotherapy (ke-mo-THER-ah-pe): Treatment with drugs. Chemotherapy is most often used in the treatment of cancer.
Cholecystectomy (ko-leh-sis-TEK-to-me): Removal of the gallbladder.
Choledochoduodenostomy (ko-led-oh-ko-doo-o-deh-NOS-to-me): New surgical attachment of the common bile duct to the duodenum; an anastomosis.
Choledochotomy (ko-led-o-KOT-o-me): Incision of the common bile duct.
Cholelithiasis (ko-leh-lih-THI-ah-sis): Abnormal condition of gallstones.
Cholesterol (ko-LES-ter-ol): Fatty substance made in the liver and found in the bloodstream. It is an important part of all cells and is necessary for creating hormones.

It may accumulate in the lining of arteries, such as in the heart, causing heart disease, or in the gallbladder to form gallstones. Normal adult levels are 120 to 200 mg/dL.

Chondroma (kon-DRO-mah): Benign tumor of CARTILAGE.

Chondrosarcoma (kon-dro-sar-KO-mah): Malignant tumor of CARTILAGE.

Chronic (KRON-ik): Lasting a long time.

Chronic obstructive pulmonary disease (KRON-ik ob-STRUK-tiv PUL-mo-na-re dih-ZEEZ): Chronic limitation in airflow into and out of the body; includes chronic bronchitis, ASTHMA, and EMPHYSEMA. Also called COPD.

Chronic traumatic encephalopathy (CTE) (KRON-ik traw-MAT-ik en-sef-ah-LOP-ah-the): A serious disease condition of the brain caused by repeated (chronic) high-impact trauma such as in boxing or football.

Circulatory system (SER-ku-lah-tor-e SIS-tem): Organs (heart and blood vessels) that carry blood throughout the body.

Cirrhosis (seh-RO-sis): Liver disease with deterioration of the liver cells. Cirrhosis is often caused by alcoholism and poor nutrition.

Clavicle (KLAV-ih-kul): Collarbone.

Clinical (KLIN-ih-kal): Pertaining to the bedside or clinic; involving patient care.

Coccygeal (kok-sih-JE-al): Pertaining to the tailbone (coccyx).

Coccygeal region (kok-sih-JE-al RE-jun): Four fused (joined-together) bones at the base of the spinal column (backbone).

Coccyx (KOK-siks): Tailbone.

Cochlear (KO-kle-er): Pertaining to the spiral-shaped cavity (cochlea) of the inner ear that transmits sound vibrations to the auditory nerve.

Colectomy (ko-LEK-to-me): Removal of the colon (large intestine).

Colitis (ko-LI-tis): Inflammation of the colon (large intestine).

Colocolostomy (ko-lo-ko-LOS-to-me): New surgical connection between two previously unconnected portions of the colon. This is an anastomosis.

Colon (KO-lon): Large intestine (bowel).

Colonic polyposis (ko-LON-ik pol-ih-PO-sis): Condition of growths or masses protruding from the mucous membrane lining the colon.

Colonoscopy (ko-lon-OS-ko-pe): Visual examination of the colon.

Colorectal surgeon (ko-lo-REK-tal SUR-jun): Physician specializing in operating on the colon and rectum.

Colostomy (ko-LOS-to-me): Opening of the colon to the outside of the body.

Colposcopy (kol-POS-ko-pe): Visual examination of the vagina and cervix.

Computed tomography scan (kom-PU-ted to-MOG-rah-fe skan): X-ray images taken to show the body in cross-sectional views. Also called CT SCAN.

Concussion (kon-KUSH-un): Traumatic brain injury that can cause bruising, damage to blood vessels, and injury to nerves. Loss of consciousness may result.

Congenital anomaly (con-JEN-ih-tal ah-NOM-ah-le): See ANOMALY.

Congestive heart failure (kon-JES-tiv hart FAIL-ur): Condition in which the heart is unable to pump its required amount of blood, resulting in inadequate oxygen to body cells.

Conization (ko-nih-ZA-shun): Removal of a wedge-shaped piece (cone) of tissue from the cervix for biopsy in the diagnosis and treatment of early cervical cancer.

Conjunctiva (kon-junk-TI-vah): Thin protective membrane over the front of the eye and attached to the eyelids.

Conjunctivitis (kon-junk-ti-VI-tis): Inflammation of the CONJUNCTIVA.

Connective tissue (kon-NEK-tiv TIS-u): Fibrous tissue that supports and connects internal organs, bones, and walls of blood vessels.

Contraindication (kon-tra-in-dih-KA-shun): Specific situation in which a drug, procedure, or surgery should not be used because it may be harmful to the patient.

Contralateral (kon-tra-LAT-er-al): Pertaining to the opposite side.

Core biopsy (kor BI-op-se): See BIOPSY.
Corium (KOR-e-um): Middle layer of the skin below the epidermis; DERMIS.
Cornea (KOR-ne-ah): Transparent layer over the front of the eye. It bends light to focus it on sensitive cells (retina) at the back of the eye.
Coronal plane (kor-O-nal playn): See FRONTAL PLANE.
Coronary (KOR-on-ayr-e): Pertaining to the heart. CORON/O means heart or crown. Coronary arteries are located on the outside of the heart, surrounding it like a crown. They bring oxygen-rich blood to the heart muscle.
Coronary angiogram (KOR-on-ayr-e AN-je-o-gram): X-ray record of blood vessels surrounding the heart.
Coronary arteries (KOR-on-ayr-e AR-ter-eez): Blood vessels that carry oxygen-rich blood from the aorta to the heart muscle.
Coroner (KOR-oh-ner): A person who determines the cause of death in cases where the death was sudden, unexpected, of suspicious origin, or while under police custody. Generally, coroners have legal and/or medical backgrounds.
Cortex (KOR-teks): Outer part of an organ (*plural:* cortices [KOR-tih-seez]).
Cortisol (KOR-tih-sol): Anti-inflammatory hormone secreted by the adrenal cortex.
Costochondritis (kos-to-kon-DRI-tis): Inflammation of the cartilage attached to a rib.
Costochondral (kos-to-KON-dral): Pertaining to a rib and its cartilage.
Cranial cavity (KRA-ne-al KAV-ih-te): Space surrounded by the skull and containing the brain and other organs.
Craniotomy (kra-ne-OT-o-me): Incision of the skull.
Cranium (KRA-ne-um): Skull.
Creatinine (kre-AT-tih-neen): Nitrogen-containing waste that is removed from the blood by the kidney and excreted in urine.
Crohn disease (kron dih-ZEEZ): Inflammation of the gastrointestinal tract (often the ileum) marked by bouts of diarrhea, abdominal cramping, and fever. Along with ulcerative colitis, Crohn's is a type of INFLAMMATORY BOWEL DISEASE.
Cross section (kros SEK-shun): Division of an organ or the body into upper and lower portions; TRANSVERSE PLANE.
Cryosurgery (kri-o-SUR-jeh-re): Use of cold temperatures (such as liquid nitrogen) to freeze and destroy tissue.
Cryotherapy (kri-o-THER-ah-pe): Treatment using cold (CRY/O) temperatures.
Cryptorchism (kript-OR-kizm): Undescended (CRYPT- means hidden) testicle. The testicle is not in the scrotal sac at birth. Also called *cryptorchidism*.
CT scan: Computed tomography study; series of x-ray images showing organs in cross section (transverse view). Also called a CAT SCAN.
Cusp (KUSP): Any one of the small flaps on the valves of the heart. Also, a sharp projection extending from the surface of a tooth.
Cushing syndrome (KOOSH-ing SYN-drohm): Clinical signs and symptoms produced by an excess of cortisol from the adrenal cortex. Cushing syndrome is marked by "moon face," fatty swellings, and weakness.
Cuticle (KU-ti-cul): Thin layer of dead skin at the base of the nail plate.
Cyanosis (si-ah-NO-sis): Bluish discoloration of the skin due to deficient OXYGEN in the bloodstream.
Cystitis (sis-TI-tis): Inflammation of the urinary bladder.
Cystoscope (SIS-to-skope): Instrument (endoscope) used to view the urinary bladder.
Cystoscopy (sis-TOS-ko-pe): Visual examination of the urinary bladder.
Cytology (si-TOL-o-je): Study of cells.

Debridement (de-BREED-ment): Removal of diseased tissue from the skin.
Deep vein thrombosis (deep vayn throm-BO-sis): Abnormal condition of clot formation in a deep vein, usually in the leg or pelvic (hip) region.
Defibrillation (de-fib-rih-LA-shun): Brief discharges of electricity applied to the chest to stop an abnormal heart rhythm.
Delusion (deh-LOO-zhun): A persistent belief held by a person despite evidence to the contrary.
Dementia (deh-MEN-shah): Loss of memory and mental abilities.
Dermal (DER-mal): Pertaining to the skin.
Dermatitis (der-mah-TI-tis): Inflammation of the skin.
Dermatologist (der-mah-TOL-o-jist): Physician specializing in the skin and its diseases.
Dermatology (der-mah-TOL-o-je): Study of the skin and its diseases.
Dermatosis (der-mah-TO-sis): Abnormal condition of the skin.
Dermis (DER-mis): Fibrous middle layer of the skin below the epidermis. The dermis contains nerves and blood vessels, hair roots, and oil and sweat glands.
Diabetes mellitus (di-ah-BE-teez MEL-lih-tus): Disorder marked by deficient insulin in the blood, which causes sugar to remain in the blood rather than entering cells. Diabetes is named from a Greek word meaning "siphon" (through which water passes easily). One symptom is frequent urination (polyuria). Type 1 diabetes is marked by lack of insulin, and patients need injections of insulin. In type 2 diabetes, insulin is not adequately or appropriately secreted. Type 2 diabetes has a tendency to develop later in life, and patients can be managed with diet, exercise, and oral antidiabetic drugs.
Diagnosis (di-ag-NO-sis): Complete knowledge of patient's condition (*plural:* diagnoses).
Dialysis (di-AL-ih-sis): Complete separation (-LYSIS) of wastes (urea) from the blood when the kidneys fail. See also HEMODIALYSIS and PERITONEAL DIALYSIS.
Diameter (di-AM-eh-ter): Measurement (-METER) through (DIA-) center of a circle or tube. The diameter of an artery is larger than the diameter of a vein or capillary.
Diaphragm (DI-ah-fram): Muscle that separates the chest from the abdomen.
Diarrhea (di-ah-RE-ah): Discharge of watery wastes from the COLON.
Digestive system (di-JES-tiv SIS-tem): Organs that bring food into the body and break it down to enter the bloodstream or eliminate it through the rectum and anus.
Dilation (di-LA-shun): Widening; dilatation.
Dilation and curettage (di-LA-shun and kur-eh-TAZH): Widening of the opening to the cervix and scraping (curettage) of the inner lining of the uterus; also called D&C.
Disc: Pad of cartilage that is between each backbone.
Diuretic (di-u-RET-ik): Drug that causes kidneys to allow more fluid (as urine) to leave the body. Diuretics remove fluid from the blood and are used to treat HYPERTENSION. DI- (from DIA-) means complete, and UR- means urine.
Diverticula (di-ver-TIK-u-lah): Small pouches or sacs created by herniation of mucous membrane linings, most commonly in the colon (*singular*: diverticulum).
Diverticulitis (di-ver-tik-u-LI-tis): Inflammation of diverticula. Penetration of fecal material through thin-walled diverticula causes inflammation and infection in the colon.
Diverticulosis (di-ver-tik-u-LO-sis): Abnormal condition of small pouches in the lining of the intestines.
Duodenal (do-o-DE-nal): Pertaining to the duodenum.
Duodenum (do-o-DE-num): First part of the small intestine.
Dura mater (DU-rah MAH-ter): Outermost of the three layers of the MENINGES surrounding the brain and spinal cord. The name comes from Latin, meaning "hard mother." It is the toughest of the three layers.

Dysentery (DIS-en-teh-re): Condition of painful intestines (often caused by bacterial infection).
Dysmenorrhea (dis-men-o-RE-ah): Painful menstrual flow.
Dyspepsia (dis-PEP-se-ah): Painful (DYS-) digestion (-PEPSIA).
Dysphagia (dis-FA-jah): Difficult swallowing.
Dysphasia (dis-FA-zhah): Difficult (impairment of) speech.
Dysplasia (dis-PLA-zhah): Abnormality of the development or the formation of cells. Normal cells change in size, shape, and organization.
Dyspnea (disp-NE-ah): Painful (DYS-) (labored, difficult) breathing (-PNEA).
Dysuria (dis-U-re-ah): Painful or difficult urination.

E

Ear: Organ that receives sound waves and transmits them to nerves leading to the brain.
Eardrum (EAR-drum): Membrane separating the outer and middle parts of the ear; the tympanic membrane.
Ectopic pregnancy (ek-TOP-ik PREG-nan-se): Pregnancy that is not in the uterus, usually occurring in the FALLOPIAN TUBES.
Edema (eh-DE-mah): Swelling in tissues. Edema is often caused by retention (holding back) of fluid and salt by the kidneys.
Ejaculation (e-jak-ku-LA-shun): Release of semen from the male urethra.
Electrocardiogram (e-lek-tro-KAR-de-o-gram): Record of the electricity in the heart.
Electroencephalogram (e-lek-tro-en-SEF-ah-lo-gram): Record of the electricity in the brain.
Electroencephalography (e-lek-tro-en-sef-ah-LOG-rah-fe): Process of recording the electricity in the brain.
Electrolyte (eh-LEK-tro-lite): Substance that conducts an electrical current and is found in blood (serum) and body cells. Examples are sodium (Na^+), potassium (K^+), calcium (Ca^{2+}), and chloride (Cl^-).
Embolization (em-bo-lih-ZA-shun): Use of a substance to block or reduce blood flow in a vessel.
Embolus (EM-bo-lus): Foreign object (air, tissue, tumor, or clot) that circulates in the bloodstream until it lodges in a vessel.
Embryo (EM-bre-o): A new organism in an early stage of development (2 to 8 weeks). From 6 to 38 weeks, the developing infant is a fetus.
Emergency medicine (e-MER-jen-se MED-ih-sin): Care of patients requiring immediate action.
Emphysema (em-fih-SE-mah): Lung disorder in which air becomes trapped in the air sacs and bronchioles, making breathing difficult. Emphysema is marked by the accumulation of mucus and the loss of elasticity in lung tissue.
Encephalitis (en-sef-ah-LI-tis): Inflammation of the brain.
Encephalopathy (en-sef-ah-LOP-ah-the): Disease of the brain.
Endocarditis (EN-do-kar-DI-tis): Inflammation of the inner lining of the heart (ENDOCARDIUM).
Endocardium (en-do-KAR-de-um): Inner lining of the heart.
Endocrine glands (EN-do-krin glanz): Organs that produce (secrete) hormones; examples are thyroid, pituitary, and adrenal glands.
Endocrine system (EN-do-krin SIS-tem): Endocrine glands.
Endocrinologist (en-do-krih-NOL-o-jist): Specialist in the study of endocrine glands and their disorders.
Endocrinology (en-do-krih-NOL-o-je): Study of ENDOCRINE GLANDS.

Endodontist (en-do-DON-tist): Dentist who specializes in diagnosis and treatment of the inner parts of a tooth (root canal therapy).
Endometriosis (en-do-me-tre-O-sis): An abnormal condition in which tissue from the inner lining of the uterus is found outside the uterus, usually in the pelvic cavity.
Endometrium (en-do-ME-tre-um): Inner lining of the uterus.
Endoscope (EN-do-skope): Instrument used to view a hollow organ or body cavity; a tube fitted with a lens system that allows viewing in different directions.
Endoscopic retrograde cholangiopancreatography (en-do-SKOP-ik RET-tro-grade kol-an-je-o-pan-kre-ah-TOG-rah-fe): X-ray images of bile ducts and pancreas after injection of contrast through a catheter from the mouth, esophagus, and stomach into bile and pancreatic ducts.
Endoscopy (en-DOS-ko-pe): Process of viewing the inside of hollow organs or cavities with an endoscope.
Enteric (en-TER-ik): Pertaining to the small intestine.
Enteritis (en-teh-RI-tis): Inflammation of the small intestine.
Epidermis (ep-ih-DER-mis): Outer (EPI-) layer of the skin (-DERMIS).
Epidural hematoma (ep-ih-DUR-al he-mah-TO-mah): Pathologic mass of blood above the dura mater (outermost layer of membranes surrounding the brain and spinal cord).
Epigastric (ep-ih-GAS-trik): Pertaining to above or upon the stomach.
Epiglottis (ep-ih-GLOT-tis): Flap of cartilage that covers the mouth of the trachea when swallowing occurs so that food cannot enter the airway.
Epiglottitis (ep-ih-gloh-TI-tis): Inflammation of the EPIGLOTTIS.
Epilepsy (EP-ih-lep-se): Condition in which abnormal electrical activity in the brain results in sudden, fleeting disturbances in nerve cell functioning. An attack of epilepsy is called a SEIZURE.
Epinephrine (eh-pih-NEF-rin): Hormone secreted by the adrenal gland in response to stress and physical injury. It is a drug used to treat hypersensitivity reactions (severe allergy), asthma, bronchial spasm, and nasal congestion. Also called ADRENALINE.
Epithelial (ep-ih-THE-le-al): Pertaining to skin cells. This term originally described cells upon (EPI-) the breast nipple (THELI-). Now, it indicates cells lining the inner part of internal organs and covering the outside of the body.
Epithelium (ep-ih-THE-le-um): Covering of the internal and external tissues of the body (skin, vessels, body cavities, glands, and organs).
Erythrocyte (eh-RITH-ro-site): Red blood cell.
Erythrocytosis (eh-rith-ro-si-TO-sis): Abnormal condition (slight increase in numbers) of red blood cells.
Erythromycin (eh-rith-ro-MI-sin): An antibiotic that is produced from a red (ERYTHR/O-) mold (-MYCIN).
Esophageal (eh-sof-ah-JE-al): Pertaining to the esophagus.
Esophagitis (eh-sof-ah-JI-tis): Inflammation of the esophagus.
Esophagoscopy (eh-sof-ah-GOS-ko-pe): Visual examination of the esophagus.
Esophagus (eh-SOF-ah-gus): Tube leading from the throat to the stomach.
Estrogen (ES-tro-jen): Hormone that promotes the development of female secondary sex characteristics. Examples are estradiol, estriol, and conjugated estrogen.
Eustachian tube (u-STA-she-an tube): Channel connecting the middle part of the ear with the throat.
Exacerbation (eg-zas-er-BA-shun): Increase in the seriousness of a disease, with greater intensity in the signs or symptoms.
Excision (ek-SIZH-un): Act of cutting out, removing, or resecting.
Exocrine glands (EK-so-krin glanz): Glands that produce (secrete) chemicals that leave the body through tubes (ducts). Examples are tear, sweat, and salivary glands.

Exophthalmic goiter (ek-sof-THAL-mik GOY-ter): Enlargement of the thyroid gland accompanied by high levels of thyroid hormone in the blood and protrusion of the eyeballs (EXOPHTHALMOS).
Exophthalmos (ek-sof-THAL-mos): Abnormal protrusion of eyeballs usually caused by HYPERTHYROIDISM.
Extracranial (eks-tra-KRA-ne-al): Pertaining to outside the skull.
Extrahepatic (eks-tra-heh-PAT-ik): Pertaining to outside the liver.
Extrapulmonary (eks-trah-PUL-mo-nah-re): Outside the lungs.
Eye (i): Organ that receives light waves and transmits them to the brain.

F

Fallopian tubes (fah-LO-pe-an toobz): Two tubes that lead from the ovaries to the uterus. They transport egg cells to the uterus; also called uterine tubes.
Family medicine (FAM-ih-le MED-ih-sin): Primary care of all members of the family on a continuing basis.
Family practitioner (FAM-ih-le prak-TIH-shan-er): Medical doctor responsible for primary care and treatment of patients on a continuing basis.
Fatigue (fah-TEEG): State of exhaustion or loss of strength.
Fecal transplant (FEE-kal TRANZ-plant): Procedure in which feces are taken from a healthy donor, and transferred to the colon of a patient with a serious bacterial infection. Symptoms improve within days of fecal transplant but usually need several weeks to become permanent. The fecal transplant is introduced via colonoscopy or in pill form.
Feces (FEE-seez): Waste material from the digestive tract that is expelled from the body through the rectum and anus.
Fellowship training (FEL-o-ship TRA-ning): Postgraduate training for doctors in specialized fields. The training may include CLINICAL and RESEARCH (laboratory) work.
Female reproductive system (FE-male re-pro-DUK-tiv SIS-tem): Organs (OVARIES) that produce and transport (FALLOPIAN TUBES) egg cells and secrete female hormones (ESTROGEN and PROGESTERONE). The system includes the uterus, where the embryo and fetus grow.
Femur (FE-mur): Thigh bone.
Fetus (FE-tus): Unborn offspring in the uterus after 8 weeks of pregnancy until birth.
Fibrillation (fih-brih-LA-shun): Rapid, irregular, involuntary muscular contraction. Atrial and ventricular fibrillation are cardiac (heart) ARRHYTHMIAS.
Fibroids (FI-broydz): Benign growths of muscle tissue in the uterus.
Fibrosarcoma (fi-bro-sar-KO-mah): Malignant tumor of fibrous tissue.
Fibula (FIB-u-lah): Smaller lower leg bone.
Fistula (FIS-tu-lah): Abnormal passageway from an internal organ to the body surface or between two internal organs.
Fixation (fik-SA-shun): Act of holding, sewing, or fastening a part in a fixed position.
Flutter (FLUT-er): Rapid but regular, abnormal heart muscle contraction. Atrial and ventricular flutter are heart ARRHYTHMIAS.
Follicle-stimulating hormone (FOL-ih-kl STIM-u-la-ting HOR-mone): Hormone secreted by the pituitary gland to stimulate the egg cells in the ovaries.
Fracture (FRAK-chur): Breaking of a bone.
Frontal (FRUN-tal): Pertaining to the front; anterior.
Frontal plane (FRUN-tal playn): Vertical plane that divides the body or an organ into front and back portions; the CORONAL PLANE.
Functional disorder (FUNG-shih-nal dis-OR-der): Condition in which there are clinical signs and symptoms but no evidence of a structural or biochemical cause.

G

Gadolinium (gad-o-LIN-e-um): Chemical element that is used as a contrast agent in MRI studies. Symbol is Gd.
Gallbladder (GAWL-blad-er): Sac below the liver that stores bile and delivers it to the small intestine.
Ganglion (GANG-le-on): Benign cyst near a joint (wrist); also, a group of nerve cells (*plural:* ganglia [GANG-le-ah]).
Gangrene (GANG-reen): Necrosis (death) of tissue as a result of blood vessel injury, frostbite, or conditions such as diabetes or atherosclerosis. It results from ischemia, deficiency of blood flow caused by narrowing or obstruction of blood vessels.
Gastralgia (gas-TRAL-jah): Stomach pain.
Gastrectomy (gas-TREK-to-me): Excision (removal) of the stomach.
Gastric (GAS-trik): Pertaining to the stomach.
Gastritis (gas-TRI-tis): Inflammation of the stomach.
Gastroenteritis (gas-tro-en-teh-RI-tis): Inflammation of the stomach and intestines.
Gastroenterologist (gas-tro-en-ter-OL-o-jist): Specialist in the treatment of stomach and intestinal disorders.
Gastroenterology (gas-tro-en-ter-OL-o-je): Study of the stomach and intestines.
Gastroesophageal reflux disease (gas-tro-eh-sof-ah-JE-al RE-flux dih-ZEEZ): Condition marked by backflow (reflux) of contents of the stomach into the esophagus. Abbreviation is GERD.
Gastrojejunostomy (gas-tro-jeh-joo-NOS-to-me): New, surgically created opening between the stomach and the jejunum (second part of the small intestine). This procedure is an anastomosis.
Gastroscope (GAS-tro-skope): Instrument used to view the stomach. It is passed down the throat and esophagus into the stomach.
Gastroscopy (gas-TROS-ko-pe): Visual examination of the stomach.
Gastrotomy (gas-TROT-o-me): Incision of the stomach.
GERD: See GASTROESOPHAGEAL REFLUX DISEASE.
Geriatric (jer-e-AH-trik): Pertaining to treatment of older people.
Geriatrician (jer-e-ah-TRISH-an): Specialist in the treatment of diseases of old age.
Geriatrics (jer-e-AH-triks): Treatment of disorders of old age.
Gestation (jes-TA-shun): Growth of the fetus that occurs during pregnancy.
Gland: Group of cells that secretes chemicals to the outside of the body (EXOCRINE GLANDS) or hormones directly into the bloodstream (ENDOCRINE GLANDS).
Glaucoma (glaw-KO-mah): Increase of fluid pressure within the eye. Fluid is formed more rapidly than it is removed. The increased pressure damages sensitive cells in the back of the eye, and vision is disturbed.
Glial cells (GLI-al selz): Supporting cells of nervous tissue in the brain. Examples are astrocytes and microglial and oligodendroglial cells. These cells are the source of primary brain tumors.
Glioblastoma (gli-o-blas-TO-mah): Malignant brain tumor composed of immature (-BLAST) glial (supportive nervous tissue) cells.
Globulin (GLOB-u-lin): Plasma protein; alpha, beta, and gamma globulins are examples.
Glucocorticoid (gloo-ko-KOR-tih-koyd): Hormone secreted by the adrenal gland (cortex) to raise blood sugar levels. Examples are cortisone and cortisol.
Glycosuria (gli-kos-U-re-ah): Abnormal condition of sugar in the urine.
Goiter (GOY-ter): Enlargement of the thyroid gland.

Gonorrhea (gon-oh-RE-ah): Sexually transmitted disease most often affecting the reproductive and urinary tracts and caused by infection with the bacterium *Neisseria gonorrhoeae*.
Gout (gout): See GOUTY ARTHRITIS.
Gouty arthritis (GOW-te arth-RI-tis): Deposits of uric acid crystals in joints and other tissues that cause swelling and inflammation of joints. Also called GOUT.
Graves disease (grayvz dih-ZEEZ): See HYPERTHYROIDISM.
Growth hormone (groth HOR-mone): Hormone secreted by the pituitary gland to stimulate the growth of bones and the body in general. Also called somatotropin.
Gynecologist (gi-neh-KOL-o-jist): Specialist in the study of female disorders.
Gynecology (gi-neh-KOL-o-je): Study of female disorders.

H

Hair follicle (hayr FOL-ih-k'l): Pouch-like depression in the skin in which a hair develops.
Hair root (hayr root): Part of the hair from which growth occurs.
Hallucination (hah-loo-sih-NA-shun): False sensory perception, such as hearing voices when none are present.
HDL: See HIGH-DENSITY LIPOPROTEIN.
Heart (hart): Hollow muscular organ in the chest that pumps blood throughout the body.
Heart attack (hart ah-TAK): See MYOCARDIAL INFARCTION.
Hemangioma (he-man-je-O-mah): Tumor (benign) of blood vessels.
Hematemesis (he-mah-TEM-eh-sis): Vomiting (-EMESIS) of blood (HEMAT/O-).
Hematologist (he-mah-TOL-o-jist): Specialist in blood and blood disorders.
Hematology (he-mah-TOL-o-je): Study of the blood.
Hematoma (he-mah-TO-mah): Mass or collection of blood under the skin. Commonly called a bruise or "black-and-blue" mark.
Hematuria (he-mah-TUR-e-ah): Abnormal condition of blood in the urine.
Hemigastrectomy (heh-me-gas-TREK-to-me): Removal of half of the stomach.
Hemiglossectomy (heh-me-glos-EK-to-me): Removal of half of the tongue.
Hemiplegia (hem-ih-PLE-jah): Paralysis that affects the right or left side of the body.
Hemoccult test (he-mo-KULT test): A standardized test to look for hidden (occult) blood in stool. It is a screening test for colon and rectal cancer. See also STOOL GUAIAC.
Hemodialysis (he-mo-di-AL-ih-sis): Use of a kidney machine to filter blood to remove waste materials such as urea. Blood leaves the body, enters the machine, and is carried back to the body through a catheter (tube).
Hemoglobin (HE-mo-glo-bin): Oxygen-carrying protein found in red blood cells.
Hemoptysis (he-MOP-tih-sis): Spitting up (-PTYSIS) of blood (HEM/O-) from the respiratory tract.
Hemorrhage (HEM-or-ij): Bursting forth of blood.
Hemothorax (he-mo-THOR-aks): Collection of blood in the chest (pleural cavity).
Hepatic (heh-PAT-ik): Pertaining to the liver.
Hepatitis (hep-ah-TI-tis): Inflammation of the liver. Viral hepatitis is an acute infectious disease caused by at least three different viruses: hepatitis A, B, and C viruses.
Hepatocellular carcinoma (hep-ah-to-SEL-u-lar kar-sih-NO-mah): Malignant tumor of the liver.
Hepatoma (hep-ah-TO-mah): Tumor (malignant) of the liver; HEPATOCELLULAR CARCINOMA.
Hepatomegaly (hep-ah-to-MEG-ah-le): Enlargement of the liver.

Hernia (HER-ne-ah): Bulge or protrusion of an organ or part of an organ through the wall of the cavity that usually contains it. In an INGUINAL hernia, part of the wall of the abdomen weakens and the intestine bulges outward or into the SCROTAL sac (in males).
Herpes genitalis (HER-peez jen-ih-TAL-is): Chronic sexually transmitted disease caused by type 2 herpes simplex virus.
Hiatal hernia (hi-A-tal HER-ne-ah): Upward protrusion of the wall of the stomach into the lower part of the esophagus.
High-density lipoprotein (hi DEN-sih-te li-po-PRO-teen): Combination of fat and protein in the blood. It carries cholesterol to the liver, which is beneficial.
Hilum (HI-lum): Depression at that part of an organ where blood vessels and nerves enter.
HIV: See human immunodeficiency virus.
Hodgkin lymphoma (HOJ-kin lim-FO-mah): Malignant tumor of lymph nodes.
Hormone (HOR-mone): Chemical made by a gland and sent directly into the bloodstream, not to the outside of the body. ENDOCRINE GLANDS produce hormones.
Hospitalist (HOS-pih-tah-list): A physician whose primary focus is hospital medicine. This includes patient care, teaching, and research related to hospital care.
Human immunodeficiency virus (HYOO-man im-u-no-deh-FISH-en-se VI-rus): Virus that infects white blood cells (T-cell lymphocytes), causing damage to the patient's immune system. It is the cause of AIDS. Abbreviated HIV.
Humerus (HYOO-mer-us): Upper arm bone.
Hydrocele (HI-dro-seel): Swelling of the SCROTUM caused by a collection of fluid within the outermost covering of the TESTIS.
Hyperbilirubinemia (hi-per-bil-ih-roo-bin-E-me-ah): High levels of bilirubin (pigment released from hemoglobin breakdown and processed in the liver) in the bloodstream. See JAUNDICE.
Hyperglycemia (hi-per-gli-SE-me-ah): High blood sugar.
Hyperparathyroidism (hi-per-par-ah-THI-royd-ism): Higher than normal level of parathyroid hormone in the blood.
Hyperplasia (hi-per-PLA-ze-ah): Cells increase in number. The prostate gland is enlarged in benign prostatic hyperplasia (BPH).
Hyperplastic (hi-per-PLAS-tik): Pertaining to excessive growth of normal cells in an organ.
Hypersecretion (hi-per-se-KRE-shun): Abnormally high production of a substance.
Hypertension (hi-per-TEN-shun): High blood pressure. *Essential hypertension* has no known cause, but contributing factors are age, obesity, smoking, and heredity. *Secondary hypertension* is a sign of other disorders such as kidney disease.
Hyperthyroidism (hi-per-THI-royd-izm): Excessive activity of the thyroid gland.
Hypertrophy (hi-PER-tro-fe): Enlargement or overgrowth of an organ or part of the body as a result of an increase in size of individual cells.
Hypochondriac (hi-po-KON-dre-ak): Pertaining to lateral regions of the upper abdomen beneath the lower ribs. Also, the term describes a person who has chronic concern about personal health and body functions.
Hypodermic (hi-po-DER-mik): Pertaining to under or below the skin.
Hypoglycemia (hi-po-gli-SE-me-ah): Low blood sugar.
Hypophyseal (hi-po-FIZ-e-al): Pertaining to the pituitary gland.
Hypopituitarism (hi-po-pih-TOO-ih-tah-rizm): Decrease or stoppage of hormonal secretion by the pituitary gland.
Hypoplastic (hi-po-PLAS-tik): Pertaining to underdevelopment of a tissue or organ in the body.
Hyposecretion (hi-po-se-KRE-shun): Abnormally low production of a substance.

Hypotensive (hi-po-TEN-siv): Pertaining to low blood pressure or to a person with abnormally low blood pressure.
Hypothyroidism (hi-po-THI-royd-izm): Less than normal activity of the thyroid gland.
Hypoxia (hi-POX-e-ah): Deficiency of oxygen in tissues.
Hysterectomy (his-teh-REK-to-me): Excision of the uterus, either through the abdominal wall (abdominal hysterectomy) or through the vagina (vaginal hysterectomy).
Hysteroscopy (his-ter-OS-ko-pe): Visual examination of the uterus with an endoscope inserted through the vagina and uterine cervix.

I

Iatrogenic (i-ah-tro-JEN-ik): Pertaining to an adverse condition that results from a medical or surgical treatment.
Ileostomy (il-e-OS-to-me): New opening of the ILEUM to the outside of the body.
Ileum (IL-e-um): Third part of the small intestine.
Ilium (IL-e-um): Side, high portion of the hip bone (pelvis).
Incision (in-SIZH-un): Cutting into the body or into an organ.
Infarction (in-FARK-shun): Area of dead tissue (necrosis) caused by decreased blood flow to that part of the body. Also called *infarct*.
Infectious disease specialist (in-FEK-shus dih-ZEEZ SPESH-ah-list): Physician who treats disorders caused and spread by microorganisms such as bacteria.
Infiltrate (IN-fil-trat): Material that accumulates in an organ. The term infiltrate often describes solid material or fluid collection in the lungs.
Inflammatory bowel disease (in-FLAM-ah-tor-e BOW-el dih-ZEEZ): Disorder marked by inflammation of the small and large intestines with bouts of diarrhea, abdominal cramping, and fever. Inflammatory bowel diseases include CROHN DISEASE and ULCERATIVE COLITIS.
Inguinal (IN-gwih-nal): Pertaining to the groin, or the area where the legs meet the body. Inguinal lymph nodes are located in the groin.
Insulin (IN-su-lin): Hormone produced by the pancreas and released into the bloodstream. Insulin allows sugar to leave the blood and enter body cells.
Insulin pump (IN-su-lin pump): Portable, battery-powered device that delivers insulin through the abdominal wall in measured amounts.
Internal medicine (in-TER-nal MED-ih-sin): Branch of medicine specializing in the diagnosis of disorders and treatment with drugs.
Intervertebral (in-ter-VER-teh-bral): Pertaining to lying between two backbones. A disc is an intervertebral structure.
Intra-abdominal (in-trah-ab-DOM-ih-nal): Pertaining to within the abdomen.
Intracranial (in-trah-KRA-ne-al): Pertaining to within the skull.
Intrauterine (in-trah-U-ter-in): Pertaining to within the uterus.
Intravenous (in-trah-VE-nus): Pertaining to within a vein.
Intravenous pyelogram (in-trah-VE-nus PI-eh-lo-gram): X-ray record of the kidney (PYEL/O- means renal pelvis) after contrast is injected into a vein.
Intravesical (in-trah-VES-ih-kal): Pertaining to within the urinary bladder.
Iris (I-ris): Colored (pigmented) portion of the eye.
Irritable bowel syndrome (IR-ih-tah-b'l BOW-el SYN-drohm): A FUNCTIONAL DISORDER of the bowel marked by abdominal pain, discomfort, and bloating, but without evidence of detectable lesions or cause.
Ischemia (is-KE-me-ah): Deficiency of blood flow to a part of the body, caused by narrowing or obstruction of blood vessels. Ischemia may lead to necrosis (death of cells).

J

Jaundice (JAWN-dis): Orange-yellow coloration of the skin and other tissues. A symptom caused by accumulation of BILIRUBIN (pigment) in the blood.
Jejunum (jeh-JOO-num): Second part of the small intestine.
Joint (joynt): Place where two or more bones come together (articulate).

K

Kidney (KID-ne): One of two organs located behind the abdomen that produce urine by filtering wastes from the blood.

L

Laminectomy (lah-mih-NEK-to-me): Removal of a piece of backbone (lamina) to relieve pressure on nerves from a herniating disc.
Laparoscope (LAP-ah-ro-skope): Instrument to visually examine the abdomen. An endoscope is inserted through a small incision in the abdominal wall.
Laparoscopic appendectomy (lap-ah-ro-SKOP-ik ap-en-DEK-to-me): Removal of the appendix through a small incision in the abdomen and with the use of a laparoscope.
Laparoscopic cholecystectomy (lap-ah-ro-SKOP-ik ko-leh-sis-TEK-to-me): Removal of the gallbladder through a small incision in the abdomen and with the use of a laparoscopic instrument.
Laparoscopic sleeve gastrectomy (lap-ah-ro-SKOP-ik sleeve gas-TREK-to-me): Minimally invasive weight-loss procedure performed by removing about 80% of the stomach. The remaining stomach is a small, tubular sleeve (pouch) that reduces the amount of food consumed and helps decrease appetite.
Laparoscopic surgery (lap-ah-ro-SKOP-ik SUR-jer-e): Removal of organs or tissues via instruments inserted into the abdomen through small incisions. Also called MINIMALLY INVASIVE SURGERY or keyhole surgery.
Laparoscopy (lap-ah-ROS-ko-pe): Visual examination of the abdomen. Small incisions are made near the navel, and an instrument (endoscope or laparoscope) is inserted to view abdominal organs.
Laparotomy (lap-ah-ROT-o-me): Incision of the abdomen. A surgeon makes a large incision across the abdomen to examine and operate on its organs.
Large intestine (larj in-TES-tin): Part of the intestine that receives undigested material from the small intestine and transports it out of the body; the COLON.
Laryngeal (lah-rin-JE-al): Pertaining to the LARYNX (voice box).
Laryngectomy (lah-rin-JEK-to-me): Removal of the LARYNX (voice box).
Laryngitis (lah-rin-JI-tis): Inflammation of the LARYNX.
Laryngoscopy (lar-in-GOS-ko-pe): Visual examination of the interior of the voice box (LARYNX) with an endoscope.
Laryngotracheitis (lah-ring-o-tra-ke-I-tis): Inflammation of the larynx and the trachea (windpipe).
Larynx (LAR-inks): Voice box; located at the top of the trachea and containing vocal cords.
Lateral (LAT-er-al): Pertaining to the side.
LDL: See LOW-DENSITY LIPOPROTEIN.
Leiomyoma (li-o-mi-O-mah): Benign tumor derived from smooth (involuntary or visceral) muscle, most often of the uterus (leiomyoma uteri). LEIOMY/O- means smooth muscle.
Leiomyosarcoma (li-o-mi-o-sar-KO-mah): Malignant tumor of smooth (involuntary) muscle.

Lens (lenz): Transparent elastic structure behind the iris and pupil of the eye. The lens bends light rays so that they are properly focused on the RETINA at the back of the eye.
Lesion (LE-zhun): Abnormal tissue, usually damaged by disease or trauma. From the Latin *laesio*, meaning "injury."
Leukemia (loo-KE-me-ah): Increase in malignant (cancerous) white blood cells (in blood and bone marrow).
Leukocyte (LOO-ko-site): White blood cell.
Leukocytosis (loo-ko-si-TO-sis): Abnormal condition of white blood cells. This is a slight increase in numbers of normal white blood cells in response to infection.
Ligament (LIG-ah-ment): Connective tissue that joins bones to other bones.
Ligamentous (lig-ah-MEN-tus): Pertaining to a LIGAMENT.
Liposarcoma (li-po-sar-KO-mah): Malignant tumor of fatty tissue.
Lithotripsy (LITH-o-trip-se): Process of crushing a stone in the urinary tract using ultrasonic vibrations. Also called extracorporeal shock-wave lithotripsy (ESWL).
Liver (LIV-er): Organ in the right upper quadrant of the abdomen. The liver produces BILE, stores sugar, and produces blood-clotting proteins.
Lobe (lobe): Part of an organ, especially of the brain, lungs, or glands.
Low-density lipoprotein (lo DEN-sih-te li-po-PRO-teen): Combination of lipid (fat) and protein. It has a high CHOLESTEROL content and is associated with formation of plaques in arteries.
Lower gastrointestinal (GI) series (LO-er gas-tro-in-TES-tin-al SER-eez): Barium is injected into the anus and rectum, and x-rays are taken of the colon (large intestine).
Lumbar (LUM-bar): Pertaining to the loins; part of the back and sides between the chest and the hip.
Lumbar puncture (LUM-bar PUNK-cher): Removal of cerebrospinal fluid (CSF) for diagnostic analysis or occasionally as treatment to relieve increased intracranial pressure.
Lumbar region (LUM-bar RE-jun): Pertaining to the 5 backbones that lie between the thoracic (chest) and sacral (lower back) vertebrae.
Lumbar vertebra (LUM-bar VER-teh-brah): Backbone in the region between the chest and lower back.
Lung (lung): One of two paired organs in the chest through which oxygen enters and carbon dioxide leaves the body.
Lung capillaries (lung KAP-ih-layr-eez): Tiny blood vessels surrounding lung tissue and through which gases pass into and out of the bloodstream.
Lupus erythematosus: See SYSTEMIC LUPUS ERYTHEMATOSUS.
Lymph (limf): Clear fluid that is found in lymph vessels and produced from fluid surrounding cells. Lymph contains white blood cells (lymphocytes) that fight disease.
Lymphadenectomy (limf-ah-deh-NEK-to-me): Removal of LYMPH NODES.
Lymphadenopathy (lim-fad-eh-NOP-ah-the): Disease of lymph nodes (glands).
Lymphangiectasis (limf-an-je-EK-tah-sis): Dilation (-ECTASIS) of small lymph vessels; often resulting from obstruction in large lymph vessels.
Lymphatic system (lim-FAT-ik SIS-tem): Group of organs (lymph vessels, lymph nodes, spleen, thymus) composed of lymphatic tissue that produce lymphocytes to defend the body against foreign organisms.
Lymphatic vessels (lim-FAT-ik VES-elz): Tubes that carry lymph from tissues to the bloodstream (into a vein in the neck region); lymph vessels.
Lymphedema (limf-ah-DE-mah): Accumulation of fluid in tissue spaces, causing swelling. Lymphedema is caused by the obstruction of lymph nodes or vessels.
Lymph node (limf node): Stationary collection of lymph cells, found all over the body. Lymph nodes are sometimes called lymph "glands."

Lymphocyte (LIMF-o-site): White blood cell that is found within lymph and lymph nodes. T cells and B cells are types of lymphocytes.
Lymphoid (LIM-foid): Resembling or pertaining to lymphatic tissue.
Lymphoma (lim-FO-mah): Malignant tumor of lymphatic tissue. Previously called lymphosarcoma. There are several types, including Hodgkin lymphoma and non-Hodgkin lymphoma.

M

Magnetic resonance imaging (mag-NET-ik REZ-o-nans IM-aj-ing): Image of the body with magnetic and radio waves. Organs are seen in three planes: coronal (front to back), sagittal (side to side), and transverse (cross-section). Also called MRI.
Male reproductive system (male re-pro-DUK-tiv SIS-tem): Organs that produce sperm cells and male hormones.
Malignant (mah-LIG-nant): Pertaining to cancerous tumors that invade and spread to distant organs; tending to become progressively worse.
Mammary (MAM-er-e): Pertaining to the breast.
Mammogram (MAM-o-gram): X-ray record of the breast.
Mammography (mam-MOG-ra-fe): X-ray recording (imaging) of the breast.
Mammoplasty (MAM-o-plas-te): Surgical repair (reconstruction) of the breast.
Mastectomy (mas-TEK-to-me): Removal (excision) of the breast.
Mastitis (mas-TI-tis): Inflammation of the breast.
Mediastinal (me-de-ah-STI-nal): Pertaining to the MEDIASTINUM.
Mediastinoscopy (me-de-ah-sti-NOS-ko-pe): Visual examination of the mediastinum with an endoscope.
Mediastinum (me-de-ah-STI-num): Space between the lungs in the chest. The mediastinum contains the heart, large blood vessels, trachea, esophagus, thymus gland, and lymph nodes.
Medulla oblongata (meh-DUL-ah ob-lon-GAh-tah): Lower part of the brain near the spinal cord. The medulla oblongata controls breathing and the heartbeat.
Medullary (MEH-du-lar-e): Pertaining to the inner, or soft, part of an organ.
Melanocytes (meh-LA-no-sites): Pigmented cells in the lower portion of the epidermis. They produce a dark pigment called melanin.
Melanoma (meh-lah-NO-mah): Malignant tumor arising from pigmented cells (melanocytes) in the skin. A melanoma usually develops from a NEVUS (mole).
Meninges (meh-NIN-jeez): Membranes surrounding the brain and spinal cord.
Meningitis (men-in-JI-tis): Inflammation of the meninges (membranes around the brain and spinal cord).
Menorrhagia (men-or-RA-jah): Excessive bleeding from the uterus during the time of MENSTRUATION.
Menorrhea (men-o-RE-ah): Normal discharge of blood and tissue from the uterine lining during MENSTRUATION.
Menses (MEN-seez): Menstruation; menstrual period.
Menstruation (men-stroo-A-shun): Breakdown of the lining of the uterus that occurs every 4 weeks during the active reproductive period of a female.
Mesothelioma (mez-o-the-le-O-mah): Malignant tumor of the lining tissue (mesothelium) of the pleura. A mesothelioma is associated with exposure to asbestos.
Metacarpals (met-ah-KAR-palz): Bones of the hand between the wrist bones (carpals) and the finger bones (phalanges).

Metastasis (meh-TAS-tah-sis): Spread of a cancerous tumor to a distant organ or location. *Metastasis* literally means change (META-) of place (-STASIS). *Metastatic* means pertaining to a metastasis.

Metatarsals (meh-tah-TAR-salz): Foot bones.

Microscopic discectomy (mi-cro-SCOP-ic dis-KEK-to-me): Surgical removal of a herniated intervertebral disc.

Migraine (MI-grayn): Attack of headache, usually on one side of the head, caused by changes in blood vessel size and accompanied by nausea, vomiting, and sensitivity to light (photophobia). This term is from the French word *migraine,* meaning "severe head pain."

Minimally invasive surgery (MIN-ih-mah-le in-VA-siv SUR-jer-e): Removal and repair of organs and tissues with small incisions for an endoscope and instruments. Examples are laparoscopic cholecystectomy (gallbladder removal), laparoscopic appendectomy (appendix removal), laparoscopic herniorrhaphy (repair of a hernia), and laparoscopic colectomy (removal of a portion of the colon).

Mitral valve prolapse (MI-tral valv PRO-laps): Protrusion of one or both cusps of the mitral valve back into the left atrium when the ventricles contract.

Monocyte (MON-o-site): White blood cell with one large nucleus.

Mononucleosis (mon-o-nu-kle-O-sis): Acute infectious disease with excess monocytes in the blood and usually associated with extreme fatigue. Mononucleosis is caused by the Epstein-Barr virus and is transmitted by direct oral (mouth) contact.

Mouth (mowth): The opening that forms the beginning of the digestive system.

MRI: See MAGNETIC RESONANCE IMAGING.

Mucus (MU-kus): Sticky secretion from mucous membranes and glands.

Multiple myeloma (MUL-tih-pul mi-eh-LO-mah): Malignant tumor of the bone marrow.

Multiple sclerosis (MUL-tih-pul skleh-RO-sis): Chronic neurologic disease in which there are patches of demyelination (loss of myelin sheath covering on nerve cells) throughout the brain and spinal cord. Weakness, abnormal sensations, incoordination, and speech and visual disturbances are symptoms.

Muscle (MUS-el): Connective tissue that contracts to make movement possible.

Muscular (MUS-ku-lar): Pertaining to muscles.

Muscular dystrophy (MUS-ku-lar DIS-tro-fe): Group of degenerative muscle diseases that cause impairment because muscles are gradually weakened and eventually ATROPHY (shrink).

Musculoskeletal system (mus-ku-lo-SKEL-eh-tal SIS-tem): Organs that support the body and allow it to move, including the muscles, bones, joints, and connective tissues.

Myalgia (mi-AL-jah): Pain in a muscle or muscles.

Myelitis (mi-eh-LI-tis): Inflammation of the spinal cord.

Myelin sheath (MI-eh-lin sheeth): Fatty covering around part (axon) of nerve cells. The myelin sheath insulates the nerve, helping to speed the conduction of nerve impulses.

Myelodysplasia (mi-eh-lo-dis-PLA-ze-ah): Abnormal development of bone marrow; a premalignant condition leading to leukemia.

Myelogram (MI-eh-lo-gram): X-ray image of the spinal cord after contrast is injected within the membranes surrounding the spinal cord in the lumbar area of the back.

Myelography (mi-eh-LOG-rah-fe): X-ray imaging of the spinal cord after injection of contrast material.

Myeloma (mi-eh-LO-mah): Malignant tumor originating in the bone marrow (MYEL/O-). Also called MULTIPLE MYELOMA.

Myocardial (mi-o-KAR-de-al): Pertaining to the muscle of the heart.

Myocardial infarction (mi-o-KAR-de-al in-FARK-shun): Death of tissue in heart muscle; also known as a heart attack or an MI.

Myocardial ischemia (mi-o-KAR-de-al is-KE-me-ah): Decrease in the blood supply to the heart muscle.
Myoma (mi-O-mah): Tumor (benign) of muscle.
Myomectomy (mi-o-MEK-to-me): Removal of a benign muscle tumor (fibroid).
Myosarcoma (mi-o-sar-KO-mah): Tumor (malignant) of muscle. SARC- means flesh, indicating that the tumor is of connective or "fleshy" tissue origin.
Myositis (mi-o-SI-tis): Inflammation of a muscle.
Myringotomy (mir-in-GOT-o-me): Incision of the eardrum.

N

Nasal (NA-zl): Pertaining to the nose.
Nausea (NAW-se-ah): Unpleasant sensation in the upper abdomen, often leading to vomiting. The term comes from the Greek *nausia*, meaning "seasickness."
Necropsy (NEH-krop-se): Examination of a dead body, usually in veterinary science, to determine the cause of death; POSTMORTEM.
Necrosis (neh-KRO-sis): Death of cells.
Necrotic (neh-KROT-ic): Pertaining to death of cells.
Needle biopsy (NE-d'l BI-op-se): Removal of living tissue for microscopic examination by inserting a hollow needle through the skin.
Neonatal (ne-o-NA-tal): Pertaining to new birth; the first 4 weeks after birth.
Neoplasm (NE-o-plazm): Any new growth of tissue; a tumor.
Neoplastic (ne-o-PLAS-tik): Pertaining to a new growth, or NEOPLASM.
Nephrectomy (neh-FREK-to-me): Removal (excision) of a kidney.
Nephritis (neh-FRI-tis): Inflammation of kidneys.
Nephrolithiasis (neh-fro-lih-THI-ah-sis): Condition of kidney stones.
Nephrologist (neh-FROL-o-jist): Specialist in the diagnosis and treatment of kidney diseases.
Nephrology (neh-FROL-o-je): Study of the kidney and its diseases.
Nephropathy (neh-FROP-ah-the): Disease of the kidney.
Nephrosis (neh-FRO-sis): Abnormal condition of the kidney. Nephrosis is often associated with a deterioration of the kidney tubules.
Nephrostomy (neh-FROS-to-me): Opening from the kidney to the outside of the body.
Nervous system (NER-vus SIS-tem): Organs (brain, spinal cord, and nerves) that transmit electrical messages throughout the body.
Neural (NU-ral): Pertaining to nerves.
Neuralgia (nu-RAL-jah): Nerve pain.
Neuritis (nu-RI-tis): Inflammation of nerves.
Neuroglial cells (nu-ro-GLE-al selz): See GLIAL CELLS.
Neurologist (nu-ROL-o-jist): Specialist in the diagnosis and treatment of nervous disorders.
Neurology (nu-ROL-o-je): Study of the nervous system and nerve disorders.
Neuropathy (nu-ROP-ah-the): Disease of nervous tissue.
Neurosurgeon (nu-ro-SUR-jun): Physician who operates on the organs of the nervous system (brain, spinal cord, and nerves).
Neurotomy (nu-ROT-o-me): Incision of a nerve.
Nevus (NE-vus): Pigmented lesion on the skin (plural: nevi); a mole.
Nitroglycerin (ni-tro-GLIS-er-in): Drug that relaxes muscle and opens blood vessels.
Nocturia (nok-TU-re-ah): Excessive urination at night.

Nose (noz): Structure that is the organ of smell and permits air to enter and leave the body.

Nosocomial (nos-o-KO-me-al): Pertaining to or originating in a hospital. A *nosocomial infection* is acquired during hospitalization.

O

Obstetric (ob-STEH-trik): Pertaining to pregnancy, labor, and delivery of a baby.

Obstetrician (ob-steh-TRISH-an): Specialist in the delivery of a baby and care of the mother during pregnancy and labor.

Obstetrics (ob-STET-riks): Practice or branch of medicine concerned with the management of women during pregnancy, childbirth, and the period just after delivery of the infant.

Ocular (OK-u-lar): Pertaining to the eye.

Oncogenic (ong-ko-JEN-ik): Pertaining to producing (-GENIC) tumors.

Oncologist (ong-KOL-o-jist): Physician specializing in the study and treatment of cancerous tumors.

Oncology (ong-KOL-o-je): Study of tumors.

Onycholysis (on-ih-KOL-ih-sis): Separating (-LYSIS) of a nail (ONYCH/O) from its foundation (bed).

Oocyte (o-o-site): Egg cell (ovum).

Oophorectomy (o-of-o-REK-to-me *or* oo-fo-REK-to-me): Removal of an ovary or ovaries.

Oophoritis (o-of-o-RI-tis *or* oo-pho-RI-tis): Inflammation of an ovary.

Ophthalmologist (of-thal-MOL-o-jist): Specialist in the study of the eye and the treatment of eye disorders.

Ophthalmology (of-thal-MOL-o-je): Study of the eye; the diagnosis and treatment of eye disorders.

Ophthalmoscope (of-THAL-mo-scope): Instrument used to visually examine the eyes.

Optic nerve (OP-tik nerv): Nerve in the back of the eye that transmits light waves to the brain.

Optician (op-TISH-an): Nonmedical specialist trained to provide eyeglasses by filling prescriptions.

Optometrist (op-TOM-eh-trist): Nonmedical specialist trained to examine and test eyes and prescribe corrective lenses.

Oral (OR-al): Pertaining to the mouth.

Orchidectomy (or-kih-DEK-to-me): Removal (excision) of a testis (testicle).

Orchiectomy (or-ke-EK-to-me): Removal (excision) of a testicle or testicles.

Orchiopexy (or-ke-o-PEK-se): Surgical fixation of the testicle (testis) into its proper location within the scrotum. This surgery corrects CRYPTORCHISM.

Orchitis (or-KI-tis): Inflammation of a testicle.

Organ (OR-gan): Independent part of the body composed of different tissues working together to do a specific job.

Orthodontist (or-tho-DON-tist): Dentist specializing in straightening teeth.

Orthopedist (or-tho-PE-dist): Specialist in the surgical correction of musculoskeletal disorders. This physician was originally concerned with straightening (ORTH/O) bones in the legs of children (PED/O) with deformities.

Osteitis (os-te-I-tis): Inflammation of bone.

Osteoarthritis (os-te-o-ar-THRI-tis): Inflammation of bones and joints. Osteoarthritis is a disease of older people and is marked by stiffness, pain, and degeneration of joints.

MINI-DICTIONARY

Osteogenic sarcoma (os-te-o-JEN-ik sar-KO-mah): Malignant (cancerous) tumor of bone (-GENIC means produced in).
Osteoma (os-te-O-mah): Tumor (benign) of bone.
Osteomyelitis (os-te-o-mi-eh-LI-tis): Inflammation of bone and bone marrow. Osteomyelitis is caused by a bacterial infection.
Osteopenia (os-te-o-PE-ne-ah): Deficiency (-PENIA) of bone tissue.
Osteoporosis (os-te-o-po-RO-sis): Decrease in bone mass with formation of pores or spaces in normally mineralized bone tissue. This condition is more serious than osteopenia.
Osteotomy (os-te-OT-o-me): Incision of a bone.
Otalgia (o-TAL-jah): Pain in an ear.
Otitis (o-TI-tis): Inflammation of an ear.
Otolaryngologist (o-to-lah-rin-GOL-o-jist): Specialist in the treatment of diseases of the ear, nose, and throat.
Ovarian (o-VAYR-e-an): Pertaining to an ovary or ovaries.
Ovarian cancer (o-VAYR-e-an KAN-ser): Malignant condition of the ovaries.
Ovarian cyst (o-VAYR-e-an sist): Sac containing fluid or semisolid material in or on the ovary.
Ovary (O-vah-re): One of two organs in the female abdomen that produces egg cells and female hormones.
Ovum (O-vum): Egg cell (*plural:* ova [O-vah]).
Oxygen (OK-sih-jen): Colorless, odorless gas that is essential to sustaining life.

Pancreas (PAN-kre-us): Gland that produces digestive juices (exocrine function) and the hormone INSULIN (endocrine function).
Pancreatectomy (pan-kre-ah-TEK-to-me): Removal of the pancreas.
Pancreatitis (pan-kre-ah-TI-tis): Inflammation of the pancreas.
Pandemic (pan-DEM-ik): A disease that spreads throughout a large region or through the world. PAN- means all and -DEMIC means pertaining to people.
Pap smear (PAP smeer): Insertion of an instrument (spatula) into the vagina to obtain a sample of cells from the cervix (neck of the uterus).
Paralysis (pah-RAL-ih-sis): Loss or impairment of movement in a part of the body.
Paraplegia (par-ah-PLE-jah): Impairment or loss of movement in the lower part of the body, primarily the legs and in some cases bowel and bladder function.
Parathyroid glands (par-ah-THI-royd glanz): Four endocrine glands behind the thyroid gland. These glands are concerned with maintaining the proper levels of calcium in the blood and bones.
Parathyroid hormone (par-ah-THI-roid HOR-mone): Hormone secreted by the parathyroid glands to maintain a constant concentration of calcium in the blood and bones. Also called PTH.
Patella (pah-TEL-ah): Kneecap.
Pathogen (PATH-o-jen): Disease-producing organism (such as a bacterium or virus).
Pathologist (pah-THOL-o-jist): Specialist in the study of disease. A pathologist examines biopsies and performs autopsies.
Pathology (pah-THOL-o-je): Study of disease.
Pediatric (pe-de-AT-rik): Pertaining to treatment of a child.
Pediatrician (pe-de-ah-TRISH-un): Specialist in the treatment of childhood diseases.
Pediatrics (pe-de-AT-riks): Branch of medicine specializing in the treatment of children.

Pedodontist (ped-o-DON-tist): Dentist specializing in the diagnosis and treatment of children's dental problems.
Pelvic (PEL-vik): Pertaining to the bones of the hip area.
Pelvic cavity (PEL-vik KAV-ih-te): Space contained within the hip bones (front and sides) and the lower part of the backbone (sacrum and coccyx).
Pelvic inflammatory disease (PEL-vik in-FLAM-ah-to-re dih-ZEEZ): Inflammation of the pelvic region in females, usually involving the FALLOPIAN TUBES.
Pelvic ultrasonography (PEL-vik ul-trah-so-NOG-rah-fe): Recording of sound waves as they impact organs in the region of the hip.
Pelvis (PEL-vis): Lower part of the trunk of the body.
Penicillin (pen-ih-SIL-in): Substance, derived from certain molds, that can destroy bacteria; an ANTIBIOTIC.
Penis (PE-nis): External male organ containing the urethra, through which both urine and semen (sperm cells and fluid) leave the body.
Peptic ulcer (PEP-tik UL-ser): Open sore (lesion) that develops in the lining of the stomach (gastric ulcer) or the first part of the small intestine (duodenal ulcer).
Percutaneous (per-ku-TA-ne-us): Pertaining to through the skin.
Percutaneous transhepatic cholangiography (per-ku-TA-ne-us trans-heh-PAT-ik kol-an-je-OG-rah-fe): Bile vessels are imaged after injection of contrast material through the skin into the liver.
Perianal (peh-re-A-nal): Pertaining to surrounding the ANUS.
Pericardium (peh-rih-KAR-de-um): Membrane surrounding the heart.
Periodontist (peh-re-o-DON-tist): Dentist specializing in the treatment of gum disease (surrounding a tooth).
Periosteum (peh-re-OS-te-um): Membrane that surrounds bone.
Peritoneal (peh-rih-to-NE-al): Pertaining to the PERITONEUM.
Peritoneal dialysis (peh-rih-to-NE-al di-AL-ih-sis): Process of removing wastes from the blood by introducing a special fluid into the abdomen (peritoneal cavity). The wastes pass into the fluid from the bloodstream, and then the fluid is drained from the body.
Peritoneal fluid (peh-rih-to-NE-al FLOO-id): Fluid produced in the abdominal cavity.
Peritoneoscopy (peh-rih-to-ne-OS-ko-pe): Visual examination of the peritoneal cavity with an endoscope. See LAPAROSCOPY.
Peritoneum (peh-rih-to-NE-um): Membrane that surrounds the abdomen and holds the abdominal organs in place.
Peritonitis (peh-rih-to-NI-tis): Inflammation of the peritoneum.
Phalanges (fah-LAN-jeez): Finger and toe bones.
Pharyngeal (fah-rin-JE-al): Pertaining to the pharynx (throat).
Pharyngitis (fah-rin-JI-tis): Inflammation of the pharynx (throat).
Pharynx (FAR-inks): Organ behind the mouth that receives swallowed food and delivers it into the esophagus. The pharynx (throat) also receives air from the nose and passes it to the trachea (windpipe).
Phenothiazine (fe-no-THI-ah-zeen): Substance whose derivatives are used as tranquilizers and antipsychotic agents to treat mental illness.
Phlebitis (fleh-BI-tis): Inflammation of a vein.
Phlebography (fleh-BOG-rah-fe): X-ray examination of veins after injection of contrast material.
Phlebotomy (fleh-BOT-o-me): Incision of a vein.

Photoselective vaporization of the prostate (fo-to-se-LEK-tiv va-por-ih-ZA-shun of the PROS-tate): Use of a GreenLight® laser to vaporize and remove prostatic tissue to treat benign prostatic hyperplasia.

Phrenic (FREH-nik): Pertaining to the DIAPHRAGM.

Physical medicine and rehabilitation (FIZ-ih-kal MED-ih-sin and re-hah-bil-ih-TA-shun): Field of medicine that specializes in restoring the function of the body after illness.

Pilosebaceous (pi-lo-seh-BA-shus): Pertaining to hair and its associated sebaceous gland.

Pineal gland (pi-NE-al gland): Small endocrine gland within the brain that secretes the hormone melatonin, whose exact function is unclear. In lower animals, the pineal gland is a receptor for light.

Pituitary gland (pih-TOO-ih-tar-e gland): Organ at the base of the brain that secretes hormones. These hormones enter the blood to regulate other organs and other endocrine glands.

Platelet (PLAYT-let): Clotting cell; a thrombocyte.

Pleura (PLOO-rah): Double membrane that surrounds the lungs. *Pleural* means pertaining to the pleura.

Pleural cavity (PLOO-ral KAV-ih-te): Space between each pleura surrounding the lung.

Pleural effusion (PLOO-ral e-FU-zhun): Collection of fluid between the double membrane surrounding the lungs.

Pleurisy (PLOO-rih-se): Inflammation of the PLEURA.

Pleuritis (ploo-RI-tis): Inflammation of the PLEURA.

Pneumoconiosis (noo-mo-ko-ne-O-sis): Group of lung diseases resulting from inhalation of particles of dust such as coal, with permanent deposition of such particles in the lung.

Pneumonectomy (noo-mo-NEK-to-me): Removal of a lung.

Pneumonia (noo-MO-ne-ah): Abnormal condition of the lungs marked by inflammation and collection of material within the air sacs of the lungs.

Pneumonitis (noo-mo-NI-tis): Inflammation of a lung or lungs.

Pneumothorax (noo-mo-THOR-aks): Abnormal accumulation of air in the space between the pleura.

Polycythemia (pol-e-si-THE-me-ah): Increase in red blood cells. One form is polycythemia vera, in which the bone marrow produces an excess of erythrocytes and hemoglobin level is elevated.

Polydipsia (pol-e-DIP-se-ah): Excessive thirst.

Polyneuropathy (pol-e-nu-ROP-ah-the): Disease of many nerves.

Polyp (POL-ip): A growth or mass (benign) protruding from a mucous membrane.

Polyuria (pol-e-UR-e-ah): Excessive urination.

Pons (ponz): Part of the brain containing nerve pathways connecting upper and lower areas.

Posterior (pos-TEER-e-or): Located in the back portion of a structure or of the body.

Posteroanterior (pos-ter-o-an-TEER-e-or): Pertaining to direction from back to front.

Postmortem (post-MOR-tem): After death.

Postpartum (post-PAR-tum): After birth.

Precancerous (pre-KAN-ser-us): Pertaining to a condition that may come before a cancer; a condition that tends to become malignant.

Prenatal (pre-NA-tal): Pertaining to before birth.

Proctologist (prok-TOL-o-jist): Physician who specializes in the study of the anus and rectum.

Proctoscopy (prok-TOS-ko-pe): Inspection of the anus and rectum with a proctoscope (ENDOSCOPE). Proctoscopy is often performed before rectal surgery.

Proctosigmoidoscopy (prok-to-sig-moyd-OS-ko-pe): Visual examination of the anus, rectum, and sigmoid colon with an endoscope.
Progesterone (pro-JES-teh-rone): Hormone secreted by the ovaries to prepare to maintain the uterine lining during pregnancy.
Prognosis (prog-NO-sis): Prediction that forecasts the outcome of treatment. Prognosis literally means before (PRO-) knowledge (-GNOSIS).
Prolapse (pro-LAPS): Falling down or drooping of a part of the body. Prolapse literally means sliding (-LAPSE) forward (PRO-).
Prostate gland (PROS-tayt gland): Male gland that surrounds the base of the urinary bladder. It produces fluid (semen) that leaves the body with sperm cells.
Prostatectomy (pros-tah-TEK-to-me): Removal of the prostate gland.
Prostatic (pros-TAT-ik): Pertaining to the prostate gland.
Prostatic carcinoma (pros-TAT-ik kar-si-NO-mah): Malignant tumor arising from the PROSTATE GLAND. Also called *prostate cancer*.
Prostatic hyperplasia (pros-TAT-ik hi-per-PLA-zhah): Abnormal increase in growth (benign) of the prostate gland.
Prosthesis (pros-THE-sis): Artificial substitute for a missing part of the body. Prosthesis literally means to place (-THESIS) before (PROS-).
Prosthodontist (pros-tho-DON-tist): Dentist specializing in artificial appliances to replace missing teeth.
Proteinuria (pro-teen-U-re-ah): Abnormal condition of protein in the urine (albuminuria).
Psychiatrist (si-KI-ah-trist): Specialist in the treatment of the mind and mental disorders.
Psychiatry (si-KI-ah-tre): Treatment (IATR/O-) of disorders of the mind (PSYCH/O).
Psychology (si-KOL-o-je): Study of the mind, especially in relation to human behavior.
Psychosis (si-KO-sis): Abnormal condition of the mind; a serious mental disorder that involves loss of normal perception of reality (*plural:* psychoses [si-KO-seez]).
Pulmonary (PUL-mo-nair-e): Pertaining to the lungs.
Pulmonary artery (PUL-mo-nair-e AR-ter-e): Artery carrying blood from the right ventricle to the lungs.
Pulmonary circulation (PUL-mo-nair-e ser-ku-LA-shun): Passage of blood from the heart to the lungs and back to the heart.
Pulmonary edema (PUL-mo-nair-e eh-DE-mah): Abnormal collection of fluid in the lung (within the air sacs of the lung). Fluid backs up into lung tissue commonly from congestive heart failure as the heart weakens and is unable to pump blood effectively.
Pulmonary embolism (PUL-mo-nair-e EM-bo-lizm): Blockage of blood vessels in the lung by foreign matter (clot, tumor, fat, or air). The EMBOLUS frequently arises from the deep veins of the leg.
Pulmonary specialist (PUL-mo-nair-e SPESH-ah-list): Physician trained to treat lung disorders.
Pupil (PU-pil): Black center of the eye through which light enters.
Pyelitis (pi-eh-LI-tis): Inflammation of the renal pelvis (central section of the kidney).
Pyelogram (PI-eh-lo-gram): X-ray record of the renal pelvis after injection of contrast.

Q

Quadriplegia (kwad-rih-PLE-jah): Paralysis of all four extremities and usually the trunk of the body caused by injury to the spinal cord in the cervical region of the spine.

R

Radiation oncologist (ra-de-A-shun ong-KOL-o-jist): Physician trained in the treatment of disease (cancer) with high-energy x-rays or particles.

Radiation therapy (ra-de-A-shun THER-a-pe): Treatment of disease (cancer) with high-energy x-rays or particles (photons and protons). Also called RADIOTHERAPY.

Radioisotope (ra-de-o-I-so-tope): See RADIONUCLIDE.

Radiologist (ra-de-OL-o-jist): Physician trained in the use of x-rays (such as computed tomography and also including ultrasound) to diagnose illness.

Radiology (ra-de-OL-o-je): Science of using x-rays in the diagnosis of disease.

Radionuclide (ra-de-o-NOO-klide): A chemical substance that emits radioactivity; radioisotope. Radionuclides are used in nuclear medicine to image parts of the body.

Radiotherapist (ra-de-o-THER-ah-pist): Physician trained to treat disease (cancer) with high-energy x-rays or particles. See RADIATION ONCOLOGIST.

Radiotherapy (ra-de-o-THER-ah-pe): Treatment of disease (cancer) with high-energy x-rays or particles such as photons and protons. Also called RADIATION THERAPY.

Radius (RA-de-us): One of two lower arm bones. The radius is located on the thumb side of the hand.

Rectal resection (REK-tal re-SEK-shun): Excision (resection) of the RECTUM.

Rectocele (REK-to-seel): Hernia (protrusion) of the rectum into the vagina.

Rectum (REK-tum): End of the colon. The rectum delivers wastes (feces) to the anus for elimination.

Relapse (RE-laps): Return of disease after its apparent termination.

Remission (re-MISH-un): Lessening or absence of signs and symptoms of a disease.

Renal (RE-nal): Pertaining to the kidney.

Renal calculus (RE-nal KAL-ku-lus): Kidney stone.

Renal failure (RE-nal FAIL-ur): Condition in which the kidneys no longer function.

Renal pelvis (RE-nal PEL-vis): Central section of the kidney, where urine collects.

Renal transplantation (RE-nal tranz-plan-TA-shun): A donor kidney is transferred to a recipient whose kidneys have failed.

Reproductive (re-pro-DUK-tiv): Pertaining to the process by which living things produce offspring.

Research (RE-surch): Laboratory investigation of a medical problem.

Resection (re-SEK-shun): Removal (excision) of an organ or a structure.

Residency training (RES-i-den-se TRAY-ning): Period of hospital work involving the care of patients after the completion of four years of medical school.

Respiratory system (RES-pir-ah-tor-e SIS-tem): Organs that control breathing, allowing air to enter and leave the body.

Retina (RET-ih-nah): Layer of sensitive cells at the back of the eye. Light is focused on the retina and then is transmitted to the optic nerve, which leads to the brain.

Retinopathy (reh-tih-NOP-ah-the): Disease of the RETINA.

Retrogastric (reh-tro-GAS-trik): Pertaining to behind the stomach.

Retroperitoneal (reh-tro-peh-rih-to-NE-al): Pertaining to behind the PERITONEUM.

Rhabdomyolysis (rab-do-mi-OL-o-sis): Breakdown of damaged skeletal muscle

Rhabdomyosarcoma (rab-do-mi-o-sar-KO-mah): Malignant tumor of muscle cells (skeletal, voluntary muscle) that occurs most frequently in the head and neck, extremities, body wall, and area behind the abdomen.

Rheumatoid arthritis (ROO-mah-toyd arth-RI-tis): Chronic inflammatory disease of the joints and connective tissue that leads to deformed joints.

Rheumatologist (roo-mah-TOL-o-jist): Specialist in the treatment of diseases of connective tissues, especially the joints. RHEUMAT/O- comes from the Greek *rheuma*, meaning "that which flows, as a stream or a river." Inflammatory disorders of joints are often marked by a collection of fluid in joint spaces.
Rheumatology (roo-mah-TOL-o-je): Branch of medicine dealing with inflammation, degeneration, or chemical changes in connective tissues, such as joints and muscles. Pain, stiffness, or limitation of motion are often characteristics of rheumatologic disorders.
Rhinitis (ri-NI-tis): Inflammation of the nose.
Rhinoplasty (RI-no-plas-te): Surgical repair of the nose.
Rhinorrhea (ri-no-RE-ah): Discharge from the nose.
Rhinotomy (ri-NOT-o-me): Incision of the nose.
Rib (rib): One of twelve paired bones surrounding the chest. Seven ribs (true ribs) attach directly to the breastbone, three (false ribs) attach to the seventh rib, and two (floating ribs) are not attached at all.

S

Sacral (SA-kral): Pertaining to the SACRUM.
Sacral region (SA-kral RE-jun): Five fused bones in the lower back, below the lumbar bones and wedged between two parts of the hip (ilium).
Sacrum (SA-krum): Triangular bone in the lower back, below the lumbar bones and formed by five fused bones.
Sagittal plane (SAJ-ih-tal playn): Imaginary plane that divides an organ or the body into right and left portions. The *midsagittal* plane divides a structure equally into right and left halves.
Sagittal section (SAJ-ih-tal SEK-shun): Cut (section) through the body, dividing it into a right and a left portion.
Salpingectomy (sal-pin-JEK-to-me): Removal of a fallopian (uterine) tube.
Salpingitis (sal-pin-JI-tis): Inflammation of a fallopian (uterine) tube.
Sarcoidosis (sahr-koy-DO-sis): Chronic inflammatory disorder of cells in connective tissue, spleen, liver, bone marrow, lungs, and lymph nodes. Small collections of cells (granulomas) form in affected organs and tissues. The cause is unknown but may involve malfunction of the immune system.
Sarcoma (sar-KO-mah): Cancerous (malignant) tumor of connective tissue, such as bone, muscle, fat, or cartilage. The root SARC means flesh.
Scapula (SKAP-u-lah): Shoulder bone.
Sclera (SKLE-rah): White, outer coat of the eyeball.
Scotoma (sko-TO-mah): Defect in vision in a defined area (blind spot).
Scrotal (SKRO-tal): Pertaining to the scrotum.
Scrotum (SKRO-tum): Sac on the outside of the body that contains the testes.
Sebaceous gland (seh-BA-shus gland): Oil-producing (sebum-producing) gland in the skin.
Section (SEK-shun): Act of cutting; a segment or subdivision of an organ.
Seizure (SE-zhur): Convulsion (involuntary contraction of muscles) or attack of epilepsy. A seizure can also indicate a sudden attack or recurrence of a disease.
Sella turcica (SEL-ah TUR-sih-kah): Cup-like depression at the base of the skull that holds the pituitary gland.
Semen (SE-men): Fluid composed of sperm cells and secretions from the prostate gland and other male exocrine glands.
Seminoma (sem-ih-NO-mah): Malignant tumor of the testis.

Sense organs (sens OR-ganz): Parts of the body that receive messages from the environment and relay them to the brain so that we see, hear, and feel sensations. Examples of sense organs are the eye, the ear, and the skin.
Septic (SEP-tik): Pertaining to infection.
Septicemia (sep-tih-SE-me-ah): Infection in the blood. Septicemia is commonly called blood poisoning and is associated with the presence of bacteria or their toxins in the blood.
Sexually transmitted infection (SEK-shoo-ah-le trans-MIT-ed in-FEK-shun): Contagious disease acquired through sexual intercourse or genital contact.
Shock (shok): Group of symptoms (pale skin, rapid pulse, shallow breathing) that indicate poor oxygen supply to tissue and insufficient return of blood to the heart.
Sigmoid colon (SIG-moyd KO-len): S-shaped lower portion of the colon.
Sigmoidoscopy (sig-moyd-OS-ko-pe): Visual examination of the sigmoid colon with an endoscope inserted through the anus and rectum.
Sinus (SI-nus): Cavity or space, such as in a bone. Also refers to the sinoatrial node or pacemaker of the heart.
Skin (skin): Outer covering that protects the body.
Skull (skul): Bone that surrounds the brain and other organs in the head.
Sleep apnea (SLEEP AP-nee-ah): See APNEA.
Small intestine (smal in-TES-tin): Organ that receives food from the stomach. The small intestine is divided into three sections: duodenum, jejunum, and ileum.
Sonogram (SON-o-gram): Record of sound waves after they bounce off organs in the body; an ULTRASOUND or echogram.
Spasm (SPAZ-um): Involuntary, sudden muscle contraction.
Spermatozoon (sper-mah-to-ZO-on): Sperm cell (*plural:* spermatozoa [sper-mah-to-ZO-ah]).
Spinal (SPI-nal): Pertaining to the spine (backbone).
Spinal cavity (SPI-nal KAV-ih-te): Space in the back that contains the spinal cord and is surrounded by the backbones.
Spinal column (SPI-nal KOL-um): Backbones; vertebrae.
Spinal cord (SPI-nal kord): Bundle of nerves that extends from the brain down the back. Spinal nerves carry electrical messages to and from the spinal cord.
Spinal nerves (SPI-nal nervz): Nerves that transmit messages to and from the spinal cord.
Spinal tap (SPI-nal TAP): See LUMBAR PUNCTURE.
Spirometer (spi-ROM-eh-ter): Instrument for testing lung function by measuring the volume of inspired and expired air.
Spleen (spleen): Organ in the upper left part (quadrant) of the abdomen that produces white blood cells (LYMPHOCYTES) and disposes of old, dying red blood cells. The spleen, as part of the immune system, helps fight foreign organisms.
Splenectomy (splen-EK-to-me): Removal of the spleen.
Splenomegaly (splen-o-MEG-ah-le): Enlargement of the spleen.
Spondylitis (spon-dih-LI-tis): Chronic, serious inflammatory disorder of backbones involving erosion and collapse of vertebrae. See ANKYLOSING SPONDYLITIS.
Spondylosis (spon-dih-LO-sis): Abnormal condition of a vertebra or vertebrae.
Sputum (SPU-tum): Material expelled from the lungs and expelled through the mouth.
Staging of tumors (STA-jing of TOO-murz): A system that describes the severity of a patient's cancer based on the extent of the original primary tumor and whether it has spread in the body.
Stent (stent): Tube inserted into an artery, blood vessel, or duct to keep it open.
Sternum (STER-num): Breastbone.

Stereotactic radiosurgery (steh-re-o-TAC-tic rad-e-o-SUR-je-re): This is a non-surgical type of radiation therapy used to treat abnormalities and small tumors of the brain. Also called Cyberknife©, this treatment can deliver precisely targeted radiation in fewer high-dose treatments than traditional therapy.
Stomach (STUM-uk): Organ that receives food from the esophagus and sends it to the small intestine. Enzymes in the stomach break down food particles during digestion.
Stomatitis (sto-mah-TI-tis): Inflammation of the mouth.
Stool culture (stool KUL-chur): Feces (stools) are placed in a growth medium (culture medium), which is later examined microscopically for evidence of microorganisms (such as bacteria).
Stool guaiac (stool GWI-ak) [test]: Examination of a small sample of stool for hidden traces of blood; HEMOCCULT TEST.
Stroke (strok): Condition resulting from trauma to or blockage of blood vessels within the brain; less blood arrives to nerve cells in the brain.
Stye (sti): Infection of a gland near the edge the eyelid, often caused by bacteria (staphylococci). Also spelled *sty*.
Subcostal (sub-KOS-tal): Pertaining to below the ribs.
Subcutaneous (sub-ku-TA-ne-us): Pertaining to under the skin.
Subcutaneous tissue (sub-ku-TA-ne-us TIS-u): Lower layer of the skin composed of fatty tissue.
Subdural hematoma (sub-DUR-al he-mah-TO-mah): Collection of blood under the dura mater (outermost layer of the membranes surrounding the brain).
Subgastric (sub-GAS-trik): Pertaining to below the stomach.
Subhepatic (sub-heh-PAT-ik): Pertaining to under the liver.
Subscapular (sub-SKAP-u-lar): Pertaining to under the shoulder bone.
Subtotal (sub-TO-tal): Less than total; often just under the total amount.
Subungual (sub-UN-gwal): Pertaining to under (SUB-) a nail (UNGU/O).
Suprarenal glands (soo-prah-RE-nal glanz): Two endocrine glands, each located above a kidney. See ADRENAL GLANDS.
Surgery (SUR-jer-e): Branch of medicine that treats disease by manual (hand) or operative methods.
Sweat gland (swet gland): Organ in the skin that produces a watery substance containing salts.
Symptom (SIMP-tum): An indication of disease observed by the patient such as abdominal pain, fatigue, or loss of appetite. The medical term asymptomatic means without symptoms.
Syncope (SING-koh-pe): Fainting; sudden loss of consciousness.
Syndrome (SYN-drohm): Set of symptoms and signs that occur together to indicate a disease condition.
Syphilis (SIF-ih-lis): Sexually transmitted infection caused by spirochete (type of bacterium).
System (SIS-tem): Group of organs working together to do a job in the body. For example, the digestive system includes the mouth, throat, stomach, and intestines, all of which help to bring food into the body, break it down, and deliver it to the bloodstream.
Systemic circulation (sis-TEM-ik ser-ku-LA-shun): Passage of blood from the heart to the tissues of the body and back to the heart.
Systemic lupus erythematosus (sis-TEM-ik LOO-pus er-ih-the-mah-TO-sus): Chronic inflammatory disease affecting many systems of the body (joints, skin, kidneys, and nerves). A red (erythematous) rash over the nose and cheeks is characteristic.

T

Tachycardia (tak-eh-KAR-de-ah): Condition of a fast, rapid heartbeat.
Tachypnea (tak-ip-NE-ah): Condition of rapid breathing.
Tendinitis (ten-dih-NI-tis): Inflammation of a tendon.
Tendon (TEN-don): Connective tissue that joins muscles to bones.
Tenorrhaphy (ten-OR-ah-fe): Suture of a tendon.
Testicle (TES-tih-kl): See TESTIS.
Testicular carcinoma (tes-TIK-u-lar kar-sih-NO-mah): Malignant tumor originating in a testis. An example is a SEMINOMA.
Testis (TES-tis): One of two paired male organs in the scrotal sac. The testes (*plural*) produce sperm cells and male hormone (testosterone). Also called a testicle.
Testosterone (tes-TOS-teh-rone): A hormone that produces male secondary sex characteristics; an ANDROGEN.
Thoracentesis (tho-rah-sen-TE-sis): Puncture of the chest to remove fluid; thoracocentesis.
Thoracic (tho-RAS-ik): Pertaining to the chest.
Thoracic cavity (tho-RAS-ik KAV-ih-te): Space above the abdomen that contains the heart, lungs, and other organs; the chest cavity.
Thoracic region (tho-RAS-ik RE-jun): Twelve backbones attached to the ribs and located in the region of the chest, between the neck and the waist.
Thoracic surgeon (tho-RAS-ik SUR-jun): Physician who operates on organs in the chest.
Thoracic vertebra (tho-RAS-ik VER-teh-brah): A backbone in the region of the chest.
Thoracotomy (tho-rah-KOT-o-me): Incision of the chest.
Throat (throt): See PHARYNX.
Thrombocyte (THROM-bo-site): Clotting cell; a PLATELET.
Thrombolytic therapy (throm-bo-LIT-ik THER-ah-pe): Treatment with drugs such as streptokinase and tPA (tissue plasminogen activator) to dissolve clots that may cause a heart attack.
Thrombophlebitis (throm-bo-fleh-BI-tis): Inflammation of a vein accompanied by formation of a clot.
Thrombosis (throm-BO-sis): Abnormal condition of clot formation.
Thrombus (THROM-bus): Blood clot.
Thymoma (thi-MO-mah): Tumor (malignant) of the thymus gland.
Thymus gland (THI-mus gland): Lymphoid organ of the immune system. It is located in the chest between the lungs. It stimulates the production of LYMPHOCYTES (white blood cells).
Thyroadenitis (thi-ro-ad-eh-NI-tis): Inflammation of the thyroid gland.
Thyroidectomy (thi-roy-DEK-to-me): Removal of the thyroid gland.
Thyroid gland (THI-royd gland): Endocrine gland in the neck that produces hormones that act on cells all over the body. The hormones increase the activity of cells by stimulating metabolism and the release of energy.
Thyroid-stimulating hormone (THI-royd STIM-u-la-ting HOR-mone): Hormone secreted by the pituitary gland to stimulate the thyroid gland to produce its hormones, such as thyroxine. Also called TSH.
Thyroxine (thi-ROK-sin): Hormone secreted by the thyroid gland. Also known as T_4.
Tibia (TIB-e-ah): Larger of the two lower leg bones; the shin bone.
Tinnitus (TIN-ih-tus): Noise in the ears, such as ringing, roaring, or buzzing.
Tissue (TISH-u): Groups of similar cells that work together to do a job in the body. Examples are muscle tissue, nerve tissue, and epithelial (skin) tissue.

Tissue capillaries (TISH-u KAP-ih-lar-eez): Tiny blood vessels that lie near cells and through whose walls gases, food, and waste materials pass.
Tomography (to-MOG-rah-fe): Series of x-ray images that show an organ in depth by producing images of single tissue planes.
Tomosynthesis (to-mo-SIN-theh-sis): Mammographic technique that shows clearer and more detailed images.
Tonsillectomy (ton-sih-LEK-to-me): Removal (excision) of a tonsil or TONSILS.
Tonsillitis (ton-sih-LI-tis): Inflammation of the TONSILS.
Tonsils (TON-silz): Lymphatic tissue in the back of the mouth near the throat.
Trachea (TRA-ke-ah): Tube that carries air from the throat to the BRONCHIAL TUBES; the windpipe.
Tracheitis (tra-ke-I-tis): Inflammation of the trachea.
Tracheostomy (tra-ke-OS-to-me): Opening of the trachea to the outside of the body.
Tracheotomy (tra-ke-OT-o-me): Incision of the trachea.
Transabdominal (tranz-ab-DOM-ih-nal): Pertaining to across the abdomen.
Transdermal (tranz-DER-mal): Pertaining to through the skin.
Transgastric (tranz-GAS-trik): Pertaining to across (through) the stomach.
Transhepatic (tranz-heh-PAT-ik): Pertaining to across or through the liver.
Transurethral (tranz-u-RE-thral): Pertaining to across (through) the urethra. TURP is transurethral resection of the prostate gland by surgery through the urethra.
Transvaginal ultrasound (tranz-VAJ-in-al UL-trah-sownd): A sound probe is placed in the vagina, and ultrasound images are made of the pelvic organs (uterus and ovaries).
Transverse plane (tranz-VERS playn): Imaginary plane that divides an organ or the body into an upper and a lower portion; a cross-sectional view.
Trichotillomania (trik-o-til-o-MA-ne-ah): Obsessive-compulsive disorder marked by the urge to pull out (TILL/O) one's hair.
Tricuspid valve (tri-KUS-pid valv): Fold of tissue between the upper and lower chambers on the right side of the heart. It has three cusps or points and prevents backflow of blood into the right ATRIUM when the heart is pumping blood.
Triglyceride (tri-GLIS-eh-ride): Fat consisting of three molecules of fatty acid and glycerol. It makes up most animal and vegetable fats and is the major lipid (fat) in blood.
Tubal ligation (TOO-bul li-GA-shun): Fallopian tubes are tied off (ligated) with sutures.
Tuberculosis (too-ber-ku-LO-sis): Infectious, inflammatory disease that commonly affects the lungs, although it can occur in any part of the body. It is caused by the tubercle bacillus (type of bacterium).
Tympanic membrane (tim-PAN-ik MEM-brayn): See EARDRUM.
Tympanoplasty (tim-pan-o-PLAS-te): Surgical repair of the eardrum.

U

Ulcer (UL-ser): Sore or defect in the surface of an organ. Ulcers (hollowed-out spaces) are produced by destruction of tissue.
Ulcerative colitis (UL-seh-rah-tiv ko-LI-tis): Recurrent inflammatory disorder marked by ulcers in the large bowel. Along with Crohn disease, ulcerative colitis is an INFLAMMATORY BOWEL DISEASE.
Ulna (UL-nah): One of two lower arm bones. The ulna is located on the little finger side of the hand.
Ultrasonography (ul-trah-so-NOG-rah-fe): Recording of internal sound waves as they impact body structures.

Ultrasound (UL-tra-sownd): Sound waves with greater frequency than can be heard by the human ear. This energy is used to detect abnormalities by beaming the waves into the body and recording echoes that reflect off tissues.

Unilateral (u-nih-LAT-er-al): Pertaining to one side.

Upper gastrointestinal (GI) series (UP-er gas-tro-in-TES-tin-al SEER-eez): Barium is swallowed, and x-ray images are taken of the esophagus, stomach, and small intestine.

Urea (u-RE-ah): Chief nitrogen-containing waste that the kidney removes from the blood and eliminates from the body in urine.

Uremia (u-RE-me-ah): Abnormal condition of excessive amounts of urea (nitrogenous waste) in the bloodstream.

Ureter (YOOR-eh-ter *or* u-RE-ter): One of two tubes that lead from the kidney to the urinary bladder.

Ureterectomy (u-re-ter-EK-to-me): Removal (excision) of a ureter.

Urethra (u-RE-thrah): Tube that carries urine from the urinary bladder to the outside of the body. In males, the urethra, which is within the penis, also carries sperm from the VAS DEFERENS to the outside of the body when sperm are discharged (ejaculation).

Urethral stricture (u-RE-thral STRIK-shur): Narrowing of the urethra.

Urethritis (u-re-THRI-tis): Inflammation of the urethra.

Uric acid (U-rik acid): Nitrogen-containing waste material from breakdown of nucleic acids (DNA and RNA). It is normally filtered from the blood by the kidneys and passes out of the body in urine. High levels of uric acid in the blood are an indication of GOUT, a type of arthritis.

Urinalysis (u-rih-NAL-ih-sis): Examination of urine to determine its contents.

Urinary bladder (UR-in-air-e BLAD-er): Muscular sac that holds urine and then releases it to leave the body through the urethra.

Urinary catheterization (UR-in-air-e kath-eh-ter-ih-ZA-shun): Catheter (tube) is passed through the urethra into the urinary bladder for short- or long-term drainage of urine.

Urinary retention (UR-in-air-e re-TEN-shun): Condition in which urine is unable to leave the urinary bladder.

Urinary system (UR-in-air-e SIS-tem): Organs that produce and send urine out of the body. These organs are the kidneys, ureters, bladder, and urethra.

Urinary tract (UR-in-air-e trakt): Tubes and organs that carry urine from the kidney to the outside of the body.

Urine (UR-in): Fluid that is produced by the kidneys, passed through the ureters, stored in the bladder, and released from the body through the urethra.

Urologist (u-ROL-o-jist): Specialist in operating on the urinary tract in males and females and on the reproductive tract in males.

Urology (u-ROL-o-je): Study of the urinary tract (surgical specialty).

Uterine (U-ter-in): Pertaining to the uterus.

Uterine artery embolization (U-ter-in AR-ter-e em-bo-lih-ZA-shun): Blockage of blood flow in the uterine artery to slow the growth of uterine fibroids.

Uterine tubes (U-ter-in toobz): See FALLOPIAN TUBES.

Uterus (U-ter-us): Muscular organ in a female that holds and provides nourishment for the developing fetus; the WOMB.

Vagina (vah-JI-nah): Muscular passageway from the uterus to the outside of the body.

Vaginitis (vah-jih-NI-tis): Inflammation of the vagina.

Valve (valv): Natural structure or artificial device that prevents backward flow of fluid (such as blood).

Varicocele (VAR-ih-ko-seel): Abnormal enlargement of veins in the SCROTUM. This condition produces a swelling that feels like a "bag of worms."

Varix (VAR-iks): An enlarged, swollen, tortuous vein (*plural:* varices [VAH-rih-seez]).

Vas deferens (vas DEF-er-enz): One of two tubes that carry sperm from the testes to the urethra for ejaculation.

Vascular (VAS-ku-lar): Pertaining to blood vessels.

Vasculitis (vas-ku-LI-tis): Inflammation of blood vessels.

Vasectomy (vas-EK-to-me): Removal of a portion of the vas deferens so that sperm cells are prevented from becoming part of SEMEN.

Vasoconstrictor (vas-o-kon-STRIK-tor): Drug that narrows blood vessels, especially small arteries.

Vasodilator (vas-o-DI-la-tor): Agent that widens blood vessels.

Vein (vayn): Blood vessel that carries blood back to the heart from tissues of the body.

Ventricle (VEN-trih-kl): One of the two lower chambers of the heart. The right ventricle receives blood from the right atrium (upper chamber) and sends it to the lungs. The left ventricle receives blood from the left atrium and sends it to the body through the aorta.

Ventricular arrhythmia (ven-TRIK-u-lar ah-RITH-me-ah): Abnormal heart rhythm originating in the lower chambers of the heart.

Venule (VEN-ul): Small vein.

Venulitis (ven-u-LI-tis): Inflammation of a small vein.

Vertebra (VER-teh-brah): Backbone.

Vertebrae (VER-teh-bray): Backbones.

Vertebral (VER-teh-bral): Pertaining to a backbone.

Vertebroplasty (ver-teh-bro-PLAS-te): Surgical repair of backbone fractures by injecting cement into vertebrae to strengthen them and relieve pain.

Vesical (VES-ih-kal): Pertaining to the urinary bladder (VESIC/O).

Vitreous humor (VIT-re-us HU-mor): Transparent clear gel that fills the space between the lens and the retina of the eye.

Virus (VI-rus): Small infectious agent that can reproduce itself only when it is inside another living cell (host).

Visceral (VIS-er-al): Pertaining to internal organs.

Womb (woom): See UTERUS.

Wound (woond): Any physical injury involving a break in the skin (chest wound, gunshot wound, puncture wound, and so on).

GLOSSARY 2

Word Parts

Section I: Medical Terminology → English 400

Section II: English → Medical Terminology 408

Section I of this glossary is a list of **medical terminology word parts** and their **English meanings. Section II** is the reverse of that list, giving **English meanings** and their corresponding **medical terminology word parts.** Section II begins on page 408.

SECTION I: MEDICAL TERMINOLOGY → ENGLISH

Word Part	Meaning
a-, an-	no, not
ab-	away from
abdomin/o	abdomen; *see also* lapar/o
-ac	pertaining to
ad-	toward
aden/o	gland
adenoid/o	adenoids
adren/o	adrenal gland
-al	pertaining to
-algia	condition of pain; *see also* -dynia
alveol/o	alveolus (air sac within the lung)
amni/o	amnion (sac that surrounds the embryo)
-an	pertaining to
ana-	up, apart
an/o	anus
angi/o	vessel (blood)
ante-	before, forward
anter/o	front
anti-	against
aort/o	aorta
append/o, appendic/o	appendix
-ar	pertaining to
arteri/o	artery
arteriol/o	small artery
arthr/o	joint
-ary	pertaining to
ather/o	fatty plaque
-ation	process, condition
aur/o	ear; *see also* ot/o
aut-	self
axill/o	armpit
balan/o	penis
bari/o	weight
bi-	two
bi/o	life
blephar/o	eyelid
brady-	slow
bronch/o	bronchial tube
bronchiol/o	small bronchial tube

Word Part	Meaning
calcane/o	calcaneus (heel bone)
capillar/o	capillary
carcin/o	cancer, cancerous
cardi/o	heart
carp/o	wrist bones (carpals)
-cele	hernia
-centesis	puncture to remove fluid
cephal/o	head
cerebell/o	cerebellum (posterior part of the brain)
cerebr/o	cerebrum (largest part of the brain)
cervic/o	neck
chem/o	drug, chemical
cholecyst/o	gallbladder
choledoch/o	common bile duct
chondr/o	cartilage
chron/o	time
-cision	process of cutting
cis/o	to cut
clavicul/o	clavicle (collarbone)
-coccus	bacterium (berry-shaped); *plural:* -cocci
coccyg/o	tailbone
col/o	colon (large intestine)
colon/o	colon
colp/o	vagina
comi/o	to care for
con-	with, together
coni/o	dust
-coniosis	abnormal condition of dust
contra-	against
coron/o	heart; crown
cost/o	rib
crani/o	skull
crin/o	secrete
-crine	secretion
-crit	separation
cry/o	cold
cutane/o	skin
cyan/o	blue
cyst/o	urinary bladder
-cyte	cell
cyt/o	cell
dactyl/o	fingers or toes
de-	away from, down
dem/o	people
dent/i	tooth
dermat/o, derm/o	skin
dia-	complete, through

Word Part	Meaning
-dipsia	thirst
duoden/o	duodenum
dur/o	dura mater (outermost meningeal layer)
-dynia	pain
dys-	abnormal, bad, difficult, painful
-eal	pertaining to
ec-	out, outside
-ectasia, -ectasis	dilation, stretching, widening
ecto-	out, outside
-ectomy	excision (resection, removal); process of cutting out
electr/o	electricity
-emesis	vomiting
-emia	blood condition
en-	in, inner, within
encephal/o	brain
endo-	within, in, inner
endocrin/o	endocrine glands
endometr/o, endometri/o	endometrium (inner lining of the uterus)
enter/o	intestines (usually small intestine)
epi-	above, upon
epiglott/o	epiglottis
epitheli/o	skin (surface tissue)
erythr/o	red
esophag/o	esophagus
esthesi/o	sensation
eu-	good (normal)
ex-, exo-, extra-	out, outside
femor/o	femur, thigh bone
fibr/o	fibrous tissue
fibul/o	fibula (smaller lower leg bone)
gastr/o	stomach
gen/o	to produce
-gen	production, formation
-genesis	producing, forming
-genic	pertaining to producing, produced by
ger/o	old age
-globin	protein
glyc/o	sugar
gnos/o	knowledge
-gram	record
-graph	instrument to record
-graphy	process of recording, to record
gynec/o	woman, female

Word Part	Meaning
hemat/o, hem/o	blood
hepat/o	liver
humer/o	humerus (upper arm bone)
hydr/o	water
hyper-	excessive, more than normal, too much, above
hypo-	below, deficient, less than normal, too little
hypophys/o	pituitary gland
hyster/o	uterus
-ia	condition
-ian	practitioner
iatr/o	treatment
-ic, -ical	pertaining to
ile/o	ileum (third part of small intestine)
ili/o	ilium (upper part of hip bone)
in-	in, into
-ine	pertaining to
infra-	below
inguin/o	groin
inter-	between
intra-	within
-ior	pertaining to
isch/o	to hold back
-ism	condition, process
-ist	specialist
-itis	inflammation
jejun/o	jejunum
lapar/o	abdomen
-lapse	slide
laryng/o	larynx (voice box)
later/o	side
ligament/o	ligament
leiomy/o	visceral (smooth, involuntary) muscle
leuk/o	white
lip/o	fat
-listhesis	sliding
lith/o	stone
-lith	stone
-logist	specialist in the study of
-logy	process of study, study of
lumb/o	loin, waist region
lymph/o	lymph
lymphaden/o	lymph nodes
lymphangi/o	lymph vessel
lys/o	breakdown, destruction, separation
-lysis	breakdown, destruction, separation

Word Part	Meaning
macro-	large
mal-	bad
-malacia	softening
mamm/o	breast
mast/o	breast
mediastin/o	mediastinum
medull/o	medulla oblongata (lower part of the brain)
-megaly	enlargement
men/o	menstruation
mening/o	meninges (membranes covering brain and spinal cord)
meta-	beyond, change
metacarp/o	metacarpals (hand bones)
metatars/o	metatarsals (foot bones)
-meter	measure
metr/o, metri/o	uterus; to measure
-metry	measurement
micro-	small
-mortem	death
-motor	movement
multi-	many
muscul/o	muscle
my/o	muscle
myel/o	bone marrow (with -blast,-cyte, -genous, -oma)
myel/o	spinal cord (with -cele, -gram, -itis)
myos/o	muscle
myring/o	eardrum
nas/o	nose
nat/i	birth
necr/o	death
neo-	new
nephr/o	kidney
neur/o	nerve
norm/o	rule, order
nos/o	disease
nulli-	none
obstetr/o	midwife
ocul/o	eye
odont/o	tooth
-oid	pertaining to, resembling
ox /o	oxygen
-oma	tumor, mass, swelling
onc/o	tumor (cancerous)
onych/o	nail
o/o	egg
oophor/o	ovary
ophthalm/o	eye
-opsy	to view; process of viewing

Word Part	Meaning
opt/o, optic/o	eye
or/o	mouth
orch/o	testicle, testis
orchi/o	testicle, testis
orchid/o	testicle, testis
orth/o	straight
-osis	abnormal condition
osm/o	smell
oste/o	bone
ot/o	ear
-ous	pertaining to
ovari/o	ovary
ox/o	oxygen
pan-	all
pancreat/o	pancreas
para-	along the side of, beside, near
parathyroid/o	parathyroid gland
-partum	birth
path/o	disease
-pathy	disease condition
ped/o	child
pelv/o	pelvis; hip area
-penia	deficiency
per-	through
peri-	surrounding
peritone/o	peritoneum (membrane around abdominal organs)
perone/o	fibula
-pexy	fixation (surgical)
phak/o	lens of the eye
phalang/o	phalanges (finger and toe bones)
pharyng/o	pharynx, throat
-phasia	speech
-philia	attraction to
phleb/o	vein
phren/o	diaphragm
phren/o	mind
physi/o	function
pituitar/o	pituitary gland
plas/o	development, formation, growth
-plasm	development, formation, growth
-plasia	formation, growth
-plasty	surgical repair
-plegia	paralysis
pleur/o	pleura (membranes surrounding the lungs)
-pnea	breathing
pneum/o	air, lung
pneumon/o	lung
-poiesis	formation
poly-	many, much

Word Part	Meaning
post-	after, behind
poster/o	back, behind
pre-	before
pro-, pros-	before, forward
prosth/o	artificial replacement
proct/o	anus and rectum
prostat/o	prostate gland
psych/o	mind
-ptom	a happening
-ptosis	prolapse, sagging
-ptysis	spitting
pulmon/o	lung
pyel/o	renal pelvis (central section of the kidney)
radi/o	x-ray; radius (lateral lower arm bone)
re-	back
rect/o	rectum
ren/o	kidney
retin/o	retina of the eye
retro-	behind
rhabdomy/o	skeletal (striated, voluntary) muscle
rheumat/o	flow, fluid
rhin/o	nose
-rrhage	excess flow of blood
-rrhagia	excess flow of blood
-rrhaphy	suture
-rrhea	discharge, flow
sacr/o	sacrum
salping/o	fallopian (uterine) tube; eustachian tube
-salpinx	fallopian (uterine) tube; eustachian tube
sarc/o	flesh
scapul/o	shoulder blade (bone)
-sclerosis	hardening
-scope	instrument to view or visually examine
-scopy	process of visual examination
scrot/o	scrotal sac, scrotum
-section	process of cutting into
sept/o	infection
septic/o	infection
-sis	state of; condition
-somatic	pertaining to the body
son/o	sound
-spasm	constriction
spin/o	backbone, spine, vertebra
splen/o	spleen
spondyl/o	backbone, vertebra
-stasis	control, stop; place, to stand
-stat	stop, control
-stenosis	narrowing
stern/o	sternum (breastbone)

Word Part	Meaning
stomat/o	mouth
-stomy	opening
sub-	below, under
supra-	above
sym-	with, together (use before b, p, and m)
syn-	with, together
tachy-	fast
tendin/o, ten/o	tendon
-tension	pressure
theli/o, thel/o	nipple
-therapy	treatment
-thesis	put, place
thorac/o	chest
thromb/o	clotting, clot
thym/o	thymus gland
thyr/o, thyroid/o, thyroaden/o	thyroid gland
tibi/o	tibia or shin bone (larger lower leg bone)
-tic	pertaining to
-tomy	process of cutting into, incision
tonsill/o	tonsils
top/o	to put, place
trache/o	trachea, windpipe
trans-	across, through
tri-	three
troph/o	development, nourishment
-trophy	development, nourishment
tympan/o	eardrum
uln/o	ulna (medial lower arm bone)
ultra-	beyond
-um	structure
ungu/o	nail
uni-	one
ureter/o	ureter
urethr/o	urethra
ur/o	urine, urinary tract
-uria	urine condition
uter/o	uterus
vagin/o	vagina
vas/o	vas deferens, vessel
vascul/o	blood vessel
ven/o	vein
venul/o	venule
vertebr/o	backbone, vertebra
vesic/o	urinary bladder
-y	condition, process

SECTION II: ENGLISH → MEDICAL TERMINOLOGY

Meaning	Word Part
abdomen	abdomin/o (*use with* -al, -centesis) lapar/o (*use with* -scope, -scopy, -tomy)
abnormal	dys-
abnormal condition	-osis
abnormal condition of dust	-coniosis
above	epi-, hyper-, supra-
across	trans-
adenoids	adenoid/o
adrenal gland	adren/o
after	post-
against	anti-, contra-
air	pneum/o
air sac	alveol/o
all	pan-
along the side of	para-
alveolus	alveol/o
amnion	amni/o
anus	an/o
anus and rectum	proct/o
aorta	aort/o
apart	ana-
appendix	append/o (*use with* -ectomy) appendic/o (*use with* -itis)
armpit	axill/o
artery	arteri/o
artificial replacement	prosth/o
attraction to	-philia
away from	ab-, de-
back	poster/o, re-, retro-
backbone	spin/o (*use with* -al) spondyl/o (*use with* -itis, -listhesis, -osis, -pathy) vertebr/o (*use with* -al)
bacterium (berry-shaped)	-coccus (*plural:* -cocci)
bad	dys-, mal-
before	ante-, pre-, pro-, pros-
behind	post-, poster/o, re-, retro-
below	hypo-, infra-, sub-
beside	para-
between	inter-
beyond	meta-, ultra-
birth	nat/i, -partum
bladder (urinary)	cyst/o (*use with* -ic, -itis, -cele, -gram, -scopy) vesic/o (*use with* -al, -stomy, -tomy)

Meaning	Word Part
blood	hem/o (*use with* -cyte, -dialysis, -globin, -lysis, -philia, -ptysis, -rrhage, -stasis, -stat)
	hemat/o (*use with* -crit, -emesis, -logist, -logy, -oma, -poiesis, -salpinx, -uria)
blood condition	-emia
blood flow, excess	-rrhage, -rrhagia
blood vessel	angi/o (*use with* -ectomy, -dysplasia, -genesis, -gram, -graphy, -oma, -plasty, -spasm)
	vas/o (*use with* -constriction, -dilation, -dilatation, -motor)
	vascul/o (*use with* -ar, -itis)
blue	cyan/o
body	-somatic
bone	oste/o
bone marrow	myel/o
brain	encephal/o
breakdown	-lysis, lys/o
breast	mamm/o (*use with* -ary, -gram, -graphy, -plasty)
	mast/o (*use with* -algia, -ectomy, -itis)
breastbone	stern/o
breathing	-pnea
bronchial tube	bronch/o
bronchiole	bronchiol/o
calcaneus	calcane/o
cancer	carcin/o
cancerous	carcin/o
capillary	capillar/o
care for (to)	comi/o
carpals	carp/o
cartilage	chondr/o
cell	-cyte, cyt/o
cerebellum	cerebell/o
cerebrum	cerebr/o
change	meta-
chemical	chem/o
chest	thorac/o
child	ped/o
clavicle	clavicul/o
clotting, clot	thromb/o
cold	cry/o
collarbone	clavicul/o
colon	col/o (*use with* -ectomy, -itis, -stomy)
	colon/o (*use with* -pathy, -scope, -scopy)
common bile duct	choledoch/o
complete	dia-
condition	-ation, -ia, -ism, -osis, -sis, -y
condition of blood	-emia
constriction	-spasm
control	-stasis, -stat

Meaning	Word Part
crown	coron/o
cut	-cision, cis/o, -section, -tomy
death	-mortem, necr/o
deficiency	-penia
deficient	hypo-
destruction	lys/o, -lysis
development	plas/o, -plasm, troph/o, -trophy
dilation	-ectasia, -ectasis
diaphragm	phren/o
difficult	dys-
discharge	-rrhea
disease	nos/o; path/o, -pathy
drug	chem/o
duodenum	duoden/o
dura mater	dur/o
dust	coni/o
dust condition	-coniosis
ear	aur/o, ot/o
eardrum	myring/o (*use with* -ectomy, -itis, -tomy)
	tympan/o (*use with* -ic, -metry, -plasty)
egg	o/o
electricity	electr/o
endocrine gland	endocrin/o
endometrium	endometri/o
enlargement	-megaly
epiglottis	epiglott/o
esophagus	esophag/o
eustachian tube	salping/o, -salpinx
excessive	hyper-
excision	-ectomy
eye	ocul/o (*use with* -ar, -facial, -motor)
	ophthalm/o (*use with* -ia, -ic, -logist, -logy, -pathy, -plasty, -plegia, -scope, -scopy)
	opt/o (*use with* -ic, -metrist)
	optic/o (*use with* -ian)
eyelid	blephar/o
fallopian tube	salping/o, -salpinx
fast	tachy-
fat	lip/o
fatty plaque	ather/o
female	gynec/o
femur	femor/o
fibrous tissue	fibr/o
fibula	fibul/o, perone/o
fingers	dactyl/o
fixation (surgical)	-pexy

Meaning	Word Part
flesh	sarc/o
flow	-rrhea, rheumat/o
fluid	rheumat/o
foot bones	metatars/o
formation	-genesis, -plasia, plas/o, -plasm, -poiesis
forward	ante-, pro-, pros-
front	anter/o
function	physi/o
gallbladder	cholecyst/o
gland	aden/o
good	eu-
groin	inguin/o
growth	plas/o, -plasm
hand bones	metacarp/o
happening	-ptom
hardening	-sclerosis
head	cephal/o
heart	cardi/o (*use with* -ac, -graphy, -logy, -logist, -megaly, -pathy, -vascular) coron/o (*use with* -ary)
heel bone	calcane/o
hernia	-cele
hip area	pelv/o
hold back (to)	isch/o
humerus	humer/o
ileum	ile/o
ilium	ili/o
in, into	in-, en-, endo-
incision	-section, -tomy
infection	sept/o, septic/o
inflammation	-itis
inner	en-, endo-
instrument to record	-graph
instrument to visually examine	-scope
intestines (small)	enter/o
jejunum	jejun/o
joint	arthr/o
kidney	nephr/o (*use with* -algia, -ectomy, -ic, -itis, -lith, -logy, -megaly, -oma, -osis, -pathy, -ptosis, -sclerosis, -stomy, -tomy) ren/o (*use with* -al, -gram)
kidney (central section)	pyel/o
knowledge	gnos/o
large	macro-

Meaning	Word Part
larynx	laryng/o
lens of the eye	phak/o
less than normal	hypo-
life	bi/o
ligament	ligament/o
liver	hepat/o
loin	lumb/o
lung	pneum/o (*use with* -coccus, -coniosis, -thorax) pneumon/o (*use with* -ectomy, -ia, -ic, -itis, -pathy) pulmon/o (*use with* -ary)
lymph	lymph/o
lymph node	lymphaden/o
lymph vessel	lymphangi/o
mass	-oma
many	poly-, multi-
measure (to)	meter, metr/o, metry
mediastinum	mediastin/o
medulla oblongata	medull/o
meninges	mening/o
menstruation	men/o
metacarpals	metacarp/o
metatarsals	metatars/o
midwife	obstetr/o
mind	psych/o, phren/o
more than normal	hyper-
mouth	or/o (*use with* -al) stomat/o (*use with* -itis)
movement	-motor
much	poly-
muscle	muscul/o (*use with* -ar, -skeletal) myos/o (*use with* -itis) my/o (*use with* -algia, -ectomy, -oma, -gram, -neural)
nail	onych/o (*use with* -lysis), ungu/o (*use with* -al)
narrowing	-stenosis
near	para-
neck	cervic/o
nerve	neur/o
new	neo-
nipple	thel/o, theli/o
no, not	a-, an-
none	nulli-
nose	nas/o (*use with* -al) rhin/o (*use with* -itis, -rrhea, -plasty)
nourishment	troph/o, -trophy

Meaning	Word Part
old age	ger/o
one	uni-
opening	-stomy
order	norm/o
out, outside	ec-, ecto-, ex-, exo- extra-
ovary	oophor/o (*use with* -itis, -ectomy, -pexy, -plasty, -tomy) ovari/o (*use with* -an)
oxygen	ox/o
pain	-algia, -dynia
painful	dys-
pancreas	pancreat/o
paralysis	-plegia
parathyroid gland	parathyroid/o
pelvis	pelv/o
pelvis (renal)	pyel/o
penis	balan/o
people	dem/o
peritoneum	peritone/o
pertaining to	-ac, -al, -an, -ar, -ary, -eal, -ic, -ine, -ior, -oid, -ous, -tic
pertaining to the body	-somatic
phalanges	phalang/o
pharynx	pharyng/o
pituitary gland	hypophys/o, pituitar/o
place	top/o, -stasis
pleura	pleur/o
practitioner	-ian
pressure	-tension
process	-ation, -ism, -y
process of cutting into	-cision, -tomy, -section
process of cutting out	-ectomy
process of recording	-graphy
process of viewing	-opsy
produce (to)	-gen, gen/o
produced by	-genic
producing	-genic, -genesis
prolapse	-ptosis
prostate gland	prostat/o
puncture to remove fluid	-centesis
put, place (to)	-thesis, top/o
radius (lower arm bone)	radi/o
record	-gram
recording (process)	-graphy
rectum	rect/o
red	erythr/o
removal	-ectomy
renal pelvis	pyel/o

Meaning	Word Part
repair	-plasty
resection	-ectomy
resembling	-oid
retina of the eye	retin/o
rib	cost/o
rule	norm/o
sacrum	sacr/o
sagging	-ptosis
scapula	scapul/o
scrotum, scrotal sac	scrot/o
secrete, secretion	-crine, crin/o
self	aut-
sensation	esthesi/o
separation	-crit, -lysis, lys/o
shin bone	tibi/o
shoulder blade	scapul/o
side	later/o
skin	cutane/o (*use with* -ous) derm/o (*use with* -al); dermat/o (*use with* -itis, -logy, -osis) epitheli/o (*use with* -al)
skull	crani/o
sliding	-lapse, -listhesis
slip (to)	-listhesis
slow	brady-
small	micro-
small artery	arteriol/o
small bronchial tube	bronchiol/o
small intestine	enter/o
smell	osm/o
smooth muscle	leiomy/o
softening	-malacia
sound	son/o
specialist	-ist
specialist in the study of	-logist
speech	-phasia
spinal cord	myel/o
spine	spin/o
spitting	-ptysis
spleen	splen/o
stand (to)	-stasis
state of	-sis
sternum	stern/o
stomach	gastr/o
stone	lith/o, -lith
stop	-stasis, -stat
straight	orth/o
stretching	-ectasia, -ectasis

Meaning	Word Part
striated (skeletal) muscle	rhabdomy/o
structure	-um
study of	-logy
sugar	glyc/o
surgical repair	-plasty
surrounding	peri-
suture	-rrhaphy
swelling	-oma
tailbone	coccyg/o
tendon	tendin/o, ten/o
testicle, testis	orch/o, orchi/o, orchid/o
thigh bone	femor/o
thirst	-dipsia
throat	pharyng/o
three	tri-
through	dia-, per-, trans-
thymus gland	thym/o
thyroid gland	thyr/o, thyroid/o, thyroaden/o
tibia	tibi/o
time	chron/o
toes	dactyl/o
together	con-, syn-, sym-
tonsil	tonsill/o
too much	hyper-
too little	hypo-
tooth	dent/i, odont/o
toward	ad-
trachea	trache/o
treatment	iatr/o, -therapy
tumor	-oma, onc/o
two	bi-
ulna	uln/o
under	hypo-, sub-
up	ana-
upon	epi-
ureter	ureter/o
urethra	urethr/o
urinary bladder	cyst/o, vesic/o
urinary tract	ur/o
urine	ur/o
urine condition	-uria
uterus	hyster/o (*use with* -ectomy, -graphy, -gram) metr/o (*use with* -itis, -rrhagia) metri/o (*use with* -al) uter/o (*use with* -ine)
uterus (inner lining)	endometr/o, endometri/o

Meaning	Word Part
vagina	colp/o (*use with* -pexy, -plasty, -scope, -scopy, -tomy)
	vagin/o (*use with* -al, -itis)
vas deferens	vas/o
vein	phleb/o (*use with* -ectomy, -itis, -lith, -thrombosis, -tomy)
	ven/o (*use with* -ous, -gram)
venule	venul/o
vertebra	spin/o (*use with* -al)
	spondyl/o (*use with* -itis, -listhesis, -osis, -pathy)
	vertebr/o (*use with* -al)
vessel	angi/o (*use with* -ectomy, -dysplasia, -genesis, -gram, -graphy, -oma, -plasty, -spasm)
	vas/o (*use with* -constriction, -dilation, -motor)
	vascul/o (*use with* -ar, -itis)
view (to)	-opsy
visual examination	-scopy
voice box	laryng/o
vomiting	-emesis
waist region	lumb/o
water	hydr/o
weight	bari/o
white	leuk/o
widening	-ectasia, -ectasis
windpipe	trache/o
with	con-, syn-, sym-
within	en-, endo-, intra-
woman	gynec/o
wrist bones	carp/o
x-ray	radi/o

GLOSSARY 3

English → Spanish Terms*

* Diagrams of the body labeled with Spanish terms are on pages 424 and 425.

Here is a list of **English → Spanish terms** that will help you communicate with Spanish-speaking patients in offices, hospitals, and other medical settings. Included are parts of the body and other medical terms as well.

abdomen	abdomen (ahb-DOH-mehn)
acne	acné (ahk-NEH)
acoustic	acústico (ah-KOOS-tee-ko)
adenoid	adenoide (ah-deh-NOH-ee-deh)
allergy	alergia (AL-ehr-ge-ah)
amebic	amébico (ah-MEH-bee-ko)
analgesic	analgésico (ah-nahl-HEH-see-koh)
anemia	anemia (ah-NEH-mee-ah)
anesthesia	anestesia (ah-nehs-TEH-see-ah)
angina	angina (ahn-HEE-na)
angioma	angioma (ahn-hee-OH-mah)
ankle	tobillo (toh-BEE-yoh)
antacid	antiácido (ahn-tee-AH-see-doh)
antiarrhythmic	antiarrítmico (ahn-tee-ah-RREET-mee-koh)
antibiotic	antibiótico (ahn-tee-bee-OH-tee-koh)
anticonvulsant	anticonvulsivante (ahn-tee-kohn-bool-SEE-ban-teh)
antidiarrheal	antidiarrético (ahn-tee-dee-ah-RREH-tee-koh)
antiemetic	antiemético (ahn-tee-eh-MEH-tee-koh)
antiepileptic	antiepiléptico (ahn-tee-eh-pee-LEHP-tee-koh)
antihistamine	antihistamínico (ahn-tee-ees-tah-MEE-nee-koh)
antiviral	antivirus (ahn-tee-BEE-roos)
anus	ano (AH-no)
appendix	apéndice (ah-PEHN-dee-seh)
arm	brazo (BRAH-soh)
armpit	axila (ahk-SEE-lah)
arteriogram	arteriograma (ahr-teh-ree-oh-GRAH-mah)
arthritis	artritis (ahr-TREE-tees)
asthma	asma (AHS-mah)
bacteria	bacteria (bahk-TEH-ree-ah)
barbiturates	barbitúricos (bahr-bee-TOO-ree-kohs)
birthmark	lunar (loo-NAHR)
bleeding	sangrado (sahn-GRAH-doh)
blood	sangre (SAHN-greh)
blood count	biometría hemática (bee-oh-meh-TREE-ah eh-MAH-tee-kah)
bone	hueso (hoo-A-so)
bradycardia	bradicardia (brah-dee-KAHR-dee-ah)
brain	cerebro (seh-REH-bro)
breast/chest	seno (SEH-noh), pecho (PEH-choh)
bronchial tube	bronquio (BROHN-kee-oh)
bronchitis	bronquitis (brohn-KEE-tees)
bruises	moretónes (moh-reh-TOH-nehs)
burn	quemadura (keh-mah-DOO-rah)
buttocks	nalgas (NAHL-gahs)
calf	pantorrilla (pahn-toh-RREE-yah)
callus	callo (KAH-yoh)
calm	calma (KAHL-mah)

cardiac	cardiaco (kahr-DEE-ah-koh)
cataract	catarata (kah-tah-RAH-tah)
cervix	cuello uterino (KOO-eh-yoh) (oo-teh-REE-noh), cerviz (SERH-bees)
chancre	chancro (CHAHN-kroh)
cheek	mejilla (meh-HEE-yah)
chemotherapy	quimioterapia (kee-mee-oh-teh-RAH-pee-ah)
chin	barbilla (bar-BEE-yah)
cholesterol	colesterol (koh-lehs-teh-ROHL)
cirrhosis	cirrosis (see-RROH-sees)
claustrophobia	claustrofobia (klah-oos-troh-FOH-bee-ah)
coagulation	coagulación (koh-ah-goo-lah-see-OHN)
collar bone	clavícula (klah-VEE-kuh-la)
colon	colon (KOH-lohn)
constipation	estreñimiento (ehs-treh-nyee-mee-EHN-toh)
cortisone	cortisona (kohr-tee-SOH-nah)
cough	tos (tohs)
cyanotic	cianótico (see-ah-NOH-tee-ko)
decongestants	descongestionantes (dehs-kohn-hehs-tee-oh-NAHN-tehs)
dehydrated	deshidratado (deh-see-drah-TAH-doh)
delirious	delirio (deh-LEE-ree-oh)
depressed	deprimido (deh-pree-MEE-doh)
diabetes	diabetes (dee-ah-BEH-tehs)
diarrhea	diarrea (dee-ah-RREH-ah)
digitalis	digital (dee-hee-TAHL)
ear (inner)	oído (oh-EE-do)
ear (outer)	oreja (oh-REH-hah)
ecchymosis	equimosis (eh-kee-MOH-sees)
eczema	eccema (ehk-SEH-mah)
elbow	codo (KOH-doh)
embolism	embolia (ehm-boh-LEE-ah)
emetic	emético (eh-MEH-tee-koh)
enteritis	enteritis (ehn-teh-REE-tees)
epilepsy	epilepsia (eh-pee-LEHP-see-ah)
euphoric	eufórico (eh-oo-FOH-ree-koh)
exudate	exudado (ehk-soo-DAH-doh)
eye	ojo (OH-hoh)
eyebrow	ceja (SEH-hah)
eyelash	pestaña (pehs-TAH-nyah)
eyelids	párpados (PAHR-pah-dohs)
fatigue	fatiga (fah-TE-gah)
fibroid	fibroma (fee-BROH-mah)
finger	dedo (DEH-doh)
fingernail	uña (OO-nyah)
fist	puño (POO-nyoh)
fistula	fístula (FEES-too-lah)
flu	gripe (GRE-pa)
foot	pie (pee-EH)
forearm	antebrazo (an-teh-BRAH-zoh)
forehead	frente (FREN-teh)

fracture	fractura (frak-TOO-rah)
fungus	hongo (OHN-goh)
gallbladder	vesícula biliar (beh-SEE-koo-lah bee-lee-AHR)
gangrene	gangrena (gahn-GREH-nah)
gastroenteritis	gastroenteritis (gahs-troh-ehn-teh-REE-tees)
gastroenterology	gastroenterología (gahs-troh-ehn-teh-roh-loh-HEE-ah)
genital organs	órganos genitales (ORH-gah-nohs heh-nee-TAH-lehs)
glaucoma	glaucoma (glah-oo-KOH-mah)
groin	ingle (EEN-gleh)
gums	encías (ehn-SEE-ahs)
gynecologist	ginecólogo (hee-neh-KOH-loh-goh)
hair	cabello (kah-BEH-yoh)
hand	mano (MAH-noh)
head	cabeza (kah-BEH-sah)
heart	corazón (koh-rah-SOHN)
heel	talón (tah-LOHN)
hematology	hematología (eh-mah-toh-loh-HEE-ah)
hematoma	hematoma (eh-mah-TOH-mah)
hemolysis	hemólisis (eh-MOH-lee-sees)
hemorrhage	hemorragia (eh-moh-RRAH-hee-ah)
hepatitis	hepatitis (eh-pah-TEE-tees)
hernia	hernia (EHR-nee-ah)
hip	cadera (kah-DEH-rah)
hypertension	hipertensión (ee-pehr-tehn-see-OHN)
icteric	ictérico (eek-TEH-ree-koh)
infection	infección (een-fehk-see-OHN)
inflammation	inflamación (een-flah-mah-see-OHN)
insulin	insulina (een-soo-LEE-nah)
intestine	intestino (een-tes-TEE-noh)
intramuscular	intramuscular (een-trah-moos-koo-LAHR)
intravenous	intravenoso (een-trah-beh-NOH-soh)
irradiate	irradiar (ee-rrhah-dee-AHR)
jaw	mandíbula (mahn-DEE-boo-lah)
kidney	riñón (ree-NYON)
knee	rodilla (ro-DEE-yah)
laparoscopy	laparoscopia (lah-pah-rohs-KOH-pee-ah)
laryngitis	laringitis (lah-reen-HEE-tees)
laxative	laxante (lahk-SAHN-teh)
left	izquierdo (ees-kee-EHR-doh)
leg	pierna (pee-EHR-nah)
ligament	ligamento (lee-gah-MEHN-toh)
lingual	lingual (leen-GUAHL)
lip	labio (LAH-bee-oh)
lithium	litio (LEE-tee-oh)
liver	hígado (EE-gah-doh)
low cholesterol	bajo colesterol (bah-hoh koh-lehs-teh-ROHL)

ENGLISH-SPANISH

low fat	bajo grasa (bah-hoh GRAH-sah)
low sodium	bajo sodio (bah-hoh soh-dee-oh)
lung	pulmón (pool-MOHN)
meningitis	meningitis (meh-neen-HEE-tees)
morphine	morfina (mohr-FEE-nah)
mouth	boca (BOH-kah)
muscle	músculo (MOOS-koo-loh)
narcotics	narcóticos (nahr-KOH-tee-kohs)
nasal	nasal (nah-SAHL)
nausea	náusea (NAH-oo-seh-ah)
navel	ombligo (ohm-BLEE-goh)
neck	cuello (koo-EH-yoh)
neonatal	neonatal (neh-oh-nah-TAHL)
nephrologist	nefrólogo (neh-PHROH-lo-goh)
nephrology	nefrología (neh-phroh-lo-HEE-ah)
nervous	nervioso (nehr-bee-OH-soh)
neurotic	neurótico (neh-oo-ROH-tee-koh)
nipple	pezón (peh-SOHN)
nitroglycerin	nitroglicerina (nee-troh-glee-seh-REE-nah)
nose	nariz (nah-REES)
nostrils	fosas nasales (foh-SAHS na-SAH-lehs)
Novocain	novocaína (noh-boh-kah-EE-nah)
nuclear medicine	medicina nuclear (meh-dee-SEE-nah NOO-kleh-ahr)
obstetrics	obstetricia (ohbs-teh-TREE-see-ah)
oncology	oncología (ohn-koh-loh-HEE-ah)
ophthalmic	oftálmico (ohf-TAHL-mee-koh)
ophthalmology	oftalmología (ohf-tahl-moh-loh-HEE-ah)
optic	óptico (OHP-tee-koh)
orthopedics	ortopedia (ohr-toh-PEH-dee-ah)
orthopedic surgeon	cirujano ortopédico (see-roo-HAH-noh ohr-toh-PEH-dee-koh)
otic	ótico (OH-tee-koh)
ovary	ovario (oh-BAH-ree-oh)
pain	dolor (DO-lor)
palate	paladar (pah-lah-DAHR)
palpation	palpación (pahl-pah-see-OHN)
palpitation	palpitación (pahl-pee-tah-see-OHN)
pancreas	páncreas (PAHN-kreh-ahs)
pancreatitis	pancreatitis (pahn-kreh-ah-TEE-tees)
paralytic	paralítico (pah-rah-LEE-tee-koh)
pathogen	patógeno (pah-TOH-hen-oh)
pathologic	patológico (pah-toh-LOH-hee-koh)
pathology	patología (pah-toh-loh-HEE-ah)
pediatrics	pediatría (peh-dee-ah-TREE-ah)
pelvis	pelvis (PEHL-bees)
penis	pene (PEH-neh), miembro viril (mee-EHM-broh vee-REEL)
pharmacy	farmacia (far-mah-SE-ah)

pneumonia	pulmonía/neumonía (pool-moh-NEE-ah/neh-oo-moh-NEE-ah)
prescription	receta (re-SE-tah)
pruritic	prurito (proo-REE-toh)
psoriasis	psoriasis (soh-ree-AH-sees)
psychiatrist	psiquiatra (see-kee-AH-trah)
psychiatry	psiquiatría (see-kee-ah- TREE-ah)
psychologist	psicólogo (see-KOH-loh-goh)
pubic	púbico (POO-bee-koh)
pulse	pulso (POOL-so)
pyorrhea	piorrea (pee-oh-RREH-ah)
radiologist	radiólogo (rah-dee-OH-loh-goh)
radiology	radiología (rah-dee-oh-loh-HEE-ah)
rectum	recto (REHK-toh)
rheumatic	reumático (reh-oo-MAH-tee-koh)
rib	costilla (kohs-TEE-yah)
right	derecho (deh-REH-choh)
roseola	roseola (roh-seh-OH-lah)
rubella	rubéola (roo-BEH-oh-lah)
scalp	cuero cabelludo (KOO-eh-roh kah-beh-YOO-doh)
sebaceous	sebáceo (seh-BAH-seh-oh)
sedatives	sedativos/sedantes (seh-dah-TEE-bohs/seh-DAHN-tehs)
shin	espinilla (ehs-pee-NEE-yah), canilla (kah-NEE-yah)
shoulder	hombro (OHM-bro)
skin	piel (pee-EHL)
skull	cráneo (KRAH-ne-oh)
spinal column	columna vertebral (koh-LUHM-nah behr-teh-BRAHL)
spleen	bazo (BAH-soh)
stethoscope	estetoscopio (ehs-teh-tohs-KOH-pee-oh)
stitches	puntos (POON-tohs)
stomach	estómago (ehs-TOH-mah-goh)
stool sample	muestra – fecal (moo-EHS-trah -feh-KAHL)
straight	derecho (deh-REH-choh)
subaxillary	subaxilar (soob-AHK-see-lahr)
subcutaneous	subcutáneo (soob-koo-TAH-neh-oh)
sublingual	sublingual (soob-LEEN-goo-ahl)
substernal	subesternal (soob-ehs-TEHR-nahl)
surgeon	cirujano (see-roo-HAH-noh)
surgery	cirugía (see-roo-HEE-ah)
symptoms	síntomas (SEEN-toh-mahs)
syncope	síncope (SEEN-koh-peh)
systole	sístole (SEES-toh-leh)
teeth	dientes (dee-EHN-tehs)
temple	sien (see-EHN)
testicles	testículos (tehs-TEE-koo-lohs)
tetanus	tétano (TEH-tah-noh)
therapy	terapia (teh-RAH-pee-ah)
thigh	muslo (MOOS-loh)
throat	garganta (gahr-GAHN-tah)

thumb	pulgar (POOL-gahr)
thyroid	tiroide (tee-ROY-deh)
toes	dedos (DEH-dos), del pié (dehl PEE-eh)
tongue	lengua (LEHN-goo-ah)
tonsillitis	tonsilitis/amigdalitis (tohn-see-LEE-tees/ah-meeg-dah-LEE-tees)
tonsils	amígdalas (ah-MEEG-da-las)
ulcer	úlcera (OOL-seh-rah)
ulnar	ulnar (OOL-nahr)
ultrasound	ultrasonido (ool-trah-soh-NEE-doh)
uremia	uremia (oo-REH-mee-ah)
urinary bladder	vejiga (beh-HEE-gah)
urine	orina (oh-REE-nah)
urticaria	urticaria (oor-tee-KAH-ree-ah)
uterus	útero (OO-teh-roh)
uvula	úvula (OO-boo-lah)
vaginitis	vaginitis (bah-hee-NEE-tees)
vagus	vago (BAH-goh)
valve	válvula (BAHL-boo-lah)
varicocele	varicocele (bah-ree-koh-SEH-leh)
vertigo	vértigo (BEHR-tee-goh)
waist	cintura (sin-TOO-rah)
womb	vientre (bee-EHN-treh)
wrist	muñeca (moo-NYEH-kah)
x-rays	rayos equis (rah-YOHS EH-kees)
zygomatic	cigomático (see-goh-MAH-tee-koh)

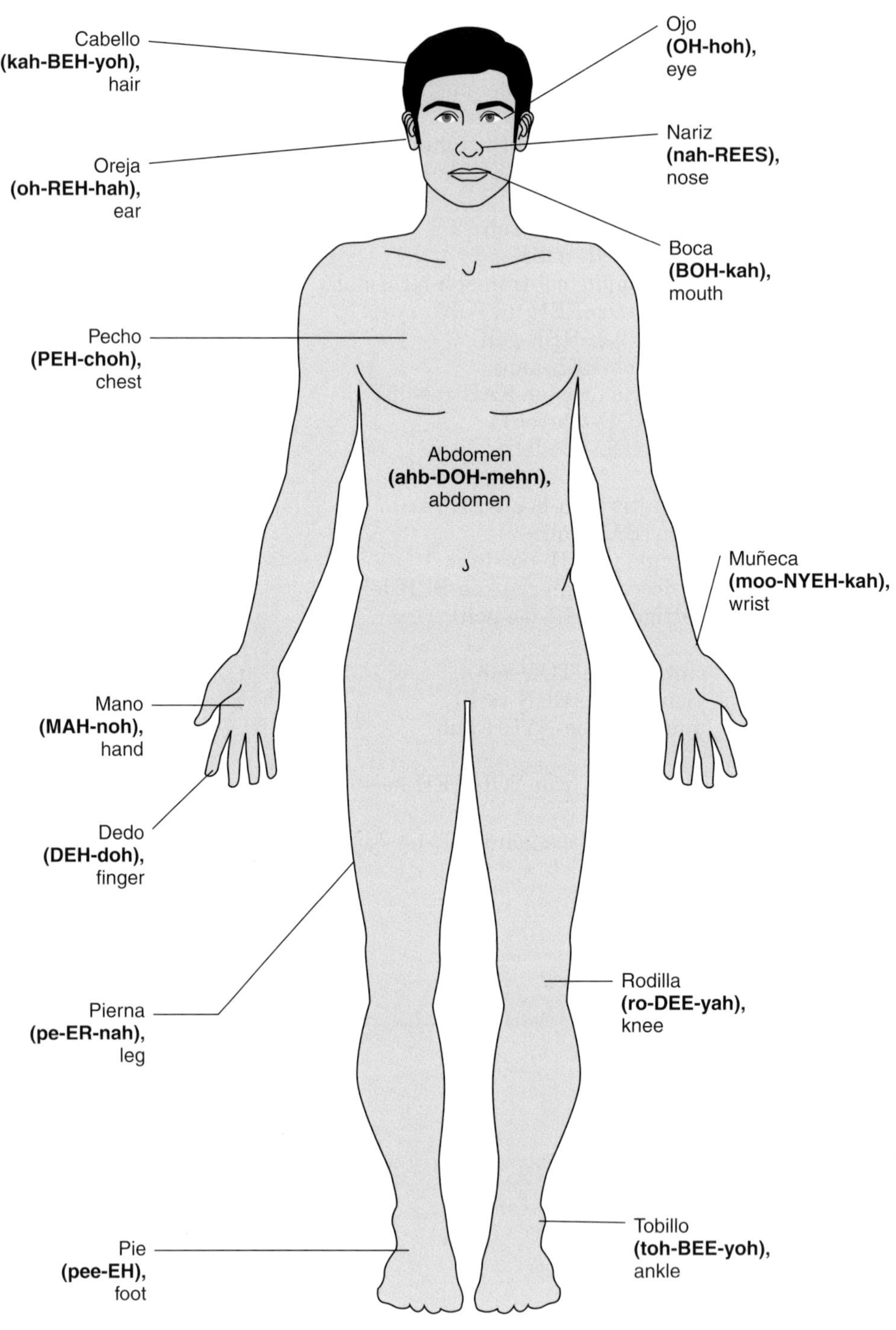

The body/El cuerpo (ehl KWEHR-poh).

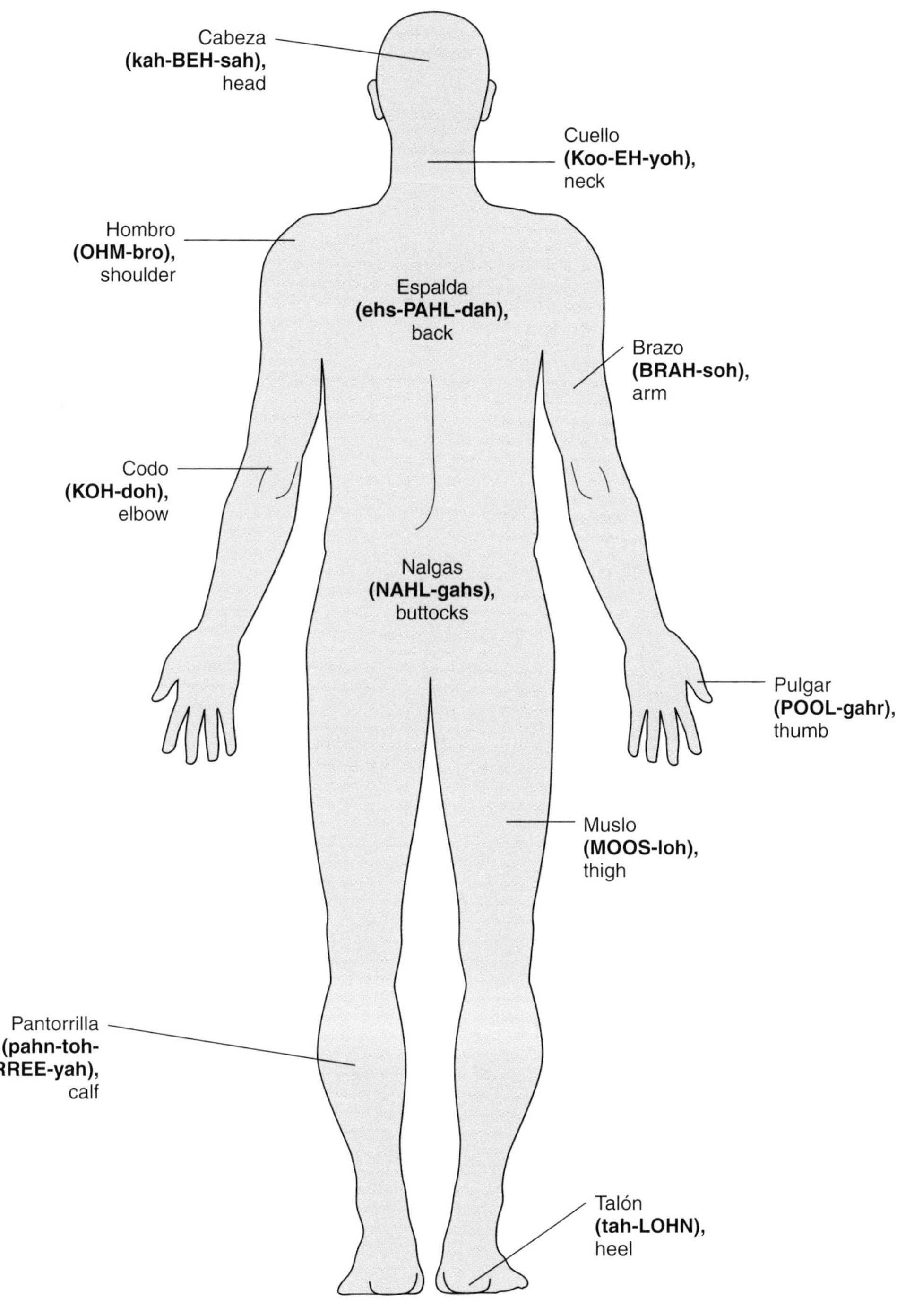

Posterior View

The body/El cuerpo (ehl KWEHR-poh).

Illustration Credits

Figure 2-9, Unnumbered Figure 3-4, courtesy of Beatrix Bess Thompson.

Figure 2-8A, Modified from Black JM, Matassarin-Jacobs E: *Medical-Surgical Nursing: Clinical Management for Continuity of Care*, ed 5, Philadelphia, 1997, Saunders.

Figure 3-22, from Bonewit-West K: *Clinical Procedures for Medical Assistants*, ed 6, Philadelphia, 2004, Elsevier.

Unnumbered Figure 1-9, modified from Carr JH, Rodak BF: *Clinical Hematology Atlas*, ed 5, Philadelphia, 2017, Elsevier.

Appendix 2 Unnumbered Figure 2-9A, courtesy Centers for Disease Control and Prevention: Atlanta, Georgia.

Figures 1-17, 2-8C, 3-9B, 3-15, 5-8, 5-14, Appendix 2 Unnumbered Figure 2-5, from Chabner D-E: *The Language of Medicine*, ed 12, St. Louis, 2021, Elsevier.

Unnumbered Figure 1-14, from Chabner D-E: *The Language of Medicine*, ed 12, St. Louis, 2021, Elsevier. Courtesy of Dr. Elizabeth Chabner.

Figures 1-2, 1-3, 1-4, 1-5, 1-15, 2-2, 2-6, 2-12, 2-14, Unnumbered Figure 2-2, Unnumbered Figure 2-3, 3-1, 3-18, 3-20, Unnumbered Figure 3-2, Unnumbered Figure 3-6, 4-1, 4-2, 4-15, 5-3, Appendix 1 Unnumbered Figure 1-2, Appendix 1 Unnumbered Figure 1-3, Appendix 1 Unnumbered Figure 1-4, Appendix 1 Unnumbered Figure 1-5, Appendix 1 Unnumbered Figure 1-6, Appendix 1 Unnumbered Figure 1-7, Appendix 1 Unnumbered Figure 1-8, Appendix 1 Unnumbered Figure 1-12, Appendix 1 Unnumbered Figure 1-13, Appendix 1 Unnumbered Figure 1-14, Appendix 2 Unnumbered Figure 2-1B, Appendix 2 Unnumbered Figure 2-2B, Appendix 2 Unnumbered Figure 2-4B, Appendix 2 Unnumbered Figure 2-6, modified from Chabner D-E: *The Language of Medicine*, ed 12, St. Louis, 2021, Elsevier.

Figure 5-5, from Currie G, Douglas G: *The Flesh and Bones of Medicine*. St. Louis, 2011, Elsevier.

Figure 1-16, courtesy of Michael J. Curtin, MD, St. Luke's Clinic, Boise, Idaho.

Figures 3-5A, 3-6B, from Damjanov I: *Pathology for the Health-Related Professions*, ed 5, Philadelphia, 2017, Elsevier.

Unnumbered Figure 1-13B, from Dinulos JGH: *Habif's Clinical Dermatology*, ed 7, Philadelphia, 2021, Elsevier.

Figure 2-10B, from Ehrlich RA, Coakes DM: *Patient Care in Radiography*, ed 10, St. Louis, 2021, Elsevier.

Figure 4-17A, and **unnnumberd Figures A,B,C on page 42 of chapter 1** courtesy Dr. Elizabeth Chabner.

Unnumbered Figure 1-12, from Forbes CD, Jackson WF: *Color Atlas and Text of Clinical Medicine*, ed 3, London, 2003, Elsevier.

Figure 3-13, from Frank ED, et al: *Merrill's Atlas of Radiographic Positions and Radiologic Procedures*, ed 11, vol 2. St. Louis, 2007, Elsevier.

Figure 3-14A, from Frank ED, et al: *Merrill's Atlas of Radiographic Positions and Radiologic Procedures*, ed 14, St. Louis, 2019, Elsevier.

Figure 3-2B, from Goldman L, Schafer AI: *Goldman-Cecil Medicine*, ed 26, Philadelphia, 2020, Elsevier.

Figure 3-11A,B, courtesy Dr. A.K. Goodman, Massachusetts General Hospital, Boston, Massachusetts.

Figure 4-17B, from Hagen-Ansert SL: *Textbook of Diagnostic Ultrasonography*, ed 6, St. Louis, 2006, Elsevier.

Appendix 2 Unnumbered Figure 2-7A, from Helbert, M: *Immunology for Medical Students*, ed 3, Philadelphia, 2017, Elsevier. Courtesy Dr. Stella Knight, London, United Kingdom.

Figure 1-12A, courtesy Dr. Francis Hornicek, Department of Orthopedics, Massachusetts General Hospital, Boston.

Figure 5-16, from Huether SE, McCance KL: *Pathophysiology: The Biologic Basis for Disease in Adults and Children,* ed 8, St. Louis, 2019, Elsevier.

Figure 3-5B, from Hunt RB: *Text and Atlas of Female Infertility Surgery*, ed 3, St. Louis, 1999, Mosby.

Figure 1-6B, 3-21B, from Ignatavicius D, et al: *Medical-Surgical Nursing*, ed 10, St. Louis, 2021, Elsevier.

Appendix 2 Unnumbered Figure 2-9B, modified courtesy of iStock #1268666422, blueringmedia.

Appendix 2 Unnumbered Figure 2-3, courtesy iStock #595762986, #595763016, #595763060, Dr_Microbe.

Appendix 2 Unnumbered Figure 2-7B, modified courtesy of iStock #1253217171, Dr_Microbe.

Unnumbered Figure 4-2, image from iStock.com/Johnny Greigi.

Unnumbered Figure 4-7, courtesy iStock #1294974306, Indra Purnama.

Appendix 2 Unnumbered Figure 2-10, modified courtesy of iStock #536807380, ttsz.

Figure 1-13, courtesy iStock #1172668129, urfinguss.

Figure 1-10B, from Jarvis C: *Physical Examination and Health Assessment*, ed 3, Philadelphia, 2000, Elsevier.

Figure 1-10A, modified from Jarvis C: *Physical Examination and Health Assessment*, ed 8, St. Louis, 2020, Elsevier.

Figure 3-14B, from Klatt EC: *Robbins and Cotran Atlas of Pathology*, ed 2, Philadelphia, 2010, Elsevier.

Figure 5-7B, from Kumar V, et al: *Robbins & Cotran Pathologic Basis of Disease*, ed 10, Philadelphia, 2021, Elsevier.

Figure 2-13, photo from Lewis SM, Heitkemper MM, Dirksen SR: *Medical- Surgical Nursing*, ed 9, St. Louis, 2014, Elsevier.

Unnumbered Figure 3-3, Figure 5-10, from Lewis SM, Heitkemper MM, Dirksen SR: *Medical-Surgical Nursing: Assessment and Management of Clinical Problems*, ed 5, St. Louis, 2000, Elsevier.

Figure 2-10A, from Long BW, Rollins JH, Smith BJ: *Merrill's Atlas of Radiographic Positioning and Procedures*, ed 13, St. Louis, 2016, Elsevier.

Figure 5-6A,B, from Mann D, et al: *Braunwald's Heart Disease: A Textbook of Cardiovascular Medicine*, ed 9, Philadelphia, 2019, Elsevier.

Unnumbered Figure 2-4B, from Mason RJ, et al: *Clinical Respiratory Medicine*, ed 4, Philadelphia, 2008, Elsevier.

Figure 3-2A, from Mason RJ, et al: *Murray and Nadel ' s Textbook of Respiratory Medicine*, ed 4, Philadelphia, 2005, Elsevier.

Unnumbered Figure 1-11, courtesy Dr. Robert W. McKenna, Department of Pathology, University of Texas Southwestern Medical School, Dallas, Texas; from Kumar V: *Robbins Basic Pathology*, ed 10, Philadelphia, 2018, Elsevier.

Figure 5-2, provided by Medtronic.

Figures 4-14C, 5-9A, 5-11A-C, from Mettler FA: *Essentials of Radiology*, ed 3, Philadelphia, 2014, Elsevier.

Unnumbered Figure 1-10, from Miller MD, Howard RF, Plancher KD: *Surgical Atlas of Sports Medicine*. Philadelphia, 2003, Elsevier.

Appendix 1 Unnumbered Figure 1-9, Appendix 1 Unnumbered Figure 1-10, modified from *Miller-Keane Encyclopedia & Dictionary of Medicine, Nursing, & Allied Health*, ed 7, Philadelphia, 2003, Elsevier.

Figure 1-8B, from the National Institute of Allergy and Infectious Diseases, Bethesda, MD.

Figure 5-9B, from National Kidney and Urologic Diseases Information Clearinghouse. In Rakel D: *Integrative Medicine*, ed 4, Philadelphia, 2018, Elsevier.

Unnumbered Figure 4-5, from Perry AG, et al: *Nursing Interventions & Clinical Skills*, ed 6, St. Louis, 2016, Elsevier.

Figure 1-10C, courtesy of Dr. Jay Rosen, The Eye Gallery, Scarsdale NY, and Louisa Thompson.

Figure 5-7A, modified from Salem S: The uterus and adnexa. In: Rumack CM, Wilson SP, Charboneau JW, editors: *Diagnostic Ultrasound*, ed 2, St. Louis, 1998, Mosby.

Figure 1-14, modified from Seidel H, et al: *Mosby's Guide to Physical Examination*, ed 5, St. Louis, 2003, Elsevier.

Unnumbered Figure 3-5, courtesy Dr. Daniel Simon and Mr. Paul Zampino.

Unnumbered Figure 4-4, modified from Sorrentino SA: *Mosby's Textbook for Nursing Assistants*, ed 10, St. Louis, 2021, Elsevier.

Figure 1-12B, from Soyer HP: *Dermoscopy*, ed 2, Philadelphia, 2012, Elsevier.

Figure 5-2, figure from stanley45/E + / Getty Images.

Figure 1-8A, from U.S. Centers for Disease Control and Prevention, Atlanta, GA.

Figure 3-4, courtesy Dr. Erik-Jan Wamsteker: Gastroenterology. In Rakel RE, editor: *Textbook of Family Medicine*, ed 7, Philadelphia, 2007, Elsevier.

Unnumbered Figure 4-6, from Weinstein WM, Hawkey CJ, Bosch J: *Clinical Gastroenterology and Hepatology*. St. Louis, 2005, Elsevier.

Figure 2-8B, modified from Weir J, Abrahams PH: *An Imaging Atlas of Human Anatomy*, ed 2, London, 2000, Mosby.

Figure 5-13, Courtesy Dr. Barbara Weissman, Brigham and Women's Hospital, Boston, Massachusetts. From Kumar V, Abbas A, Aster J: *Robbins & Cotran Pathologic Basis of Disease*, ed 9, Philadelphia, 2015, Elsevier.)

Figure 5-15, From Yanoff M, Duker JS: *Ophthalmology*, ed 5, St. Louis, 2019, Elsevier.

Unnumbered Figure 4-3, from Zitelli BJ, Davis HW: *Campbell's Operative Orthopaedics*, ed 4, St. Louis, 2008, Elsevier.

Index

A

AAA (abdominal aortic aneurysm), 221
abbreviations, comprehensive list of, 320–330
  cardiovascular system, 218
  digestive system, 226
  ears/hearing, 281
  endocrine system, 234
  eyes/vision, 280
  female reproductive system, 240
  male reproductive system, 250
  musculoskeletal system, 255
  urinary system, 287
abdomen, 8f, 52f, 53, 54f, 61
  CT scan of, 228
  laparoscopy and, 12, 12f, 18, 18f, 48
  laparotomy and, 12, 12f, 48
  MRI of, 228
  ultrasonography for, 228
abdominal aortic aneurysm (AAA), 221
abdominal cavity, 8f, 52f, 53, 54f
abdominal pain, 191
abdominal x-ray, 190f
abdominocentesis (paracentesis), 308, 322
abdominopevic quadrants, 81f
abdominopelvic regions, 80f
ABG (arterial blood gas), 274
Achilles tendon, 257f, 343
acid reflux, 189, 343
ACL (anterior cruciate ligament), 260
acquired immunodeficiency syndrome (AIDS), 149t, 176, 247–248
acromegaly, 235
acronyms, comprehensive list of, 341–342
ACS (acute coronary syndrome), 221
ACTH (adrenocorticotropic hormone), 138t, 236
acute conditions, 97

Page numbers followed by "*f*" indicate figures, "*t*" indicate tables, and "*s*" indicates spotlights.

acute coronary syndrome (ACS), 221
acute myocardial infarction (AMI), 221
acute myocardial ischemia, 186
acute renal failure (ARF), 289
acute respiratory distress syndrome (ARDS), 149t, 274, 304
AD (Alzheimer disease), 266, 267, 343
adductor magnus, 256f, 257f
adenectomy, 101t
adenitis, 5
adenocarcinoma, 48, 93, 93f
adenoidectomy, 98, 99f, 101t
adenoids, 99f, 101t, 271f, 272
  excision of, 98, 99f, 101t
adenoma, 5, 93
adenopathy, 95t
adjective suffixes, 96–97
adrenal glands, 7f, 48, 234f, 287f
  diseases of, 95t
  hormones of, 138t
  location of, 234f
adrenaline (epinephrine), 138t
adrenocorticotropic hormone (ACTH), 138t, 236
adrenopathy, 95t, 235
AED (automated external defibrillator), 221
AFP (alpha-fetoprotein) tests, 308
AIDS (acquired immunodeficiency syndrome), 10s, 148t, 176, 247
air sacs (alveoli), 271f
alanine transaminase (ALT), 229, 308
albumin tests, 308
albuminuria, 288
alkaline phosphatase tests, 229, 308
allergist, 179t
allergy test, 283, 308
allied health careers, 354–362
alopecia, 282
alpha-fetoprotein (AFP) tests, 308
ALT (alanine transaminase), 229, 308
alveoli (air sacs), 271f

Alzheimer disease (AD), 266, 267, 343
ambulatory electrocardiography. *See* Holter monitoring
amenorrhea, 134, 241
AMI (acute myocardial infarction), 221
amniocentesis, 98, 99f, 242, 308
amnion sac, 88t, 99f, 308
ANA (antinuclear antibody) test, 259, 260, 309
analysis of urine (urinalysis), 135s, 289, 327
anastomoses (anastomosis), 105, 106f, 130, 229
anemia, 19, 48, 134
  case report, 188, 191
  forms of, 134t
  menorrhagia and, 96s
anesthesiologists, 179t
anesthesiology, 178
aneurysm, 219
angina, 186, 219
angiography (angiogram), 102, 220, 309
  cerebral, 267, 309
  cholangiography, 228, 312
  coronary, 124f, 186, 186f, 220
  digital subtraction, 314
  fluorescein, 283, 317
  magnetic resonance, 320
  pulmonary, 273, 324
angioplasty, 104, 104f, 124f, 221
ankylosing spondylitis, 259
anterior, definition of, 58–60, 61, 62t
anterior cruciate ligament (ACL), 260
antiarrhythmic drugs, 186
antibiotics, 136, 176
antibody/antibodies, 64, 135, 176, 185s, 299–305, 299f–304f
anticoagulant drugs, 186
antigen, 135, 176, 298–305, 298f–300f
antigen-presenting cell (APC)/ dendritic, 300, 300f
antihypertensive medications, 195
antinuclear antibody (ANA) tests, 259–260, 309
anuria, 288
anus, 54f, 132, 184f, 226f
aorta, 86, 97f, 150f, 192, 192f, 218f
Apgar score, 341
aphasia, 6s, 134
aplastic anemia, 134t
apnea, 134, 169f
appendectomy, 101, 229
appendicitis, 92t
appendix, 226f
  excision of, 101t
ARDS (acute respiratory distress syndrome), 274
areola, 240f
ARF (acute renal failure), 289
armpit (axillary) lymph nodes, 182, 246f
arrhythmias, 219, 220
  ventricular, 186
arterial blood gas (ABG), 274
arteries, 96, 97f, 97s, 104f, 124f, 218f, 219
arteriography, 309
arterioles, 218f, 219
arteriosclerosis, 96, 97f
arteriovenous fistula, 195, 195f
arthralgia, 16, 90
arthritis, 5
  ankylosing spondylitis, 259
  gouty, 259
  osteoarthritis, 13, 13f, 43f, 185s
  rheumatoid, 185, 185f, 185s, 259
arthrocentesis, 98, 259, 309
arthrography/arthrogram, 16, 259, 309
arthroplasty, 260
arthroscopy, 18, 138t, 259
  of knee, 40f
  of shoulder, 19f
ascites, 54s, 64, 65f
aspartate transaminase (AST) test, 229, 309
Asperger syndrome, 333
asphyxia, 273
aspiration, 242, 309
AST (aspartate transaminase) test, 229, 309
asthma, 273
atelectasis, 273
atheroma, 96, 96f
atherosclerosis, 96, 97f, 219
atherosclerotic aorta, 97f
atrophy, 134, 140, 140f, 185f
  of bone, 185f
audiologist, 354
audiometry, 309
auditory canal, 281f
auditory nerve, 281f
auras, with migraines, 196
auscultation, 309
autoimmune diseases
  antibodies and, 185s
  Sjögren syndrome, 345
automated external defibrillator (AED), 221
autopsy, 14, 19, 216
  images of brain, 124f
axial (transverse) plane, 58f, 59, 59f, 60f, 73f, 86
  MRIs of, 60f
axilla (underarm), 240f
axillary, 97, 182
axillary (armpit) lymph nodes, 182, 246f

back, structures of, 56, 55f -56f
backbone, 54, 54f
bacteremia, 90s
bacterial tests, 283, 309
baldness, 282
balloon angioplasty, 104, 104f, 221
bariatric surgery, 122, 122f
barium, 191
barium enema (BE), 228, 229, 309, 320
barium swallow, 191, 228, 309
barium tests, 228, 310
Barlow syndrome, 343
Barrett esophagus, 343
basophil, 9f
BE (barium enema), 228, 229, 309, 320
Bell palsy, 343
Bence Jones protein test, 310
benign prostatic hyperplasia (BPH), 140, 149, 251, 252
  treatment for (TURP), 21, 21s, 21f

benign tumors, 93, 94f, 130, 142s, 188, 188f. *See also* cancer/malignant tumors
biceps brachii, 256f–257f
biceps femoris, 257f
bilateral oophorectomy, 100f, 130
bile emulsification, 108
bilirubin, 228–229
bilirubin tests, 229, 310
biology, 5
biopsy, 5, 14, 17, 216, 242, 310
  bone marrow, 311
  muscle, 259, 321
  skin, 283, 325
  stereotactic breast, 320
  types of, 310
bladder, urinary, 7, 7f, 21f, 54, 54f, 135f, 184f, 250f, 287f
blood, 11
  circulation of, 218f
  infections of, 90
  travel (heart), 149, 150f
  urea in, 96, 96f
  in urine, 96s
  withdrawing, 107, 107f, 322
blood bank technologists, 354
blood cells, 9, 9f
blood chemistry profile, 310
blood cultures, 310
blood differential tests, 310
blood pressure (hypertension), 140, 145s, 219, 221
blood sugar, 20, 20s, 22
blood urea nitrogen (BUN), 288, 310
blood vessels, 6, 86, 89, 186, 279f
  dilation of, 196
body cavities, 52f, 53
  abdominal, 8f, 52f, 53, 54f, 55
  cranial, 6f, 52f, 53
  thoracic, 53, 52f, 53f
  pelvic, 52f, 54, 255f
  spinal, 52f, 54, 56f, 86
body planes, 58–61, 58f, 59f, 60f
body systems
  definition of, 50
  groups of cells, tissues, organs, and, 50f
  overview of, 50–51
bolus, food, 65f
bone density test (DEXA), 259, 260, 311
bone marrow, 89, 258, 299
  biopsy, 311
  inflammation of, 92t
  malignant tumor of, 94t
  multiple myeloma, 93, 94t, 130
bone scan, 259, 311
bones. *See also* musculoskeletal system
  cancer of, 94t
  carpal, 142, 143f, 255f
  diseases of, 95t
  finger, 143f, 255f
  fracture of, 143f, 194, 194f, 259, 260
  metacarpal, 142, 143f, 255f
  of middle ear, 281f
  of the body, 235f
  of spinal column, 52f, 54, 56, 56f, 86
Paget disease and, 345
BP (blood pressure), 140, 145s, 219, 221
BPH (benign prostatic hyperplasia), 140, 149, 251, 252
  treatment for (TURP), 21, 21s, 21f
brachialis, 256f–257f
brachioradialis, 257f
brain, 6, 6f, 9, 266
  Alzheimer disease and, 266, 267, 343
  anatomy of, 265f
  concussion and, 266
  CTE (chronic traumatic encephalopathy), 95, 124f
  disease condition of, 95, 124f
  epilepsy and, 266
  glioblastoma and, 266
  Reye syndrome and, 345
  surrounding anatomy and structures of, 92
  syncope and, 266
brain scan, 311
breast bone, 52f
breast cancer, 102f, 176
  metastasis of, 142f
  breast, 89, 240f, 241
  anatomy of, 240f
  aspiration of, 242
  mammography of, 102, 102f, 242, 308
  stereotactic biopsy of, 320
bronchial tubes, 53f, 61, 86, 88, 91, 271f, 272
bronchioles, 271f, 272
bronchitis, 91, 273
bronchoscope, 82f
bronchoscopy, 61, 82f, 138t, 272, 311
buccinator, 257f
BUN (blood urea nitrogen), 288, 289, 310
Burkitt lymphoma, 343
bursitis, 92t

CA-125 tests, 311
CABG (coronary artery bypass grafting), 220–221
CAD (coronary artery disease), 221
calcium (Ca), 260
calcium levels, 259
calcium tests, 311
calculus/calculi
  renal, 190, 190f
callus formation, 194, 194f
cancer/malignant tumors
  adenocarcinoma, 48, 93, 93f
  adenoma, 5, 93
  benign tumors compared to, 142s
  of bones, 94t
  breast, 89, 102f, 142f, 176, 240f, 241
  Burkitt lymphoma, 343
  carcinoma, 5, 17, 48, 93, 94t, 102f, 192, 192f, 228
  chemotherapy for, 105, 189, 248
  chondroma, 62, 258
  chondrosarcoma, 62, 94t
  diagnosis of lung cancer, case study, 79, 192, 192f
  Ewing sarcoma, 344
  fibrosarcoma, 94t
  glioblastoma, 266
  hepatoma, 94t
  Hodgkin lymphoma, 189, 189f, 247–248
  Kaposi sarcoma, 344
  leiomyomas, 94t
  leiomyosarcoma, 94t, 258
  leukemia, 16, 41, 41f, 48, 95s, 328
    case study, 38

cancer/malignant tumors *(Continued)*
liposarcoma, 94t
lung, 53f, 192, 192f
lymphoma, 94t, 189, 247–248
melanoma, 94t, 283
mesothelioma, 94t
metastasis of, 142, 142f, 176
multiple myeloma, 93, 94t, 248
myosarcoma, 93, 130
names without carcin/o and sarc/o, 94t
non-Hodgkin lymphoma, 248
osteogenic sarcoma, 94t
osteosarcomas, 15f, 48
primary, 176
prostatic carcinoma, 251
radiotherapy for, 105s, 184, 184f, 189, 248
rhabdomyosarcoma, 92t
sarcoma, 14, 15f, 48, 66s, 94t
seminoma, 251
testicular carcinoma, 251
thymoma, 94t
Wilms tumor, 346
CAPD (continuous ambulatory peritoneal dialysis), 289
carbon dioxide (CO_2), 272
carbon dioxide test, 311
carcinoembryonic antigen (CEA) test, 312
carcinomas, 5, 14, 15f, 16, 48, 93, 93f, 102f, 192, 192f, 228, 229, 251
hepatocellular, 16, 94t, 229
prostatic, 251
testicular, 251
cardiac (coronary) care unit (CCU), 186, 221
cardiac catheter ablation, 220
cardiac catheterization, 220, 312
cardiac enzyme tests, 220, 312
cardiologists, 179t, 216
cardiology, 5, 17t
case report for, 186–187
cardiomyopathy, 95, 95s
cardiopulmonary resuscitation (CPR), 221, 274
cardiovascular surgeons, 179t, 216
cardiovascular system, 218–221
abbreviations for, 221
anatomy of, 218, 218f
diagnostic procedures and laboratory tests for, 220
pathology of, 219
terminology of, 219
treatment procedures for, 220–221
cardiovascular technician, 356
cardioversion, 220
carpal bones, 142, 143f, 255f
carpal tunnel syndrome, 149t, 176, 259
cartilage, 13, 13f, 14, 56, 56f, 62, 258
arthritis and, 13, 13f, 185, 185f
cancer of, 14, 62, 94t
of ribs, 80f
thyroid, 66f, 107f, 140f
tracheal and laryngeal, 66f
cataract, 282, 321
catheterization, 312
cardiac, 220, 312
urinary, 289
catheter
cardiac, 104f
Foley, 312, 344
intra-abdominal, 289
intravenous feeding and, 169f
nephrostomy and, 182, 182f
peritoneal dialysis and, 103f
cauda equine, 64f, 265f
cauterization, 242
cavities. *See* body cavities
CBC (complete blood count), 313
CCU (cardiac care unit), 186, 221
CEA (carcinoembryonic antigen) tests, 312
cecostomy, 106f
cells, 50, 50f
cellulitis, 92t
central nervous system (CNS), 265f, 267
cephalgia, unilateral frontal, 196
cephalic, definition of, 6
cerebellum, 6f, 265f, 266
cerebral, definition of, 6
cerebral angiography, 267, 309
cerebrospinal fluid (CSF)
analysis of, 267, 312
lumbar puncture and, 64f
cerebrovascular accident (CVA), 6, 6s, 73f, 96, 116, 130, 266, 267
cerebrum, 6, 6f, 265f, 266
cervical, definition of, 62
cervical (neck) lymph nodes, 182, 246f
cervical nerves, 265f
cervical spine, 56, 86
cervical vertebra, 56, 56f, 255f, 260
cervix, 62, 63f, 100f, 240f, 241
cauterization of, 242
conization of, 242, 313
Cesarean section (CS), 243
chemotherapy, 105, 189, 248
chest x-rays, 59, 59f, 192, 192f, 273, 312
Cheyne-Stokes respiration, 343
CHF (congestive heart failure), 219, 221
chiropractor, 354
chlamydial infection, 251
cholangiography, 228, 312. *See also* endoscopic retrograde cholangiography
cholecystectomy, laparoscopic, 100, 101f, 108, 130, 229
cholelithiasis, 228
cholesterol tests, 312–313
chondroma, 62
chondrosarcoma, 62, 94t
chorionic villus sampling, 313
chronic bronchitis, 273
chronic conditions, 97
chronic kidney disease (CKD), 289
chronic obstructive pulmonary disease (COPD), 273–274
chronic renal failure, 195
chronic traumatic encephalopathy (CTE), 95, 124, 124f

circulatory system, 50, 218–221, 218f
cirrhosis, 228
CK (creatine kinase) test, 313
CKD (chronic kidney disease), 289
clavicle (collarbone), 148f, 255f
clinical laboratory technologist (CLT), 355
CLT (clinical laboratory technologist), 355
CNS (central nervous system), 265f, 267
CO_2 (carbon dioxide), 274
  blood test measuring, 311
coccygeal, definition of, 62
coccygeal nerve, 265f
coccygeal division (section) of spine, 56, 56f, 86
cochlea, 281f
colectomy, 101t
colitis, ulcerative, 181, 181s, 228, 229
collarbone (clavicle), 148f, 255f
Colles fracture, 343
colocolostomy, 105
colon, 8f, 9, 54f, 181, 226f, 227
  excision of, 101t
  polyposis of, 228
  polyp in, 204f
  stomas of, 106f
colonoscopy, 138t, 170, 170f, 228, 312
  polyps found during, 145, 204f
colorectal surgeons, 179t
colostomy, 105, 106f, 229
colposcopy, 242, 312
combining forms, 3–4
  definition of, 3
  for medical specialists, 181–186
combining vowels, 2–3
common bile duct, 101f
complete blood count (CBC), 313
computed tomography (CT scan), 59, 59f, 192f, 313
  abdominal, 228
  definition of, 313
  description of procedure, 67
  for endocrine system, 236
  for lymphatic system, 247
computed tomography (CT scan) *(Continued)*
  of brain, 7ef
  of nervous system, 267
  for respiratory system, 273
concussion, 266
congenital anomaly, 136
  webbed toes as example of, 136f
  polyactyly as example of, 168f
congestive heart failure (CHF), 219, 221
conization, 242, 312
conjunctiva, 280f, 282
conjunctivitis, 282
continuous ambulatory peritoneal dialysis (CAPD), 289
continuous positive airway pressure (CPAP), 169, 169f, 274
COPD (chronic obstructive pulmonary disease), 273–274
core biopsy, 310
cornea, 280f
coronal (frontal) plane, 58, 58f, 59f, 60f, 86
  MRIs of, 60f
coronary, 97
coronary angiography, 186, 186f, 309
coronary arteriography, 309
coronary artery, 90, 90f, 97, 97s
  angiography of, 124f, 186, 186f
  angioplasty and, 104, 104f
  atherosclerosis and, 90s
  ischemia of, 90f, 124f, 186, 186f
  occlusion of, 90f, 124f
coronary artery bypass grafting (CABG), 220–221
coronary artery disease (CAD), 220
coronary artery spasm, 186, 186f
coronavirus, 11s, 11f, 149t
  asymptomatic transmission of, 149s
  COVID-19 and, 11, 39, 141, 149t, 302, 302f
  electron micrograph of, 11f
  hypoxia and, 141s
  pneumonia and, 91, 91f
coronavirus *(Continued)*
  spike proteins and, 11f, 302, 302f, 304
  vaccines for, 302–306, 302f–305f
coroner, 14s
cortisol, 235
COVID-19, 11s, 11f, 20
  asymptomatic transmission of, 149s
  case study of, 39
  fever and, 39
  hypoxia and, 141s
  pneumonia and, 91, 91f
  vaccines and, 302–306, 302f–305f
CPAP (continuous positive airway pressure), 169, 169f, 274
CPR (cardiopulmonary resuscitation), 221, 274
cranial cavity, 6f, 52f, 53, 55
cranial nerves, 265f
cranium, 255f
creatine kinase (CK) test, 313
creatinine clearance test, 313
creatinine tests, 289, 314
Crohn disease, 181s, 197–198, 228, 229
cross section, 59, 86
cryosurgery, 242
cryotherapy, 105
cryptorchism, 251
CS (Cesarean section), 243
CSF (cerebrospinal fluid) analysis, 267, 312
CST (surgical technologist), 362
CT. *See* computed tomography
culdocentesis, 314
culture, 314
Cushing syndrome, 235, 343
cuticle, 279f
CVA (cerebrovascular accident), 6, 6s, 73f, 96, 116, 130, 266, 267
CyberKnife, 267
cystography, 314
cystoscopy, 7, 7f
cystoscopy, 7, 138t, 288, 314
cytology, 8

D&C (dilation and curettage), 242–243, 315

deep, definition of, 62f
deep vein thrombosis, 41, 41f
venography and, 328
defibrillation, 220
degenerative disorders
Huntington disease, 344
osteoarthritiis, 13, 13f, 185s
Parkinson disease, 345
Tay-Sachs disease, 345
degenerative joint disease (DJD), 260
delayed-onset muscle soreness (DOMS), 260
deltoid, 256f–257f
delusions, 14
dementia, irreversible, 266
dental assistant, 355
dental hygienist, 355
dental laboratory technician, 355
dental specialists, 183s, 355
dermal, 8
dermatitis, 8, 92t
dermatologists, 179t
dermatology, 17t, 178
dermis, 139, 279f, 282
DEXA (dual-energy x-ray abdorptiometry; bone density test), 259, 260, 311
diabetes mellitus (DM), 20, 235
insulin pump and, 193f
glucose test for, 236, 318
glycosuria and, 135s
hyperglycemia and, 20, 20s, 140
insulin and, 140, 235
insulin pump and, 193f
living with type, 1, 22–23
pancreas and, 20s
polydipsia and, 145, 193
polyuria and, 145, 193
type, 1, 20, 20s, 22–23, 193, 235
type, 2, 2, 20, 20s, 235
diagnosis, 10, 19, 48
of acute migraine case, 196
of fibroids in uterus case, 121, 188, 188f
of Hodgkin lymphoma case, 189, 189f
of leukemia case, 38
of lung cancer case, 79, 192, 192f
of osteoarthritis, 42, 42f
of toxic shock syndrome case, 166
diagnostic medical sonographer, 356
diagnostic suffixes, 89–96
dialysis, 103, 103f, 130, 289
hemodialysis, 103, 123f, 130, 195
peritonieal, 103, 103f, 130
diameter, 19
diaphragm, 8f, 52f, 53, 53f, 55, 271f, 272, 328f
diarrhea, 136, 136s, 181s, 197
dietitian, 356
digestive system, 51, 226–233
abbreviations for, 229
anatomy of, 226, 226f
definition and role of, 51
diagnostic procedures and laboratory tests for, 228–229
pathology of, 228
terminology of, 227
treatment procedures for, 229
digital rectal examination (DRE), 251, 312
digital subtraction angiography, 314
dilation, of blood vessels, 196
dilation and curettage (D&C), 242–243, 315
discectomy, microscopic, 260
disease conditions (-pathies), 95t
discs, 56, 56f, 57f
herniated (L4-L5), 57f
distal, definition of, 62t
diuretics, 145s, 186
diverticula, 228
diverticulitis, 228
diverticulosis, 228
DJD (degenerative joint disease), 260
DM. *See* diabetes mellitus
DOMS (delayed-onset muscle soreness), 260
Doppler ultrasound, 220–315
double membranes, 54s, 86
Down syndrome, 149t
DRE (digital rectal examination), 251, 312
drug-eluting stents, 104f
drugs, reference guide for top 50 prescribed, 350t–352t
dual-energy x-ray abdorptiometry (bone density test; DEXA), 259, 260, 311
DUB (dysfunctional uterine bleeding), 243
Duchenne muscular dystrophy, 344
Duodenum, 8f, 122f, 226f
dura mater, 92f, 132t, 139f
dysentery, 19
dysfunctional uterine bleeding (DUB), 243
dysmenorrhea, 137, 188, 241
dyspepsia, 191
dysuria, 137, 190, 288

eardrum, 281, 281f, 282
ears, nose, throat (ENT), 283
ears/hearing
anatomy of, 281f
audiologist for, 354
Ménière disease and, 345
Rinne tests for, 345
tinnitus of, 283
tuning fork tests and, 283, 327
ECG. *See* electrocardiogram
ECG technician, 356
Echocardiography, 220–221, 315
ectopic pregnancy, 137, 137f, 241
EEG. *See* electroencephalogram
EGD (esophagogastro-duodenoscopy), 316
ejaculation, 7
electrocardiogram (ECG), 8, 186, 220, 221, 315
electroencephalogram, 9, 123f
electroencephalography (EEG), 102, 123, 123f, 267, 315
electrolyte panel, 315
electrolytes, 236, 315
electromyography (EMG), 259, 260, 315
electrophoresis (serum protein electrophoresis), 324
ELISA (enzyme-linked immunosorbent assay), 247–248, 316

embryos, 240f
emergency medical technician (EMT), 356
emergency medicine, 178
emergency practitioners, 179t
EMG (electromyography), 259–260, 315
emphysema, 273
EMTs (emergency medical technician), 356
endarterectomy, 221
endocarditis, 92t
endocardium, 20
endocrine glands, 20, 48, 138, 145f, 234f
  adrenal glands as, 135f
  major types of, 138t
endocrine system, 51, 234–239
  abbreviations for, 236
  anatomy of, 234, 234f
  definition and role of, 51
  diagnostic procedures and laboratory tests for, 236
  pathology of, 235–236
  terminology of, 235
endocrinologists, 179t
endocrinology, 17t
  case report for, 193
endodontists, 183s
endometriosis, 241
endometrium, 241
endoscopic retrograde cholangiography (ERCP), 228–229, 316
endoscopic ultrasonography (E-US), 228, 316
endoscopy, 316
  gastrointestinal, 10, 10f, 229, 318
  of the colon, 170f
  types of, 138t, 316
endotracheal intubation, 274
endotracheal tubes, 144f
ENT (ears, nose, throat), 283
enteritis, 9, 181
enzyme-linked immunosorbent assay (ELISA), 247–248, 316
eosinophil, 9
epidemic, 20
epidermis, 139, 279f
epidural hematoma, 139, 139f
epigastric, 20, 80f
epiglottis, 65f, 65s, 99f, 107f
epiglottitis, 92t
epilepsy, 266
epinephrine (adrenaline), 138t
epithelial, 63, 93
eponyms, comprehensive list of, 343–346
Epstein-Barr virus, 344
ERCP (endoscopic retrograde cholangiography), 228–229, 316
erythrocyte sedimentation rate (ESR), 259–260, 316
erythrocytes (red blood cells), 9, 9f, 40f, 48, 259, 316, 324
erythrocytosis, 95
erythromycin, 136
esophagogastroduodenoscopy (EGD), 316
esophagogastroscopy, 138t
esophagography, 316
esophagoscopy, 228, 316
esophagus, 8f, 53f, 63, 65f, 86, 145f, 226f
  abnormal changes in lining of, 343
  adenocarcinoma of, 93, 93f
  definition of, 86
ESR (erythrocyte sedimentation rate), 259–260, 316
estradiol assays, 316
estrogen, 138t
estrogen receptor assays, 317
ESWL (extracorporeal shock wave lithotripsy), 190, 190f, 289
ETTs (exercise tolerance tests), 220, 325, 326
E-US (endoscopic ultrasonography), 228, 316
eustachian tube, 281f, 344
Ewing sarcoma, 344
exacerbation, definition of, 147
excision procedures, 101t
excisional biopsy, 317
exercise tolerance tests (ETTs), 220, 325, 326
exocrine glands, 20, 48
exophthalmic goiter, 236
exophthalmometry, 236, 317
exophthalmos, 236
exploratory laparotomy, 12, 12f
external oblique, 256f, 257f
extracorporeal shock wave lithotripsy (ESWL), 190, 190f, 289
eye care professionals
  ophthalmologists, 13, 13f, 179, 183
  opticians, 183
  optometrists, 183
eyes/vision
  anatomy of, 280f
  cataracts and, 282
  conjunctivitis and, 282
  exophthalmic goiter and, 236
  exophthalmometry and, 236, 317
  fluorescein angiography and, 283, 317
  glaucoma and, 282
  ophthalmic professionals for, 359
  ophthalmologists fort, 13, 13f, 179
  ophthalmology for, 17t, 178
  ophthalmoscope and, 13, 13f
  ophthalmoscopy for, 283, 321
  path of light through, 280f
  retinopathy of, 95t
  scotomas and, 196, 196f
  slit-lamp microscopy and, 283, 325
  stye of, 283
  visual acuity, 283

facial nerve paralysis, 343
fainting, 266
fallopian tubes, 89t, 240f, 241, 344
  ectopic pregnancy and, 137f, 214
  salpingectomy and, 100f
  salpingitis and, 241, 243
  tubal ligation and, 18f
family practitioners, 179t
fasting blood sugar (glucose) tests, 236, 318
fatty tissue, cancer of, 94t
fecal transplant, 136, 136s
feces, 136, 136s, 229
fellowship training, 178
female reproductive system
  abbreviations for, 243
  anatomy of, 240, 240f
  definition and role of, 51
  diagnostic procedures and laboratory tests for, 242
  pathology of, 241
  terminology of, 241
  treatment procedures for, 242
femur, 194, 194f, 255f
fetus, 10s, 99f, 149, 150f, 240f, 242
fibrillation, 219
fibroids, uterine, 93, 94f, 96s, 101t, 188, 188f, 241–242
  case study of, 121

fibrosarcomas, 94t
fibrous tissue, cancer of, 94t
fibula, 194, 194f, 255f
finger bones (phalanges), 143f, 255f
fingers
  RA and, 185f
fixation, of fractures, 194
fluorescein angiography, 283, 317
fluoroscopy, 317
flutter, 219
Foley catheters, 312, 344
follicle-stimulating hormone (FSH), 138t
food bolus, 65f
food tube. *See* esophagus
forceps, 18f
fracture (Fx), 259, 260
  callus formation in, 194f
  Colles, 343
  fixation of, 194
  of metacarpal, 143f
  of fibula, 194, 194f
frontal (coronal) plane, 58, 58f, 59f, 60f, 86
  MRIs of, 60f
frozen section technique, 317
FSH (follicle-stimulating hormone), 138t
fungal tests, 283, 309
Fx (fracture), 259, 260

G

gallbladder (GB), 8f, 101f, 226f, 227
  removal of, 100, 101f, 108, 130, 229
  stones in, 108, 130, 228
  ultrasound of, 317
gallium scans, 317
gangrene, 95, 125f
gastrectomy, 16, 101t
  laparoscopic sleeve, 104, 122f, 319
  peptic ulcer and, 191
gastric, definition of, 15
gastric (peptic) ulcers, 191, 191f, 228
gastritis, 92t
gastrocnemius, 256f–257f
gastroenteritis, 16
gastroenterologists, 179t
gastroenterology, 17t
  case report for, 191, 191f
gastroesophageal reflux disease (GERD), 228–229
gastrointestinal (GI), 227
  test, lower GI, 320
  test, upper GI, 327
gastrointestinal endoscopy, 229
gastroscope (endoscope), 10, 10f, 18
gastroscopy, 10, 10f, 18, 191, 318
GB. *See* gallbladder
GERD (gastroesophageal reflux disease), 228–229
geriatricians, 179t
GFR (glomerular filtration rate), 289
GH (growth hormone), 138t, 236
GI (gastrointestinal), 227
  test, lower GI, 320
  test, upper GI, 327
Giardia, 344
glands, excision of, 101t
glaucoma, 282
glial cells, 266
glioblastoma, 266
glomerular filtration rate (GFR), 289
glucometer, 22–23
glucose (fasting blood sugar) tests, 236, 318
glucose tolerance tests (GTTs), 236, 318
gluteus maximus, 257f
gluteus medius, 256f
glycosuria, 288
goiter, 236
gonorrhea, 251, 345
gouty arthritis (gout), 259
  uric acid levels and, 259, 328
gracilis, 254f–255f
Graves disease (hyperthyroidism), 16, 140, 140f, 165–166, 236
  exophthalmos and, 17f
GreenLight PVP (photoselective vaporization of prostate), 252
groin (inguinal) lymph nodes, 182, 246f
growth hormone (GH), 138t, 236
GTTs (glucose tolerance tests), 236, 318
gynecologists, 179t, 216
gynecology (GYN), 10, 10s, 17t, 216, 243
  case report for, 188, 188f

HAART (highly active antiretroviral therapy), 248
hair
  alopecia and, 282
  fiber, 279f
  follicle, 279f
  melanocytes, 279f
  root, 279f
hallucinations, 14
hand
  bones of, 255f
  RA and, 195f, 259
  x-ray of, 143f
HbA1c (hemoglobin A1c), 236
HCC (hepatocellular cardinoma), 94t, 228, 229
HCG (human chorionic gonadotropin), 242, 318, 323
Hct (hematocrit), 318
HD. *See* hemodialysis
HDL (high-density lipoprotein), 220, 221, 312–313
head, 6, 139f
head, eyes, ears, nose, throat (HEENT), 283
headaches, migraine, 196
health information administrator (HIA), 357
health information technician (HIT), 357
heart, 218f, 219–221
  congestive heart failure, 219, 221
  ischemia of, 90, 90f, 85s, 96, 97s, 124f, 130, 186, 186f
  occlusions of, 90f
  transplantation, 221
  tricuspid and mitral valves of, 149, 150f
heart attack (myocardial infarction), 90, 95s, 96, 97s, 116, 130, 186, 219, 220–221

HEENT (head, eyes, ears, nose, throat), 283
hematemesis, 191
hematocrit (Hct), 318
hematologist, 179t, 216
hematology, 2, 17t
hematoma, 11, 11f
epidural and subdural, 139, 139f
hematuria, 96, 96s, 116, 135s, 190, 288
hemigastrectomy, 139
hemiplegia, 139, 176, 266
hemoccult test, 229, 318
hemodialysis (HD), 103, 123f, 130, 195, 289
arteriovenous fistula for, 195, 195f
hemoglobin, 11, 16
hemoglobin A1c (HbA1c), 236
hemoglobin assay, 318
hemolytic anemia, 134t
hemoptysis, 273
hemothorax, 273
hepatitis, 11, 92t, 228
hepatocellular carcinoma (HCC), 16, 94t, 228, 229
hepatoma (hepatocellular carcinoma), 16, 94t
hepatopathy, 95t
herniated intervertebral disc, 56, 57f, 260
herpes genitalis, 251
HIA (health information administrator), 357
high blood pressure. *See* hypertension
high-density lipoprotein (HDL), 220, 221, 312–313
highly active antiretroviral therapy (HAART), 248
hilum, 192, 192f
hip bone, 184f
HIT (health information technician), 357
HIV (human immunodeficiency virus), 247–248
viral load test for, 328
Hodgkin lymphoma, 189, 247, 344
holter monitoring, 229, 318
home health aide, 357
hordeolum, 283
hormone replacement therapy (HRT), 243
hormones, 236
secretion of, 48, 234f
endocrine glands and, 138
Horner syndrome, 344
Hospitalists, 179t
HRT (hormone replacement therapy), 243
human chorionic gonadotropin (HCG), 242, 318, 323
human immunodeficiency virus (HIV), 247–248
viral load test for, 328
humerus, 148f, 255f
Huntington disease, 344
hydrocele, 251
hyperbilirubinemia, 228
hyperglycemia, 20, 20s, 140, 235, 318
hyperplasia, 140, 140f
hypertension (high blood pressure), 140, 145s, 186, 196, 219, 221
hyperthyroidism (Graves disease), 16, 17f, 140, 140f, 165–166, 236
hypertrophy, 140, 140f
hypoglycemia, 20, 23, 141
hypothalamus, 236
hypoxia, 141, 141s
hysterectomy, 100, 100f, 188, 241–242
hysterosalpingography, 242, 319
hysteroscopy, 138t, 319

I

iatrogenic, definition of, 182
IBD (inflammatory bowel disease), 181s, 228, 229
IBS (irritable bowel syndrome), 228–229
ICD (implantable cardioverter-defibrillator), 221
ileostomy, 106f, 229
ileum, 8f, 226f, 229
stomas of, 108f
ilium, 255f
IM (intramuscular), 260
immunoassays, 319
immunoglobulin test, 319
immunoglobulins, 136s, 248, 299, 299f
immunohistochemistry, 319
implantable cardioverter-defibrillator (ICD), 221
in vitro fertilization (IVF), 243
incisional biopsy, 319
infarct, 73f, 219
infarction, 96. *See also* myocardial infarction
infections
blood, 90
chlamydial, 251
nosocomial, 183
sexually transmitted, 243, 251
urinary tract, 137
infectious disease specialists, 179t
inferior, definition of, 62t
inflammation/inflammatory conditions, 91, 92t
Crohn disease, 181s, 197–198, 228, 343
gouty arthritis, 259
inflammatory bowel disease, 181s, 228, 229
of meninges, 266
PID, 241, 243
RA, 185s, 185f, 259
sarcoidosis, 247
inflammatory bowel disease (IBD), 181s, 228, 229
inguinal lymph nodes, 246f
inguinal (groin) lymph nodes, 182
insulin, 20, 20s, 22–23, 138t, 140, 141, 235
insulin pump, 22, 193, 193f
intensive care units, 143s
internal medicine, 178
internists, 178, 178t
intervenous urography, 328
intervertebral discs, 56f, 141
intra-abdominal catheter, 289
intra-abdominal injuries, 194
intracoronary artery stents, 104f, 124f
intramural masses, 94f
intramuscular (IM), 260
intrauterine, 141
intravenous (IV), 141, 141f, 169f
intravenous pyelography (IVP), 328
intravenous urography, 328
iris, 280f
iron deficiency anemia, 134t

irreversible dementia, 266
irritable bowel syndrome (IBS), 228–229
ischemia, 90, 90f, 95–96, 130
  acute myocardial, 186, 186f
  coronary artery and, 90f, 124f
  gangrene and, 125f
  Raynaud phenomenon and, 345
ischium, 255f
IV (intravenous), 141, 141f, 169f
IVF (in vitro fertilization), 243
IVP (intravenous pyelography, urography), 328

J

jaundice, 228–229
jejunum, 8f, 122f, 226f, 227
joint, 5, 255f, 258
  arthritis and, 13, 13f, 185, 185f, 185s
  arthroplasty of, 147f, 151, 260
  degenerative disorders of, 13, 13f, 185, 185f
  hip, 42, 42f, 147f
  knee, 13, 13f, 147, 147f, 151
  RA and, 185s, 185
  shoulder, 19f
  subluxation of, 185f

K

K^+ (potassium), 236, 315, 323
Kaposi sarcoma, 149t, 344
keyhole surgery, 229
kidney, 7f, 14, 54f, 287f
  adrenal glands and, 135f
  anatomy of, 287f
  dialysis procedures for, 103, 103f, 123f, 289
  failure of, 288
  nephrostomy and, 182, 182f
  stones in, 190f
  transplantation of, 289
  Wilms tumor of, 346
  x-ray of, 190f
kidneys, ureters, bladder (KUB) x-rays, 288, 289, 319
knee joint
  arthroscopy of, 40, 40f
  osteoarthritis of, 13, 13f
  total replacement of, 146, 147f, 151
KUB (kidneys, ureters, bladder) x-ray, 288, 289, 319

laminectomy, 101t, 260
laparoscopic appendectomy
laparoscope, 12, 2f, 18f, 319
laparoscopic appendectomy, 229
laparoscopic cholecystectomy, 100, 101f, 108, 130, 229
laparoscopic oophorectomy, 100, 100f, 130
laparoscopic sleeve gastrectomy, 104, 122, 122f, 319
laparoscopic surgery, 229
laparoscopy, 12, 12f, 138t, 229, 319
  definition of, 46, 229
  for tubal ligation, 18f
laparotomy, 12, 12f, 48
large intestine, 8f, 9, 54f, 181, 226f
laryngectomy, 63, 107f
laryngoscopy, 104, 105f, 138t, 273, 320
larynx, 53f, 63, 105f, 107f
  cartilage of, 66f
  definition of, 63, 86
  location of, 63, 86, 271
lateral
  definition of, 62t
  view, 192, 192f
lateral (sagittal) plane, 59, 59f, 60f, 86
  MRIs of, 60f
latissimus dorsi, 256f, 257f
LDL (low-density lipoprotein), 220–221, 312–313
left atrium, 150f, 218f
left ventricle, 150f, 218f
leg prosthesis, 146, 146f, 168f
leiomyoma (fibroid), 93, 94f, 96s, 101t, 188, 188f, 241
leiomyosarcoma, 94t, 258
lens, 280f
leukemia, 16, 41f, 48, 90
  diagnosis case study for, 36
  leukocytosis compared to, 95s
leukocytes, 9f, 12, 16, 41f
  immunity and, 298, 298f
  leukemia and, 90
  tonsillitis and, 99f
  white blood cell (WBC) count test, 328
leukocytosis, 17, 48, 95, 116
  leukemia compared to, 95s
levator scapulae, 256f
LFTs (liver function tests), 229, 230. *See also* alanine transaminase; alkaline phosphatase tests; aspartate transaminase tests; bilirubin
licensed practical nurse (LPN), 357
lipid tests, 220, 320
lipoprotein tests, 220. *See also* cholesterol tests
liposarcoma, 94t
lithotripsy, 190, 190f, 289
liver, 8f, 11, 54f, 63, 65f, 226f
  bile production of, 101f, 108
  cirrhosis of, 228
  diseases of, 95t
  hepatitis of, 11, 92t, 228
  malignant tumor of, 94t
liver function tests (LFTs), 229. *See also* alanine transaminase; alkaline phosphatase tests; aspartate transaminase tests; bilirubin
lobectomy, 274
low-density lipoprotein (LDL), 220–221, 312–313
lower gastrointestinal examination, 320
LPN (licensed practical nurse), 357
lumbar nerves, 265f
lumbar puncture (spinal tap), 64, 64f, 267, 320
lumbar section of spine, 56, 56f, 64, 64f, 86, 255f
lumbar vertebra, 255f, 260
lung capillaries, 218f

lungs, 8f, 53f, 271f
  blood travel to, 150f
  cancer of, 192
collapsed (atelectasis), 273
  CT scab of, 192f
  diagnosis of cancer in, case study, 79
removal of, 274
  x-ray of carcinoma in, 192f
  x-ray of pneumonia compared to normal, 91f
lunula, 279
lymph, 50, 98
lymph nodes, 86, 182, 240f
  anatomy of, 246f
  diseases of, 95t
  malignant tumor of, 94t, 247, 343t
lymph vessels, 246f
lymphadenopathy, 95t, 182, 187
lymphatic system
  abbreviations for, 248
anatomy of, 246, 246f
  definition and role of, 50
  diagnostic procedures and laboratory tests for, 247
  pathology of, 247
  terminology of, 247
  treatment procedures for, 247
lymphedema, 247
lymphocytes, 9f, 64, 299, 299f
  AIDS and, 149t, 247
  B cell and T cell, 64, 299, 299f, 300f, 301, 304, 304f, 305t
  immunity and, 64, 299, 299f
  lymph and, 246f
  mononucleosis and, 247
  spleen and, 246f
lymphoma, 94t
  Burkitt, 343
  definition of, 247
  Hodgkin, 189, 247, 248
  non-Hodgkin, 248

M

MAC (*Mycobacterium avium* complex), 248
magnetic resonance angiography (MRA), 308
magnetic resonance imaging (MRI), 60, 60f, 61f, 220
  abdominal, 228
  definition of, 320
  description of procedure, 67
  for endocrine system, 236
  for nervous system, 267
  for respiratory system, 273
mediastinal masses and, 289f
of herniated disc, 57f
of upper body, 189f
male reproductive system
  abbreviations for, 252
  anatomy of, 250, 250f
  definition and role of, 51
  diagnostic procedures and laboratory tests for, 251
  pathology of, 251
  terminology of, 251
  treatment procedures for, 252
malignant tumors, benign compared to, 142s. *See also* cancer/malignant tumors
mammary papilla, 240f
mammography (mammogram), 102, 102f, 242, 320
  tomosynthesis and, 102, 102f
Marfan syndrome, 344
masseter, 257f
MDI (metered-dose inhaler), 274
M.E. *See* medical examiner
medial, definition of, 62t
medial malleolus, 255f
mediastinal lymph nodes, 182, 246f
mediastinal structures, 192
mediastinoscopy, 138t, 321
mediastinum, 53, 53f, 55, 86
medical assistants, 357
medical examiner (M.E.), 14s
medical intensive care unit (MICU), 143s
medical laboratory technologist, 358
medical specialists, 178–181
  areas of practice for, 179t
  case reports for, 186–196
  residency training for, 178
medical/surgical intensive care unit (MSICU), 143s
medications, reference guide for top 50 prescribed, 350t–352t
medulla oblongata, 265f
melanocytes, melanocytes (in hair), 279f
melanoma, 94t, 283t
Ménidisease, 345
meninges, 86, 92f, 139f
  inflammation of, 91, 266
meningitis, 91, 266
  meninges and, 92f
menorrhagia, 96, 96s, 188, 241
menorrhea, 96s
menstruation, 96, 241
mesothelioma, 94t
metacarpal bones, 142, 143f, 255f
metastasis, 142, 142f, 176
metatarsals, 255f
metered-dose inhaler (MDI), 274
MI. *See* myocardial infarction
microscopic discectomy, 260
MICU (medical intensive care unit), 143s
middle ear, bones of, 280
midsagittal plane, 59
migraine, 196, 266
milk glands, 240f
minimally invasive surgery, 229
mitral valve, 149, 150f
mitral valve prolapse syndrome, 149t, 176
molds, 136
mole, 283
monocytes, 9f, 247
mononucleosis, 247
mouth, 226f
MRA (magnetic resonance angiography), 320
MS (multiple sclerosis), 266–267
MSICU (medical/surgical intensive care unit), 143s
mucus, hypersection of, 91
MUGA (multiple-gated acquisition) scans, 220, 321
multiple myeloma, 93, 94t, 248
multiple myomas, 94f

multiple sclerosis (MS), 266–267
multiple-gated acquisition (MUGA) scans, 220, 321
muscle biopsy, 259, 321
muscles
 anterior superficial, 256f
 atrophy of, 134, 140, 140f, 185f
 biopsy of, 259
 diseases of, 95t
 posterior superficial, 257f
muscular dystrophy, 259, 344
musculoskeletal system, 51, 255–264
 abbreviations for, 260
 anatomy of, 255–257, 255f–257f
 anterior superficial muscles of, 257
 definition and role of, 51
 diagnostic procedures and laboratory tests for, 260
 pathology of, 260
 posterior superficial muscles of, 257f
 terminology of, 258
 treatment procedures for, 260
Mycobacterium avium complex (MAC), 248
myelin sheath, 266
myelography/myelograms, 101, 130, 267, 321
myeloma
 definition of, 130
 multiple, 93, 94t, 248
 myocardial infarction (heart attack), 90f, 95s, 96, 97s, 130, 219, 221
 prevention of, 186
myomas, 93, 94f, 130, 242
myomectomy, 101t, 242
myopathy, 95t
myosarcomas, 93, 130
myositis, 92t

N

Na+ (sodium), 236, 315, 325
nail plates, 279f
nail, 279f
 cuticle, 279f
 lunula, 279f
 nail plate, 279f
 paronychium, 279f
nasogastric intubation, 321
nausea, 196
neck (cervical) lymph nodes, 182, 246f
necrosis, 95, 97s, 125f, 130
necrotic tissue, 125f, 219
needle biopsy, 189, 310
Neisseria gonorrhoeae, 345
neonatal intensive care unit (NICU), 143, 143s, 144f
neonates, 134, 144f
 Apgar score, 343
 PKU tests and, 322
nephrectomy, 12
nephritis, 92t
nephrolithiasis, 190, 190f, 288
nephrologists, 179t, 216
nephrology, 15
 case report for, 195
nephrosis, 17, 95
nephrostomy, 182, 182f
nerve ending, 279f
nerves
 cranial, 265f
 diseases of, 95t, 266
 Horner syndrome of, 344
 spinal, 64f, 86, 265f
nervous system
 abbreviations for, 276
 anatomy of, 265, 265f
 central, 265f, 267
 definition and role of, 51
 diagnostic procedures and laboratory tests for, 267
 pathology of, 266
 peripheral, 265f
 terminology of, 266
 treatment procedures for, 267
neural, 16
neurologists, 16, 179t, 216
neurology, 17t
neuropathy, 95t
neurosurgeons, 179t, 216
neurotomy, 18
neutrophil, 9f, 298, 298f
nevus, 283
NICU (neonatal intensive care unit), 143, 143s, 144f
nitroglycerin, 186
non-Hodgkin lymphoma, 248
nonsteroidal anti-inflammatory drugs (NSAIDs), 260
nose, 14, 65f, 271, 272
nosocomial infections, 183
nothing by mouth (NPO), 229
NSAIDs (nonsteroidal anti-inflammatory drugs), 260
nuclear medicine technologist, 358
nurse anesthetist, 358
nursing aide, 359
nutritionist, 356

O

O_2 (oxygen), 132m, 274
 asphyxia and, 273
 ischemia and, 90, 90f, 97s, 130
 hypoxia and, 141s
 measure levels in body, 141s
 blood cells and, 9f
 blood circulation and, 218f
 breathing and, 271f
 hemoglobin and, 11, 318
 therapy in COVID-19, 91
 stroke and, 6s, 130
obstetricians, 179t, 216
obstetrics (OB), 11s, 243
occlusions (blockages), heart muscle, 90f
occult blood tests. *See* Hemoccult tests
occupational therapist assistant (OTA), 359
occupational therapist (OT), 359
oncogenic viruses, 183
oncologists, 12, 179t, 216
oncology, 17t
 case report for, 189s
oophorectomy, laparoscopic, 100, 100f, 130, 243
ophthalmic professionals, 359
ophthalmologists, 13, 13f, 179t
ophthalmology, 17t, 178
ophthalmoscope, 13, 13f
ophthalmoscopy, 283, 321
optic nerve, 280f
opticians, 183
optometrists, 183
orbicularis oculi, 256f–257f
orbicularis oris, 256f
orchiopexy, 272

organs, 50, 50f
orthodontists, 183
orthopedics, case report for, 194
orthopedists, 179t, 183, 216
osteoarthritis, 13, 13f, 42, 42f, 185s
  degeneration from, 13, 13f, 185s
  of the hip, 42, 42f
  of the knee, 13, 13f
  vesus normal joint, 13f
osteogenic sarcoma, 94t
osteomyelitis, 92t
osteopathy, 95t
osteoporosis, 235, 259
osteosarcoma, 15f, 48
OTA (occupational therapist assistant), 359
otitis, 92t
otolaryngologists, 179t, 216
otoscopy, 283, 321
OTs (occupational therapist), 359
ovaries, 234f, 240f, 241
  hormones of, 138t
ovum, 10t, 240f
oxygen (O_2), 274, 218
  blood cells and, 9, 9f, 40f
  deficiency of, 141, 141s
  hemoglobin and, 11, 19
  ischemia and, 90, 90f, 130
  pulse oximeter and, 141s, 141f

P

PA (pulmonary artery), 192, 192f
PACU (post anesthesia care unit), 143s
Paget disease, 345
palpation, 322
pancreas, 8f, 19s, 226f, 234f
hormones of, 139t
  location of, 101f
  Whipple procedure for, 334
pandemic, 20
COVID-19 vaccines and, 302–306
Pap smear (test), 242, 322, 345
paracentesis (abdominocentesis), 322
paralysis
  definition of, 144, 176
paralysis *(Continued)*
  facial nerve (Bell Palsy), 343
  hemiplegia, 139, 176, 266
  paraplegia, 144, 176, 266
  quadriplegia, 147, 176
paraplegia, 144, 176, 266
parathyroid glands, 138t, 144, 145f, 234f
parathyroid hormone (PTH), 138t
Parkinson disease, 345
paronychium, 279f
PA (physician assistant), 360
patella, 255f
pathologists, 14, 14s, 179t, 216
pathology, 17t, 178
PCI (percutaneous coronary intervention), 221
PCP (Pneumocystis pneumonia), 248
PCR (polymerase chain reaction) tests, 322
PE (pulmonary embolism), 274
pectoralis major, 256f
pediatric or psychiatric care unit (PICU), 143s
pediatricians, 170t
pediatrics, 179
pedodontists, 183s
pedunculated fibroid growth, 94f
pedunculated polyp, 204f
PEEP (positive end-expiratory pressure), 274
pelvic cavity, 52f, 54, 255f
pelvic exam, 322
pelvic injuries in case report, 194
pelvic inflammatory disease (PID), 241, 243
pelvic ultrasonography, 242
pelvis, 54, 55, 255f
  injuries to, 194
penicillin, 136
penis, 250f
peptic (gastric) ulcers, 191, 191f, 228
percussion, 322
percutaneous coronary intervention (PCI), 221
percutaneous transhepatic cholangiography, 228
pericardium, 20, 86
periodontists, 183s
peripheral nervous system, 265f
peritoneal cavity, 54, 54f, 54s, 64, 65f, 103f
peritoneal dialysis, 103, 103f, 116, 130
peritoneal fluid, 64, 65f
  ascities and, 64, 65f
peritoneum, 54–55, 54f, 86, 241
peritonitis, 92t
pernicious anemia, 134t
peroneus longus, 256f
PERRLA (pupils equal, round, reactive to light and accommodation), 283
PET (positron emission tomography) scans, 220, 267, 323
PFTs (pulmonary function tests), 273–274, 324
phalanges (finger bones), 143f, 255f
pharmacy technician, 359
pharyngeal, definition of, 65
pharyngitis, 92t
pharynx (throat), 84, 145f, 226f, 271f
  anatomy and physiology of, 65f
  phenylalanine, 322
phenylketonuria (PKU) tests, 322
phlebotomist, 360
phlebotomy, 107f, 322
photoselective vaporization of prostate (GreenLight PVP), 252
physiatrists, 179t, 216
physical therapist (PT), 360
physical therapy (PT), 260
physical therapy assistants (PTA), 360
physician assistant (PA), 360
PICU (pediatric or psychiatric care unit), 143s
PID (pelvic inflammatory disease), 241, 243
pigmented cells in skin, malignant tumor of, 94t
pineal gland, 234f
pituitary gland, 48, 52f, 53, 234f, 235
  hormones of, 138t

PKU (phenylketonuria) tests, 322
planes of body, 58–60, 58f
combining forms for, 61–66
platelet count, 322
platelets, 9f, 15, 40f
platysma, 256f
pleura, 53, 53f, 55, 64, 86, 271f
pleural cavity, 53, 53f
pleural cells, malignant tumor of, 94t
pleural effusion, 54s, 98f, 274, 326
drainage of, 98f
pleural membranes, 273
pleural space, 271f
plural formations, 10s
pneumoconiosis, 273
Pneumocystis pneumonia (PCP), 248
pneumonectomy, 101t, 274
pneumonia, 91, 91f, 149t, 273, 302
polydipsia, 143, 191
polymerase chain reaction (PCR) tests, 310
polyp, 145, 170f, 204f, 228
polyuria, 145s, 193
pons, 265f
positional and directional terms list, 62tf
positive end-expiratory pressure (PEEP), 274
positron emission tomography (PET) scans, 220, 267, 323
post anesthesia care unit (PACU), 143s
posterior, definition of, 58–59, 62t
posteroanterior chest x-rays, 192, 192f
potassium (K^+), 236
potassium tests, 323
precancerous lesions, 145
prefixes
definition of, 4–5
pregnancy
amniocentesis and, 98, 99f, 242, 308
ectopic, 137, 137f, 241
tests, 242, 323
prescribed medications, reference guide for top, 50, 350–352
primary malignant tumors, 174
procedural suffixes, 98–107
proctosigmoidoscopy, 323
progesterone, 138t
progesterone receptor assays, 323
prognosis, definition of, 10, 18, 48
prolapse, uterine, 146, 146f
prone, definition of, 62t
prostate gland, 7f, 250f
excision of, 101t
photoselective vaporization of, 252
transurethral resection of, 21s, 21f, 149
prostatectomy, 101t
prostate-specific antigen (PSA), 251, 323
prostatic carcinoma, 251
prosthesis, 146, 146f, 147f, 168f, 260
prosthodontists, 183s
protein electrophoresis. *See* serum protein electrophoresis
prothrombin time, 323
proximal, definition of, 62t
PSA (prostate-specific antigen), 251, 252, 323
psychiatrists, 178t, 179t, 216
psychiatry, 178
psychology, 17t
PT (physical therapy), 260
PTA (physical therapy assistant), 360
PTH. *See* parathyroid hormone
PT (physical therapist), 360
pubis, 255f
pulmonary angiography, 273, 324
pulmonary artery (PA), 190, 190f
pulmonary circulation, 218f
pulmonary edema, 218
pulmonary embolism (PE), 274
pulmonary function tests (PFTs), 273–274, 324
pulmonary perfusion scans, 324
pulmonary ventilation scan, 324
pulmonologists, 179t, 216
pulse oximeter, 141s, 141f
pupil, 280f, 283
pupils equal, round, reactive to light and accommodation (PERRLA), 283
pyelography. *See* urography

Q

quadriceps femoris, 256f
quadriplegia, 147, 176

R

RA (rheumatoid arthritis), 185s, 185f, 259, 324
radiation iodine uptake (RAIU), 236, 326
radiation oncologists, 105s, 179t, 216
radiation therapist, 361
radiation therapy (radiotherapy), 105, 105s, 184, 184f, 189, 248
radioactive iodine uptake, 236, 326
radiographer, 361
radiography. *See also* x-ray films
definition of, 66
radiologic technologist, 361
radiologists, 105s, 179t, 216
radiology, 66, 105s, 178t, 307
case report for, 192–193
radiotherapy (radiation therapy), 105, 105s, 184, 184f, 189, 248
radius, 255f
RAIU (radiation iodine uptake), 236, 326
range of motion (ROM), 260
Raynaud phenomenon, 345
rectocele, 184, 184f
rectum, 7f, 18f, 54f, 63f, 65f, 146f, 159f, 184, 184f, 226f, 250f
rectus abdominis, 256f
red blood cell (RBC) count, 324
red blood cells (erythrocytes), 9, 9f, 11, 19, 40f, 134t
registered nurse (RN), 361
relapse, 147, 176
remission, 147, 176
renal, definition of, 14

renal calculi, 190, 190f
lithotripsy to treat, 190f
renal failure, 288, 289
chronic renal failure, 195
renal pelvis, 287f, 288
renal transplantation, 289
research skills, 178
resections, 21, 101t, 130
residency training, for medical specialists, 178
respiratory system, 51, 271–278
abbreviations for, 274
anatomy of, 271, 271f
definition and role of, 51
diagnostic procedures and laboratory tests for, 273
pathology of, 273
terminology of, 272
treatment procedures for, 274
respiratory therapist, 362
retina, 13f, 280f, 282
retinopathy, 95t, 282
retrogastric, 21
retrograde pyelogram (RP), 288, 189, 328
retroperitoneal area, 54f, 148
Reye syndrome, 345
rhabdomyolysis, 259
rhabdomyosarcoma, 94t
rheumatoid arthritis (RA), 185s, 185f, 259, 324
rheumatoid factor assays, 324
rheumatologists, 179t, 216
rheumatology, 17t, 185
rhinitis, 14
rhomboideus major, 257f
ribs, 132, 255f
abdominopelvic regions and, 80f
hematoma from broken, 11f
x-ray views of, 59f, 91f
right atrium, 150f, 218f
right ventricle, 150f, 218f
Rinne tests, 345
RN (registered nurse), 361
ROM (range of motion), 260
roots of words, 2–4
definition of, 2
suffixes containing, 19s
Rorschach test, 345
RP (retrograde pyelogram), 288, 189, 328

S

sacral nerves, 265f
sacral spine, 56, 57f, 86
sacrum, 56, 57f, 66, 66s, 255f
sagittal (lateral) plane, 59, 59f, 60f, 86
MRIs of, 60f
salivary glands, 48
Salmonella, 345
salpingectomy, 100, 100f, 241
salpingitis, 241, 243
sarcoidosis, 247
sarcoma, 14, 15f, 66s, 93, 94t, 258
Ewing, 344
Kaposi, 149t, 344
of bone, 15f, 48, 94t
of cartilage, 62, 94t
of muscle, 42f
Ewing, 344
Kaposi, 344
SARS, 149t, 176
SARS CoV-2 (COVID-19), 149t, 302
sartorius, 256f
scalenes, 256f
scapula (shoulder bone), 132t, 148f, 255f–256f
sclera, 280f
scotoma, 196, 196f
scrotum, 250f, 251
sebaceous glands, 279
seizures, 266
semen, 7, 250f
semen analysis, 251, 324
seminomas, 251
sense organ system, 51
abbreviations for, 283
anatomy of, 279–281
diagnostic procedures and laboratory tests for, 283
pathology of, 282–283
terminology of, 282
sensitivity tests, 314, 325
septicemia (sepsis), 90, 90s
sequential multiple analysis (SMA), 310
serum enzyme tests. *See* cardiac enzyme tests
serum protein electrophoresis (electrophoresis), 324
serum tests, 236
sestamibi scan, 326
sexually transmitted diseases (STDs), 243, 251, 252
sexually transmitted infections (STIs), 243, 251, 252
Shigella, 345
shock, 219
shortness of breath (SOB), 274
shoulder bone (scapula), 132t, 148f, 255f–256f
sickle cell anemia, 132t
SICU (surgical intensive care unit), 143s
sigmoid colon, 224f
sigmoidoscopy, , 138t, 227, 229, 323 *See also* proctosigmoidoscopy
Sjögren syndrome, 345
skeletal muscles, cancer of, 94t
skin and sense organ system, 51
abbreviations for, 283
anatomy of, 279f, 282
biopsy of, 283, 325
dermis, 279
diagnostic procedures and laboratory tests for, 283
epidermis, 139, 279f, 282
melanoma and, 283
nevus of, 283
pathology of, 282–283
pigmented cells in, malignant tumor of, 924
terminology of, 282
skin lesions, removal of, 105, 325
skin tests, 325
skull, cranial cavity, 6f, 52f, 53, 55
sleep apnea, 132
slit-lamp microscopy, 281, 312
SMA (sequential multiple analysis), 310
small bowel follow-through. *See* barium tests; upper gastrointestinal examination

small intestine, 8f, 9, 54f, 226f
  bariatric surgery and, 122, 122f
  Crohn Disease and, 181s, 197–198
  inflammation of, 9, 181
Snellen test, 345
SOB (shortness of breath), 274
sodium (Na^+), 236
sodium level test, 325
soft tissue, swelling of, 185f
soleus, 256f–257f
sonography. *See* ultrasonography
spasm, coronary artery, 186, 186f
speculum, vaginal, 18f
speech-language pathologist, 362
sperm, 7, 250f
spinal cavity, 52f, 54–55, 56f
spinal column, 56, 57f, 86
  divisions of, 56, 57f, 86
spinal cord, 54, 56, 56f, 64f, 86, 265f
  myelograms for, 101, 130, 321
  surrounding anatomy and structures of, 92f
spinal nerves, 265f
spinal tap (lumbar puncture), 64, 64f, 101, 267, 320
spirometer, 273, 324
spleen, 8f, 80f, 101f, 130, 246f, 247
  excision of, 101t
splenectomy, 101t, 130
sputum tests, 271, 312
Staphylococcus aureus, 149t, 166
STDs (sexually transmitted diseases), 243, 251, 252
stents, arterial, 104, 104f, 124f, 186, 221
stereotactic breast biopsies, 320
stereotactic radiosurgery, 267
sternocleidomastoid, 256f–257f
sternum, 255f
STIs (sexually transmitted infections), 241, 249
stomach, 8f, 10, 54f, 65f, 226f
  bariatric surgery and, 122, 122f
  excision of, 101t
  gastroscopy and, 10, 10f, 318
  inflammation of, 92t
  peptic ulcer in, 191, 191f, 228
  subtotal gastrectomy and, 16, 122f, 148
  visual examination of, 10, 10f, 318
stomas, 105, 106f
stool culture, 229, 325
stool guaiac tests. *See* Hemoccult tests
stress tests, 220, 325
stroke (cerebrovascular accident), 6, 6s, 73f, 96, 116, 130, 266, 267
stye, 283
subclavian artery, 104f
subcutaneous tissue, 279f
subdural hematoma, 139f
subhepatic, 21
subluxation, of joints, 185f
subserosal masses, 94f
subtotal gastrectomy, 146
subtotal hysterectomy, 100
suffixes, 2–4
  adjective, 96–97
  commonly confused, 137s
  definition of, 2
  diagnostic, 89–97
  forming plural, 10s
  procedural, 98–107
  roots of words in, 19s
superficial, definition of, 62t
superior, definition of, 62t
supine, definition of, 62t
surfactant, 142f
surgury, residenct program in, 178
surgical intensive care unit (SICU), 143s
surgical technologist (CST), 362
swallowing process, 65f, 65s
sweat glands, 48, 279f
symbols, list of, 342
symptom, 149s
  remission and relapse of, 147, 176
syncope, 266
syndrome, 148, 149t, 176
  acquired immunodeficiency syndrome (AIDS), 149t, 176, 247, 248
  acute coronary syndrome (ACS), 221
  acute respiratory distress syndrome (ARDS), 274
  carpal tunnel syndrome, 149t, 259
  Cushing syndrome, 235
  Down syndrome, 149t
  irritable bowel syndrome (IBS), 228, 229
  mitral valve lapse syndrome, 149t, 176
  severe acute respiratory syndrome (SARS), 149t, 176, 304
  toxic shock syndrome (TSS), 149t, 166
synovial membrane, 185f
syphilis, 251
systemic circulation, 218f
systems. *See* body systems

T3 (triiodothyronine), 236, 326
T4 (thyroxine), 138t, 236, 326
T&A. *See* tonsillectomy and adenoidectomy
TAH. *See* total abdominal hysterectomy
TAH-BSO (total abdominal hysterectomy with bilateral salpingo-oophorectomy), 100, 100f, 243
tarsals, 255f
Tay-Sachs disease, 345
tear glands, 20, 48
technetium Tc 99m sestamibi scan, 220, 326
teeth, dental specialists for, 183s
tendons, atrophy of, tendons, 255f
  atrophy of, 185f
TENS (transcutaneous electrical nerve stimulation), 267
testes, 138t, 234f, 250f–251f
  cryptorchism of, 251
  hormone of, 138t
  orchiopexy and, 252
testicular carcinoma, 251

testosterone, 138t
thallium-201 scans, 220, 326
thoracentesis, 98, 98f, 274, 326
thoracic cavity, 52f, 53, 53f, 55
thoracic nerves, 265f
thoracic spine, 56, 57f, 66, 86
thoracic surgeons, 179t, 216
thoracic vertebra, 255f, 260
  x-ray of, 59f
thoracocentesis. *See* thoracentesis
thoracocoscopy, 326
thoracotomy, 66, 186, 274
THR (total hip replacement), 42, 42f, 147f, 260
throat. *See* pharynx
thrombocytes, 9f, 15, 40f
thrombolytic therapy, 221
thrombophlebitis, 92t
thrombosis, thrombosis, 15, 15f
  deep vein, 41f, 328
thrombus, 15, 15f
thymoma, 94t
thymus gland, 246f
  tumor of, 94t
thyroid cartilage, 66f, 107f, 140f
thyroid function tests, 236, 326
thyroid gland, 48, 145f, 234f, 235
  hormones of, 138t
  location of, 142f
thyroid scan, 236, 326
thyroid-stimulating hormone (TSH), 138t, 236, 326
thyroxine (T4), 138t, 236, 326
TIA (transient ischemic attack), 267
tibia, 147f, 255f, 256f
tibialis anterior, 256f
tinnitus, 283
tissue capillaries, 218f
tissue plasminogen activator (tPA), 220
tissues, 50, 50f
TKR (total knee joint replacement), 147f, 151, 260
toes, webbed, 136, 136f
tomography/tomograms, 326
tomosynthesis, 102, 102f
tonsillectomy, 98, 99f
tonsillectomy and adenoidectomy (T&A), 99f
tonsils, 99f, 271f
total abdominal hysterectomy (TAH), 100, 100f
total abdominal hysterectomy with bilateral salpingo-oophorectomy (TAH-BSO), 100, 100f, 243
total hip joint replacement (THR), 42, 42f, 147f, 260
total hysterectomy, 100, 100f
total knee joint replacement (TKR), 147f, 151, 260
total parenteral nutrition (TPN), 229
Tourette syndrome, 346
toxic shock syndrome (TSS), 149t, 166
tPA (tissue plasminogen activator), 221
TPN (total parenteral nutrition), 229
trachea, 8f, 53f, 65f, 65s, 66f, 86, 99f, 145f, 271f
  cartilage of, 66f
  definition of, 86
tracheostomy, 105, 107f, 274
tracheotomy, 66f
transcutaneous electrical nerve stimulation (TENS), 267
transdermal, 21
transient ischemic attack (TIA), 267
transurethral, 21
transurethral resection of prostate gland (TURP), 21, 21f, 149, 252
transverse (axial) plane, 58f, 59, 59f, 60f, 73f, 86
  MRIs of, 60f
trapezius, 256f–257f
triceps brachii, 256f–257f
tricuspid valve, 147, 148f
triglycerides tests, 326
triiodothyronine (T3), 236, 326
troponin tests, 326
TSH (thyroid-stimulating hormone), 138t, 236, 326
TSS. *See* toxic shock syndrome
tubal ligation, 18, 18f, 242
tuberculin tests, 273, 327
tuberculosis, 273, 327
tumors, benign, 62, 93, 94f, 130, 142s, 188f, 241. *See also* cancer/malignant tumors
tuning fork tests, 283, 327
TURP. *See* transurethral resection of prostate gland

UA (urinalysis), 135s, 289, 327
ulcerative colitis, 181s, 228, 229
ulcers, peptic, 191, 191f, 228
ulna, 255f
ultrasonography, 188, 188f, 327
  abdominal, 228
  definition of, 327
  Doppler, 220, 315
  endoscopic, 228, 316
  fetal, 150f
  gallbladder, 108, 317
  pelvic, 188f, 242
underarm (axilla), 88, 240f
unilateral frontal cephalgia, 196
upper gastrointestinal examination (series), 191, 327
upper respiratory infection (URI), 274
urea, 91, 96s, 103, 103f, 288, 289, 310
uremia, 91, 96s, 116, 288
ureters, 7f, 135f, 182f, 190f, 250f, 287f
urethra, 7f, 54f, 63f, 250f, 287f
URI (upper respiratory infection), 274
uric acid, 289
  gouty arthritis and, 259
uric acid test, 259, 327
urinalysis (UA), 135s, 289, 327
urinary bladder, 7, 7f, 54f, 63f, 135f, 250f, 287f
  inflammation of, 91
  nephrostomy and, 182, 182f
  urinary catheterization and, 290
  visual examination of, 7, 7f, 138t, 288, 314
urinary catheterization, 287

urinary system, 51, 287–292
  abbreviations for, 289
  anatomy of female, 287, 287f
  definition and role of, 51
  diagnostic procedures and laboratory tests for, 288–289
  pathology of, 288
  terminology of, 288
  treatment procedures for, 289
urinary tract, female, 7, 7f, 287f
urinary tract, male, 7, 7f, 287f
urinary tract infection (UTI), 137, 289
urination
  diuretics and, 145s
  excessive amount of, 145, 145s, 193
  lack of, 288
  painful, 137, 190, 288
urine, 278
  analysis of, 135s, 289, 328
  blood in, 96, 96s, 116, 190, 288
  glucose in, 135s, 140, 288
  protein in, 135s, 288
urine (serum and urine) tests, 236
urography (urogram), 289, 328
urologist, 179t, 216
urology, 17t
  case report for, 190s
uterine artery embolization, 240
uterine prolapse, 146, 146f
uterus, 7f, 54f, 63f, 240f, 241
  amniocentesis and, 99f
  fibroids in, 93, 94f, 101t, 121, 188, 188f, 241
  hysterectomy and, 100, 100f, 188, 242, 243
  hysteroscopy and, 138t, 319
  implantation in pregnancy and, 137f
  prolapse and, 146f
  ultrasound of, 327
UTI (urinary tract infection), 135, 287

V

VA (visual acuity), 283
vagina, 7f, 18f, 54f, 63f, 94f, 100f, 146f, 184f, 240f
vaginal speculum, 18f
varicocele, 251
vas deferens, 159f, 250f, 251
vasectomy, 252
vasoconstrictor, 196
VATS (video-assisted thoracic surgery), 274, 326
VCUG (voiding cystourethrogram), 289, 314, 328
vein, 218f, 219
  blood clot within, 15f
  imaging of, 102, 124f, 220, 309
  withdraw blood from, 107f, 322
  within a, 141, 141f, 169f
venea cavae, 86, 150f
venipuncture. *See* phlebotomy
venography, 309, 328
ventilation-perfusion scan (VQ scan), 273–274, 328
ventricular arrhythmias, 186
venules, 218f
vertebra(e), 56, 56f, 57f, 66, 255f, 258, 260
  lumbar puncture and, 64f
  x-ray views of, 59f
vertebroplasty, 260
VF (visual field), 196f, 283
video-assisted thoracic surgery (VATS), 274, 326
viral load test, for HIV, 328
virus, 11, 11s
  antigens and, 135, 298
  antigen-presenting cell (APC) and, 300f–304f
  dendritic cell and, 300f–304f
  lymphocytes and, 300f
  replication of, 303, 303f
  vaccines against, 301f–306f
  white blood cells and, 298f
visceral muscle, cancer of, 94t, 258
vision. *See* eyes/vision
visual acuity (VA), 283
visual field (VF), 196f, 283
vitreous humour, 280f
voice box. *See* larynx
voiding cystourethrogram (VCUG), 289, 314, 328
von Willebrand disease, 346
VQs (ventilation-perfusion scan), 273–274, 328

WBC count. *See* white blood cell count
webbed toes, 136f
Weber tuning fork test, 346
Western blot tests, 247, 328
Whipple procedure, 346
white blood cell. *See* leukocyte
white blood cell (WBC) count, 328
Wilms tumor, 346
windpipe. *See* trachea
word analysis, 2–5
word parts, 4t
Wrist. *See* carpal

xiphoid process, 253f
x-ray films (radiography), 64
  angiography, 102, 220, 309
  cerebral angiography, 265
  chest, 59, 59f, 192, 192f, 273, 274, 312
  coronary angiography, 124f, 186, 186f, 309
  of hand, 143f
  hysterosalpingography, 242, 319
  KUB, 288, 289, 319
  lateral chest, 192f
  mammography, 102, 102f, 242
  myelograms, 101, 130, 267, 321
  of normal lungs and pneumonia, 91f
  posteroanterior chest, 192, 192f
  of renal calculi, 190, 190f
  for urinary system, 288–289